Rhythms of Broken Hearts

J. Anthony Gomes

Rhythms of Broken Hearts

History, Manifestations, and Treatment
of Heart Rhythm Disorders and Heart Disease

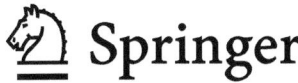 Springer

J. Anthony Gomes
Icahn School of Medicine at Mount Sinai
New York, NY
USA

ISBN 978-3-030-77381-6   ISBN 978-3-030-77382-3   (eBook)
https://doi.org/10.1007/978-3-030-77382-3

This Springer imprint is published by the registered company Springer Nature Switzerland AG
The registered company address is: Gewerbestrasse 11, 6330 Cham, Switzerland

"The heart is the only broken machine that works."

—*T.E. Kalem*

To my patients who have been the source of inspiration for this book, and to my family: my wife Margarita, my daughter Tanya, and my grandchildren, Jojo, Jayden, Jonathan, Nicholas, Gabriel, and Kai.

Praise for Rhythms of Broken Hearts

The development of the ECG marked the beginning of the recognition of the heart's electricity and heart rhythm disorders. However, more than half-a-century later, in 1967 and 1969, two monumental studies would change the course of medicine, ushering a new field in cardiology, that of clinical cardiac electrophysiology that over time, resulted in advanced treatment of the heart's rhythm maladies. In *Rhythms of Broken Hearts,* Dr. J. Anthony Gomes narrates the history, the manifestations and treatment of common cardiac diseases, and heart rhythm disorders marvelously chronicled with enticing patient anecdotes. Taken as a whole, this book is a "Tour de Force." A marvelous feat, seen through the lens of a cardiologist's and cardiac electrophysiologist's extraordinary career. In each chapter, Dr. Gomes depicts a different cardiac abnormality, with its own history, and science, expounding the narrative as a physician, novelist, and humanist. A great read for both the academician and the nonprofessional.

Benjamin Scherlag, PhD
Professor of Medicine
Regents Professor
George Lynn Professor of Research
Helen Webster Chair of Cardiac Arrhythmias
Oklahoma University Health Sciences Center
Oklahoma City, OK 73104

Like an illuminated manuscript of the heart-centered cosmos for our digitized age, *Rhythms of Broken Hearts* represents a major work by J. Anthony Gomes, MD, who in the doctor/writer tradition of Anton Chekov and William Carlos Williams, is both a renowned cardiologist and novelist. The author occupies a unique perspective, a cardiovascular researcher in the thick of the epoch's monumental discoveries, and a practitioner, translating those seismic shifts in thinking into real world utility. *"I have not forgotten that patients are human beings, whole entities rather than parts,"* he writes in the preface to this brilliant exhaustive study in which the colossal research-doctors, those explorers of the heart and its slow and fast beating, and whose breakthroughs revolutionized patient treatment, loom large. Elucidated with remarkable clarity, *Rhythms of Broken Hearts* achieves the delicate balance between writing for the layperson as well as the medical professional. Beautifully told patient anecdotes anchor the more esoteric material with the universal. The heart's territory, in Gomes' hands, becomes a mesmerizing dramatic poetry, not only a material organ, but a philosophical, spiritual, and literary essence.

Stephanie Dickinson, author of more than 9 books, including *Blue Swan Black Swan: The Trakl Diaries,* and founding editor of Rain-Mountain Press.

Dr. J. Anthony Gomes has written an important book for anyone who has a personal or professional interest in understanding the basics of heart rhythm disorders and other common maladies of the heart. His affinity and empathy for his patients and their stories make universal the experiences of illness that we all must navigate at some point in our lives. He does justice to complex science in terms that are clear and readily accessible to the layperson while avoiding oversimplification and talking down to the reader. In this book, Gomes has woven a rich tapestry of science, history, and art that makes for a rewarding journey for patients and health care providers alike.

Jeremy N. Ruskin, MD
Professor of Medicine, Harvard Medical School
Founder, Cardiac Arrhythmia Service
Alomran Endowed Chair in Cardiology
Massachusetts General Hospital

This radiant book will make you understand heart disease in the wide perspective of medicine, literature, and philosophy. Only a world-famous cardiac specialist who is also a novelist, poet, and humanist could have written this multicultural account. Dr. J. Anthony Gomes shares stories of patients struggling with heart disease, some with riveting near-death experiences. He traces views of the ancient Egyptians, Greeks, and Indians, many of which, surprisingly, jibe with modern medical concerns. The great writers he quotes have intuited much of what is known today about disorders of the heart, and the great strides in the treatment and prevention of the world's leading killer. Additionally, the book has a spiritual component, lifting it far and above the science it delivers. If you ever have a broken heart—romantic or medical—you will be totally absorbed in this dazzling multicultural read.

Grace Schulman, author of six exclaimed books of poetry, including *The Broken String, Without A Claim,* and *The Marble Bed,* and winner of the Frost Award for Lifetime Achievement in American Poetry. She is currently Distinguished Professor of English at Baruch College, C.U.N.Y.

The heart is a muscular pump and an electrical organ that provides life's rhythm through circuits tuned to the millisecond. The diseases that disturb these pathways, some common and others quite rare, cause cardiac arrhythmias with symptoms ranging from innocent palpitation to syncope to sudden death. The evaluation and management of patients with these rhythm disturbances often represent complex challenges and frequently call for referral to a cardiac electrophysiologist with specialized knowledge and experience. Dr. J. Anthony Gomes is not only a seasoned clinical electrophysiologist whose career has placed him at the forefront of the evolution of this science, but also a prolific writer whose poetry reflects keen sensitivity to the human side of every patient's story. In *Rhythm of Broken Hearts*, he distills from this multifaceted perspective a unique story that knits history, physiology, emotion, and wisdom together, into a compelling narrative that explains the inner workings of the heart and its ailments, capturing both the intellect and the imagination. This book is required reading for anyone who knows someone with heart disease or is concerned about the inner workings of their own internal metronome.

Jonathan L. Halperin, MD, FACC, FAHA, FACP, MSVM
Robert and Harriet Heilbrunn Professor of Medicine (Cardiology)
Associate Director
The Zena and Michael A. Wiener Cardiovascular Institute
Icahn School of Medicine at Mount Sinai
Mount Sinai Medical Center
New York, NY

Throughout his career, Dr. J. Anthony Gomes has witnessed major advances in our knowledge of the human heart, often participating in research that led to crucial discoveries. As a practicing cardiologist with a deep concern for his patients, he has helped develop treatments for critical malfunctions. He knows the history and the people who made it, relating the stories from an inside perspective. Moreover, these are human stories, brought to life through his depictions of scientists committed to solving mysteries and of individual patients, whose cardiac crises were the source of their concerns. In *Rhythms of Broken Hearts* Gomes explains complex technical issues with clarity and compassion, animating the excitement of unraveling an unknown and of saving a specific life, along with thousands more lives in the years to come. He speaks directly to his readers, aware each of us must cope with the vulnerabilities of our own hearts.

Walter Cummins, author of more than 10 books including *Knowing Writers*. He is an Emeritus Professor of English Literature at Fairleigh Dickinson University.

Books by J. Anthony Gomes, MD

Medicine

- *Signal Averaged Electrocardiography: Concepts, Methods and Applications.*
- *Heart Rhythm Disorders: History, Mechanisms and Treatment Perspective*
- *Rhythms of Broken Hearts*

Poetry

- *Visions from Grymes Hill*
- *Mirrored Reflection*

Fiction

- *The Sting of Peppercorns*
- *Nas Garras Do Destino*
- *Have A Heart*

Author's Note

The aim of science is to discover and illuminate truth. And that, I take it, is the aim of literature, whether biography or history... It seems to me, then, that there can be no separate literature of science.— Rachel Carson

Medicine is my lawful wife and literature my mistress; when I get tired of one, I spend the night with the other.— Anton Chekhov

This book is mostly about runaway fast and slow heart rhythm disorders that plague the old as well as the young affecting their quality of life and resulting in premature death. Like the runaway train that gains speed and cannot be controlled until it crashes, many heart rhythm disorders are uncontrollable, and in some instances, such as a rapid ventricular tachycardia and ventricular fibrillation, death comes suddenly and instantaneously. On the opposite end of the spectrum, there are slow and disconnected rhythms that are bothersome, and can sometimes result in death as well.

The book is also about stories of patients I encountered and treated—their broken hearts, their journey through the meanderings of life, and the endurance of their spirit. To them I owe a debt of gratitude. Their stories are real, with some changes, mostly to protect a patient's or a doctor's privacy in compliance with enacted federal Health Insurance Portability and Accountability (HIPAA) privacy legislation. Often, however, and where appropriate, I have used real names of my associates and co-worker physicians, and my fellows in training. My narrative also rests on past writers, and the many physicians and clinician scientists I encountered in the field of cardiology and heart rhythm disorders.

I would also like to mention that the contributions to the specialty of cardiology and heart rhythms have come over several decades from a host of individuals often working independently in different institutions mostly from Europe and the United States. Additionally, many drug and device companies here and abroad have contributed immensely to the field.

I have been fortunate to have lived to see and partake in the astronomical advances in cardiovascular medicine over the last four and a half decades and, moreover, to have been at the birth and forefront of my specialty. Although, today, we employ high-end technology—fancy machines and recording systems; cool tip, deep freeze, and laser tip catheters; metal and drug eluting stents and the recently introduced deployable artificial valves; assist devices to keep the heart pumping, complex devices and pacemakers that can shock the heart in an instant and pace different chambers of the heart at the same time—I have not abandoned the power of laying hands. I have not forgotten that patients are human beings, whole entities rather than parts, organs, and limbs of a whole. I have not abandoned the harmonious union between mind and matter, and the random ordering of their lives. This perspective I have held onto, and when possible used not only to heal the body, but to keep abreast of the psychological struggles within. I must confess, however, that I have sometimes not lived up to these ideals, but I have realized my shortfalls, and attempted to make up for my errors whenever possible.

The tragedy of human disease is not only the physical pain and loss of livelihood, but even larger struggles of guilt, acceptance, fear of death, and the re-alignment of that shattered unity: the body, mind, and spirit. No human being can recover or succumb to the devastation of disease without achieving a certain balance, and the physician needs to play an integral part in this healing process.

The medieval Sephardic Jewish philosopher and physician Maimonides said: "The physician should not treat the disease but the patient who is suffering from it." Several centuries later, the late Dr. Bernard Lown reiterated the same dictum: "Medicine is the art of engagement with the human condition rather than with disease." In today's day and age, unlike in the Middle Ages or even a few decades ago, there are curative treatments for a host of diseases. And so, these old aphorisms do not necessarily apply today.

Physicians need to treat the disease as well as the patient. Unfortunately, medical school doesn't prepare doctors to deal with the emotional and psychological elements of disease. Moreover, time factors, specialization and super-specialization, and reimbursement and insurance claims occupy the physician's mind and time. However, physicians need to constantly keep abreast of the fact that a patient typically has the highest faith and trust in their doctor. Although somewhat of a hyperbole, there is some truth in the saying of George Bernard Shaw: "We have not lost faith, but we have transferred it from God to the medical profession."

In this book, I have written about heart rhythm disorders as well as other important aspects of cardiovascular medicine such as coronary intervention in a way accessible to readers not trained in medicine. At the same time, I have also made a concerted effort not to entirely water down the science. In my own life, I have maintained a symbiotic relationship between the humanities and the sciences, and if anything, it has made me a better doctor. It has opened yet another dimension, a greater desire to know and reckon with not only the "disease element" of my patients, but also to probe into their stories: the suffering and the psychological dilemmas they and their families face exemplified in the stories of survival in this book. And so, this book also seeks to understand the impact of heart disease and the complexities of living with it. There are stories of individual patients, and although, metaphorically speaking, they all have broken hearts, fixable in some, non-fixable in others, in medical terms they are often unconnected to each other. However, in human terms of pain, suffering, and loss, of the influence of God and religion on their illness, and of death itself, their stories are intricately connected. And therefore, no matter who or what we are scientifically—atoms and molecules, products of our genetic mold, different organs of a whole—we are after all that element of a shared humanity.

I sincerely hope readers of this book will find some magic in these stories. I also anticipate that those who have gone through the trials of heart disease, and those who have suffered from a heart arrhythmia, will relate to the stories, and perhaps gain inspiration and fortitude to fight on. To those who have never experienced such maladies, I ask that they join me on life's highway, and walk with me on rounds as I talk to, examine and treat my patients and tell you their stories. Perhaps one day, if you are hit with the calamity of a heart ailment, you may be the wiser for it. *Nonetheless, I would like to point out that this book is not a substitute for your cardiologist and/or your heart rhythm expert (clinical cardiac electrophysiologist), who should render a diagnosis and treatment of your cardiac malady.*

New York, NY, USA   J. Anthony Gomes, MD, FACC, FAHA

Preface

For while knowledge defines all we currently know and understand, imagination points to all we might yet discover and create.—Albert Einstein

Change is the law of life. And those who look only to the past or the present are certain to miss the future.—John F. Kennedy

Let's walk down a busy street and glance at the adults passing by. If they are a cross-section of the US public, one out of every three will have a disease of the heart or blood vessels doctors call cardiovascular disease (CVD). If they are all non-Hispanic blacks, almost half will. On the basis of The National Health and Nutrition Examination Survey (NHANES), the prevalence of CVD (comprising coronary heart disease, heart failure, stroke, and hypertension in adults $\geq$20 years of age) was 126.9 million (in 2018) and increases with age in both males and females.

Undoubtedly, with age the danger of having heart disease rises. If that street happens to contain only people between 60 and 79 years, two out of three will have CVD. And if it has only people over 80, you'll have trouble finding anyone without it. For the aged, CVD is destiny. It has long been the leading killer in the USA, currently claiming more lives each year than all cancers and chronic lung disease combined. In 2017, 868,662 people died of CVD; it is also the leading global cause of death, and accounted for approximately 18.6 million deaths in 2019. The most common type of CVD is coronary heart disease (CHD) accounting for approximately 13% of deaths in the USA in 2018, amounting to 365,744 deaths. Although from 2008 to 2018, the actual number of CHD deaths declined by 9.8%, the burden and risk factors remain astoundingly high.

On average, one American dies of it every 39 seconds, or the maximum time between plays in the NFL. Life expectancy would increase by 7 years if we eliminated CVD, but 3 years if we eliminated all cancers. It is worrisome that 34% of these deaths occur before the age of 75, or below the current life expectancy of 78.8 years. However, it is noteworthy that since the appearance of the COVID-19 pandemic, life expectancy dropped by 1year in 2020, the largest drop since World War II; while in black-Americans the drop was 2.7years after 20 years of gains.

Rather alarmingly, people often harbor heart disease much as they do cancer, utterly unaware of it. For instance, on February 12, 2017, the 51-year-old fitness guru Bob Harper fell to the ground after a workout. "My heart stopped," he said. "Not to be dramatic, but I was dead. I was on that ground dead." Only incredible luck—the nearby presence of doctors with a defibrillator—saved his life. Harper is a man intensely aware of his health, yet he'd had no prior warning signs. Indeed, of the approximately 400,000 annual sudden cardiac deaths, nearly half of the men and two-thirds of the women had no symptoms before the tragic event.

We obviously cannot quantify the cost in life and sorrow. But we can calculate its burden in dollars, and it is enormous. In the USA, between 2016 to 2017, its direct and indirect cost amounted to about $363.4 billion, more than for any other medical condition.

Heart disease kills people of all ages, races, and nationalities, and everyone over 60 years of age must recognize that it is a potential threat. And yet, we have made great strides over the last several decades in detecting and managing heart disease, preventing sudden death, caring for survivors, and treating arrhythmias. We have seen a revolution in cardiovascular care, far beyond the imagination of our forefathers as the Internet itself. I distinctly remember how it was in the recent past.

In 1970, the USA was fighting a war in Vietnam, computer microprocessors were unknown, the Beatles were still recording together, and Jesus Christ Superstar was due to make its debut on Broadway. In that year, around 6 a.m. one morning, cabdriver Pedro Sanchez was scouting the streets of New York for a pickup when his taxi veered from the street, crashed into a fire hydrant, and landed on the sidewalk. Paramedics found him slumped on the wheel, unconscious without a pulse. They started chest compressions and cardiopulmonary resuscitation. They rushed him to a New York City hospital just two blocks away, where I was an intern.

In the emergency room, doctors found him in ventricular fibrillation, the heart rhythm of death if not terminated immediately. After three electrical shocks to his chest, Pedro recovered a normal pulse and consciousness. He was immediately transferred to the CCU, where I first met him. He was a 40-year-old immigrant who had arrived in this country about 3 years before—my first patient to survive an episode of cardiac arrest. He had recently gotten a job as a cabdriver and called for his young wife and his two kids. He was about five-foot four, with rather rugged features and a bit of a paunch, who smoked two packs of cigarettes, and drank three or four beers a day. I listened to his heart with my stethoscope and heard sounds that seemed weak and distant. I also heard a few crackles at the bases of his lungs, suggesting some lung congestion. There was no other significant finding on my physical examination. His electrocardiogram (ECG) was alarming, however. The ECG is the imprint of the electrical waves of the heart and can point to the diagnosis of an acute heart attack or myocardial infarction. Pedro's ECG indicated that he had an evolving heart attack in the front, or "anterior," part of the heart due to blockage of a main coronary artery. In those days, there was no echocardiography, and so we couldn't assess the extent of the damage.

Pedro did not speak much English, but since I was fluent in Portuguese, I could manage some Spanish or rather what the Brazilians call *Portunol*— a mixture of Portuguese and Spanish. I couldn't extract much history from him except that his father had died suddenly at the age of 49, and that just a few hours before he had felt some burning sensation beneath the breastbone that lasted for a few minutes. He attributed the pain to indigestion and swallowed a couple of Tums.

In fact, it is not uncommon to think that heart-related chest pain comes from acid reflux. For instance, on September 23, 1953, President Dwight D. Eisenhower began to experience a burning discomfort in his chest during a round of golf in Colorado. He thought it came from the onions in his lunchtime hamburger. Major General Snyder, his personal physician, came by at dinnertime and noting that the President's upset seemed minor, mixed some cocktails. The increasingly uncomfortable President was sent to bed with a bottle of Milk of Magnesia. Eisenhower woke up in the middle of the night all sweaty with excruciating chest pain. The president was having a heart attack.

Pedro grew very concerned about his family's welfare when I told him that he had a heart attack. I ordered morphine for pain and an intravenous Lidocaine drip to prevent the forms of rapid heartbeat called "ventricular tachycardia" and "ventricular fibrillation." That was all I could do for Pedro.

He was resting somewhat comfortably when I left the coronary unit. I was in the cafeteria lunching on beef stew and salad when I heard the overhead pager issue a code blue, followed by my name. I was needed in the coronary unit "stat," that is, "urgently." At about the same time my beeper went off. Along with other resident doctors, I left my half-eaten lunch and ran to the unit.

Pedro was in ventricular tachycardia. In other words, his heart was beating much too rapidly. The abnormal rapid rhythm was coming from the heart muscle that was damaged from the heart attack. He was gasping for breath and in the process of losing consciousness. Soon after, he went back into the dreaded rhythm: ventricular fibrillation. We started CPR, the anesthesiologist placed a breathing tube, and I applied paddles and electrical shocks to his chest several times. The fourth electrical shock finally worked, but this time around there was no rhythm. The electrical system was shot. Silent! The eerie silence of death. We injected a stimulant in his heart, but to no avail.

Pedro was dead.

It was the first time I had seen a fast death from a heart attack. During my residency training I would see many more. It was a sobering experience: The fragility of life. The sudden unexpected encounter with death!

The heart muscle needs blood just like every other organ, and in Pedro's case the main artery that feeds the heart muscle was blocked causing a heart attack. The rapid rhythm, ventricular tachycardia and ventricular fibrillation—its consequence— it's what killed Pedro.

I had to inform his wife of his death. It was hard to console a sobbing young immigrant woman who had come to the USA with her two little children a few months ago full of hope for a new life, now lost in this city jungle.

If Pedro had survived, he would have stayed in the hospital for at least 4 to 6 weeks in complete bed rest, and perhaps longer if he had other complications. Just before discharge, he would be allowed to dangle his legs over the bed and walk around the ward. We simply had nothing else to offer Pedro. We had no oral beta-adrenergic blockers to prevent sudden death, no lipid lowering agents to reduce cholesterol, no angiotensin-converting enzyme (ACE) inhibitors to improve heart function, no water-pills to treat heart failure, and no knowledge that aspirin was useful in preventing heart attacks. It is unlikely that Pedro would be able to continue driving his taxi, and it is highly likely that he would have continued smoking. We had no advice to give him: about what food to eat, how much to exercise (if at all), whether to stop smoking, whether to have sex or abstain for a certain length of time. We simply didn't know. Ignorance may sometimes be bliss, but it rarely is for the patient. The odds were high that Pedro would have died suddenly within the first 6 months after his heart attack or be incapacitated with heart failure.

In Pedro's time, the relationship between smoking and heart disease was not yet known, and indeed most doctors smoked even on rounds and in the wards. I distinctly remember one of my attending physicians always asking for a Marlboro from one of the doctors in training during rounds. "Can I have one of those?" he would say. And light up. He was an excellent clinician and vice chair of medicine. Unbeknownst to him, we called him the Marlboro Man: *Come where the flavor is. Come to Marlboro Country!*

Pedro had coronary artery disease, which is just one kind of heart ailment. And because it is a mouthful—nine syllables—I'll refer to it in shorthand. I'll call it CAD, as most doctors do. The much broader term is "cardiovascular disease," which is any disease associated with the circulatory system and the heart. (The "vascular" part refers to vessels that carry blood.) For instance, stroke is cardiovascular disease, but it's not CAD, since it doesn't involve a heart-serving artery. Malfunctioning heart valves, congenital heart defects, heart rhythm abnormalities, aneurysm and rupture of the aorta—all are also cardiovascular disease. I have used the standard abbreviation for this broad group of ailments: CVD.

When I think of Pedro now 51 years later, I feel confident that if we had encountered him in 2020, he would have survived. How and why, I will relate much later as we make our journey through a maze of spectacular successes over the last few decades of medical progress in CAD and heart rhythm disorders. And yet, we still have a long way to go to prevent CAD, cardiac arrhythmias, and sudden cardiac death.

Your work is going to fill a large part of your life, and the only way to be truly satisfied is to do what you believe is great work. And the only way to do great work is to love what you do.—Steve Jobs

My romance with the heart started at a very young age, when I was nine. I grew up in Goa, then a Portuguese colony in India, and during one of my visits to the general practitioner after a bout of illness, I rather boldly asked the doctor if I could listen with his stethoscope. I was surprised when he let me use it on himself. He lay on the patient's couch with his shirt off and asked me to place the diaphragm of the stethoscope on his heart. I was mesmerized by its lab-dab—lab-dab. I could feel the rhythmic beating of my own heart if I placed my hand on my chest. I soon learned that if I lay on my left side on the bed, I could hear my own heart slowing down and speeding up as I took in a deep breath. It was music to my ears. From that day on, I felt a romantic attachment to the heart. I hoped that one day I would become a heart specialist—a cardiologist. Just as kids believe in Santa Claus and the magic of moonlight, I believed that the heart was the seat of love.

When I stepped into the cardiology training program in 1973, after 3 years of internship and residency in internal medicine, it was as if I was embarking on a journey to the center of the universe. I was excited to be focusing on the heart, the most important organ of the body, the one that feeds all the others with life-sustaining blood thick with oxygen and nutrients. As I began this new adventure, I was well aware that romancing the heart did not involve poetry, but the understanding of the electrical and mechanical properties of this superb organ that nature has provided. Nonetheless, in those days, listening to the heart with the stethoscope still offered an element of mystery and wonder.

After my residency, I began a fellowship—that period when a doctor trains to be a specialist—in cardiovascular medicine. It was nothing compared to the demands of a cardiology and cardiac electrophysiology fellowship today. We had only a few drugs to treat heart disease, and no one even dreamt of powerful agents like clot busters or complex procedures such as coronary stents or the pinpoint destruction of heart tissue with electrical current to treat arrhythmias. Besides, we knew of an occasional kid dropping dead after hearing a sudden load honk of a car, of adults dying suddenly on the street pavement, of an athlete dropping dead on a basketball court, of patients with atrial fibrillation having a massive stroke, of individuals dying after a voodoo curse, of patients passing out with recurrent ventricular tachycardia, of women dying of a broken heart, and we had heard of Napoleon's French soldiers with frozen hands on their catastrophic retreat from Russia survive if they stayed away from the campfire. We looked askance at each other at these happenings. We had no answers to these unusual and bizarre occurrences. And yet, only a few decades later we were about to solve these mysteries and witness some of the greatest advances in technology and cardiac care in human history.

For instance, ultrasound had just entered the diagnostic armamentarium of the cardiologist during my fellowship. It is also known as echocardiography, and it works the same way bats "see" in the dark (echolocation). It bounces high-frequency sound waves off the inner organs and records the echoes that return. Together, they form an accurate image of the heart and as a result, we feel we are peering through solid matter. It was introduced in 1953, by the Swedish Inge Edler (1911–2001) and his physicist friend Hellmuth Hertz. It marked the beginning of a new and spectacular diagnostic noninvasive technique. For his landmark discovery, Edler is recognized as the "Father of Echocardiography."

As a fellow, I was mesmerized at the echo depiction of the wall motion of a patient whose heart function had hit the ground after a massive heart attack, and of a severely diseased and narrowed mitral valve of a patient with rheumatic heart disease. (The mitral valve lies between the upper left and the lower left chambers of the heart.) Today, with two- and three-dimensional echocardiography and Doppler flow studies, images of the heart and blood flow are breathtaking and highly precise.

During my fellowship, I took part in several research projects and initiated my own research, publishing original articles on heart rhythm abnormalities, and in the then-infant field of cardiac ultrasound with which I was enamored at the time. I worked with Dr. Howard Friedman on studies in the animal model of cardiac tamponade,[1] and with Dr. Jacob I. Haft on the role of stress and vitamin E on the aggregation of blood platelets.

Ultrasound proved every bit as rewarding as it had seemed. Utilizing it, I described for the first time the presence of dense vegetations on the aortic heart valve in a patient with fungal infection. I also was one of the first to use ultrasound to measure heart function and indices of heart muscle contractility and show the benefits of drugs in patients with heart failure. When I saw my first paper in print as the lead author, I felt a thrill, a sense that I had contributed to the medical literature. I knew then that I was cut out to pursue an academic career. Dr. Haft, who treated me with much respect and friendship during my fellowship training, recommended me to Dr. Anthony N. Damato as a research associate in the startup field of cardiac electrophysiology at the United States Public Health Service Hospital (USPHS) in Staten Island, New York. It was here that my work and those of many other pioneers in heart rhythm disorders began.

♥

New York, NY, USA   J. Anthony Gomes

---

[1] Cardiac tamponade results when a critical accumulation of fluid in the pericardial sac—the lining around the heart compresses the heart. The shrunken ventricles can't pump all the blood the body needs, and if the fluid is not removed judiciously with needle aspiration, this condition can be lethal.

Acknowledgments

First of all, I would like to thank my patients who appear in this book under a pseudonym for confiding in me their personal trials and tribulations as they and their families faced a new reality of heart disease and heart rhythm disorders.

I would like to express my gratitude to Dan McNeill for his editorial assistance in simplifying some of the science in the book to make it more accessible to a lay readership.

My profound appreciation to the editorial board at Springer Nature (Richard Lansing, Michelle Tam, Gregory Sutorius, Abha Krishnan and his Team, and Rekha Udaiyar) for acceptance of my book proposal, its contents, and formatting to my wishes, as well as their editorial assistance.

To my wife, Margarita, for her patience and encouragement as I spent hours on the computer writing and revising.

To the current members of the Two Bridges Workshop for reading some of the chapters and offering their suggestions.

To Grace Schulman for her friendship, inspiration, and for always being there.

A special thanks to Dr. Stephen Winters, my first fellow-in-training, and my first associate at The Mount Sinai Medical Center, at a difficult time in our professional lives when the management of cardiac arrhythmias was in its infancy. I would also like to express my gratitude to the cardiac surgeons: Drs. Arisan Ergin, Jorge Cammunas, Manuel Estioko, Steven Lansman, and Randall B. Griepp with whom I had the privilege of working before the era of catheter ablation, and before the implantation of pacemakers and defibrillators became the domain of the cardiac electrophysiologist.

A word of recognition for Ms. Elena Pé, the nurse-supervisor and research nurse during my directorship of the Electrophysiology and Electrocardiography Sections, for her dedication, motivation, and thoroughness in all and every endeavor.

I would like to acknowledge my ex-associates Dr. Davendra Mehta and Dr. Noelle-Marie Langan, and the many fellows-in-training for their helping hands and enthusiasm.

My spirited appreciation of my current colleagues: Drs. Vivek Y. Reddy, Srinivas Dukkipati, Marc Miller, William Wang, and Jacob Koruth for their cutting-edge approach to cardiac arrhythmias and their friendship.

Finally, I would like to thank the fulltime cardiovascular faculty at Mount Sinai Medical Center, specifically to Drs. Valentin Fuster, Samin K. Sharma, Jonathan L. Halperin, and Annapoorna S. Kini, as well as to the voluntary faculty for their support and friendship over the last 38 years.

Contents

Part I
The Mythology of the Human Heart

Chapter 1
Romanticizing the Heart

I would rather have eyes that cannot see; ears that cannot hear;
lips that cannot speak, than a heart that cannot love.

—Robert Tizon

Tears come from the heart and not from the brain.

—Leonardo da Vinci

Since time immemorial, the heart has been likened to a household divinity, the source of life, and that of the immortal soul. Throughout history, the image of the heart has been symbolized as the seat of human emotions, and this characterization continues to this day. In this chapter, I will review the interpretations of the heart since ancient times to Harvey's understanding of the heart through meticulous anatomic experimentation.

Ancient Egyptian View of the Heart

Some 2500 years ago, a woman in her late 30s or 40s died in ancient Thebes (now Luxor) in Egypt (Fig. 1.1). She was a wealthy married woman who stood about 5 feet tall. Her coffin bore the word "Nestawedjat," meaning "The one who belongs to the wedjat eye." Wedjat eyes symbolized regeneration, and the Egyptians thought that amulets depicting them helped the wearer pass safely into the afterlife. The unwrapped mummy was extremely well-preserved. CAT scans revealed her femininity and also showed the single internal organ left inside her body: *her heart.*

Why leave the heart?

For ancient Egyptians, death was not the end. Nestawedjat's soul would arise from her body and begin an extraordinary and dangerous journey through the

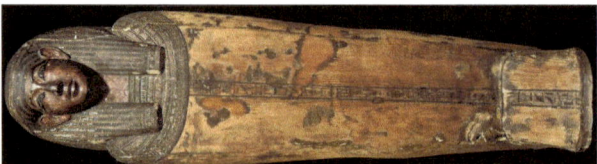

Fig. 1.1 Coffin of Nestawedjat. The coffin has a striking polychrome painted face, enlivened by the use of inlaid eyes set into bronze sockets. The wig and collar are also painted. The surface of the body is simply decorated with a line of inscription on the lid and another around the case, both texts addressing the gods. (Reprinted from the British Museum) https://www.britishmuseum.org/collection/object/Y_EA22813-b

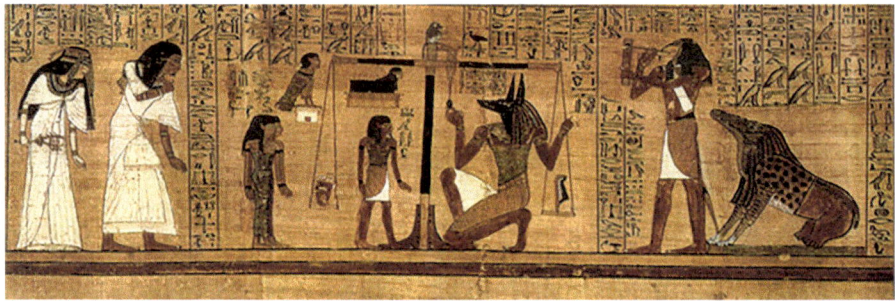

Fig. 1.2 The weighing of the heart against the feather of Ma'at. Legend: God Anubis proceeds to the weighing of the dead person's heart against the feather of Ma'at (the symbol of truth) on a balance. (Book of the Dead, circa 1250 BCE). (From: https://commons.wikimedia.org/wiki/File:BD_Weighing_of_the_Heart.jpg)

underworld. At the very end of this journey, she'd face her biggest test of all. She'd enter the Hall of Two Truths and come before god Anubis. He'd weigh her heart to see if it had become heavy with sin during her life. If it weighed less than or equal to the feather of Ma'at—an ostrich feather symbolizing the goddess of truth, balance, and morality (Fig. 1.2)—she had been virtuous. Her soul would then rejoin her body—in the mummy, which had preserved it—and she would enter Aaru,[1] the heavenly paradise. There she'd live forever.

But without her heart, she couldn't reach paradise.

The heart had paramount importance for the ancient Egyptians in earthly life as well. In their worldview, the heart, or *ib*, was actually part of the soul. It was the source of intelligence, as it was for the Mesopotamians and Babylonians. The ancient Egyptians had also linked the heart to the pulse.

---

[1] Aaru is also known as Sekhet-Aaru.

Ancient Indian View of the Heart

The oldest Hindu scriptures, the Vedic texts (c. 1500–c. 1000 BCE), considered the heart or *hridaya* (derived from *hrd*, "center") a light of consciousness, the abode of the soul and that of Brahman. In the Rig Veda, the human heart is the sacrificial fire altar, and more, the cosmic axis. In the later Hindu scriptures of the Upanishads (c. 800–c. 500 BCE), the heart is the source of the immortal soul or the Self (*Atman*):

> The shining self, dwells hidden in the heart.
> Everything in the cosmos, great and small,
> Lives in the Self—the source of life.

It is rather a majestic concept, the entire universe dwelling in one's heart. In many usages, the heart is our core, our essence.

Ancient Greek View of the Heart

Among the early Greek scientists and philosophers, the heart also had broad significance. Philosopher Empedocles (c. 492–c. 432 BCE) believed that intelligence resided in the heart. And so did one of the most famous minds of all time: Aristotle (c. 384–383 BCE). He never dissected a human, but examined animals after strangulation, when their hearts had ceased beating. He concluded that the heart was the origin of the soul, the seat of thought, reason, and emotion.

Stoic philosophy founded in Athens by Zeno of Citium (331–262 BCE) and advanced by Chrysippus of Soli (277–204 BCE), viewed the soul as the unity of thoughts, feelings, and desires all governed by a single principle, the *hegomonikon*, located in the heart. *Hegomonikon* is the source of our word "hegemony," meaning dominance.

Greek physician Aelius Galenus or Claudius Galenus, better known as Galen (129–c. 200/216 CE), challenged Aristotle's point of view. He was a brilliant man who, at age 28, became surgeon to gladiators in Pergamum, on the Aegean coast of modern Turkey. With injuries constantly before him, he learned fast. At the age of 33, he went to Rome and became physician to Emperor Marcus Aurelius. He was also a showman and a self-promoter, and he had seen how brain damage in gladiators affected the rest of the body. In Rome, he once gave a dramatic demonstration before a hall of eminent political and academic figures. He lashed down a squealing pig and cut the nerve leading to its larynx. The pig instantly stopped oinking. He thus showed that the brain controls voice and provided evidence that our thoughts, sensations, and movements arise there. The brain, he held, was the seat of the soul.

However, his views about the heart were complex and mislead physicians for centuries. He viewed the blood as moving outward in two separate systems, like rivers running into desert lakebeds and evaporating. In one, the liver turned food into the darker, venous blood, which flowed out to flesh and organs. Some of this blood, he believed, also seeped through invisible pores in the heart wall, the septum, where it mixed with air from the lungs and become the brighter arterial blood. In this second system, the arteries provided heat and motion to the rest of the body and "psychic spirits" to the brain. Galen also believed in tiny blood vessels he called *rete mirabile* ("wonderful net") at the base of the brain, where "vital spirits" changed to "animal spirits" before going throughout the body.

Ancient Islamic View of the Heart

The Persian philosopher Avicenna (Ibn Sina, 980–1037) was one of the great minds of his time. At the age of 10, he reputedly memorized the Qur'an. Then he turned his attention to medicine, and when the sultan of Bukhara (then in Iran, now in Uzbekistan) fell ill with a mysterious ailment, the young Avicenna apparently cured him. In gratitude, the sultan allowed him into his vast library and Avicenna soaked up knowledge. Because of political instability, he spent much of his life on the move. Accounts of him vary, but most suggest a brilliant wit, political shrewdness, and a sybaritic love of music and alcohol. In his *The Canon of Medicine*, he integrated Aristotle's ideas into his largely Galenic physiology. He wrote: "The heart is the root of all faculties and gives the faculties of nutrition, life, apprehension, and movement to several other members." His ideas exerted much influence on medieval Europe.

It was Arab physician Ibn al-Nafis (1210–1288) who first challenged Galen's and Avicenna's concepts of blood circulation. Born in Damascus and practicing in Cairo, he like many other great talents of the time wrote on varied topics, including law, sociology, astronomy, and fiction. But he is remembered for his *The Commentary on Anatomy in Avicenna's Canon*, written at the age of 29. In it, he became the first to describe pulmonary circulation. Blood flows from the right half of the heart to the lungs, he said, and thence down to the left half. In addition, he said that around the lungs, blood passes through minute channels from veins to arteries and turns from dark to bright. Not until the microscope and Marcello Malpighi (1628–1694) would anyone see these capillaries. Finally, al-Nafis firmly stated that Galen's invisible pores in the septum did not exist. His views were largely ignored, and his *Commentary* was only made known to the Western world around the late 1920s, when a Berlin student happened upon it in the Prussian State Library.

The Renaissance Heart

The revival of anatomy during the Renaissance period fostered the study of the basic structures of the heart. The great Leonardo da Vinci (1452–1519), who painted the Mona Lisa, the Last Supper, Salvator Mundi, and many other masterpieces, was also an architect, an engineer, and a scientist with keen interest in human anatomy. Somewhere between 1504 and 1508, the human heart occupied his interest. During this time, he met a very old man in the hospital of Santa Maria Nuova in Florence, who told him he was hundred years old and did not feel, in Leonardo's own words, "any bodily ailment other than weakness." While Leonardo was at his bedside, the centenarian suddenly died. It is then that he did something unheard of for a man with no medical background. He did an autopsy on the old man "and found that it proceeded from weakness through the failure of blood and of the artery that feeds the heart and the other lower members, which I found to be very dry, shrunken and withered." It is believed that he was the first to describe atherosclerosis of the aorta. His drawings illustrate the typical Renaissance image of the heart with two basic chambers, the ventricles, divided by the septum. He showed that the heart is a muscle and that it does not warm the blood as previously thought. He also attributed the pulse to the contraction of the left ventricle. However, Leonardo was not aware of the concept of *circulation*.

Much later, the Aragonese Michael Servetus (1509–1553) also independently identified pulmonary circulation, but his discovery, first written in the Manuscript of Paris (1546), did not reach the public. It was later incorporated into the theological work *Christianismi Restitutio* (Restoration of Christianity, 1553). In this book, he rejected the doctrine of the Trinity and the concept of predestination, both of which were fundamental to Christianity since the time of St. Augustine and reemphasized by John Calvin in his *magnum opus*, *Institutio Christianae Religionis*. It also contained by way of illustration his views on pulmonary circulation, in which he wrote: "The blood is passed through the pulmonary artery to the pulmonary vein for a lengthy pass through the lungs, during which it becomes red, and gets rid of the sooty fumes by the act of exhalation." He was soon arrested as a heretic by order of Geneva's Protestant governing council and burned at the stake near the city gates. The book was suppressed, but Servetus had been in communication with many other scholars in Europe, and possibly some of them knew of his ideas.

William Harvey's View of the Heart

It was ultimately the English physician William Harvey (1578–1657, Fig. 1.3) who overthrew Galenic circulation of blood completely. His contribution was monumental. He was born in Folkestone, England, where his father was a merchant and the town's mayor in 1600. After graduating from Cambridge, he pursued medical studies at the University of Padua at the same time Galileo was teaching there. He graduated as a doctor of Medicine in 1602, at the age of 24. He immediately returned to England and in the same year obtained his doctorate in Medicine from Cambridge University. He married the daughter of Queen Elizabeth's physician in 1604, and in 1618, he became royal physician to King James I and later King Charles I. Among his many dictums, two stand out: *All we know is still infinitely less than all that remains unknown. I profess both to learn and to teach anatomy, not from books but from dissections; not from positions of philosophers but from the fabric of nature.*

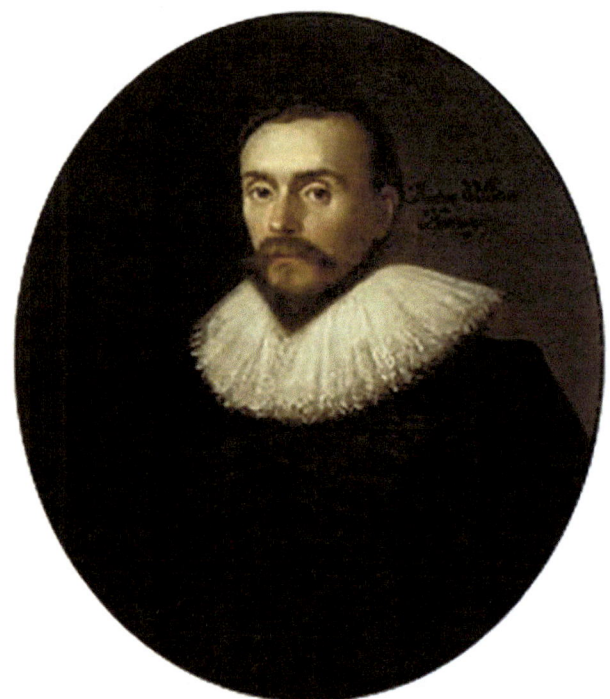

He began studying the heart and found it bewildering. He was working with small animals whose heart contractions and dilations occurred "in the twinkling of an eye, like a flash of lighting. Systole seemed at one time here, diastole there, and then all reversed, varied, and confused. So, I could reach no decision." He even wondered if God alone could understand the heart. But eventually, through patience and meticulous observation, he said, "I felt my way out of this labyrinth, and gained information, which I desired, of the motions and functions of the heart and arteries."

He described his findings in the landmark 1628 work: *Exercitatio Anatomica de Motu Cordis et Sanguinis in Animalibus.* It was in Latin, standard for scholars at the time, and the English translation appeared two decades later: *On the Motion of the Heart and Blood in Living Beings.* In it, he expounded that the heart was actively at work when it was small, hard and contracted (systole), expelling blood, and at rest when it was large and filled with blood (diastole). In his writing, William Harvey strongly refuted the Galenic concept of passage of blood through pores in the interventricular septum.

"The heart's one role," Harvey said, "is the transmission of the blood and its propulsion, by means of the arteries, to the extremities everywhere." Yet, he did not entirely challenge the metaphysical interpretation of the heart. He also wrote: "The heart, consequently, is the beginning of life; the sun of the microcosm, even as the sun in his turn might well be designated the heart of the world; for it is the heart by whose virtue and pulse the blood is moved, perfected, and made nutrient, and is preserved from corruption and coagulation; it is the household divinity which, discharging its function, nourishes, cherishes, quickens."

French philosopher René Descartes (1596–1650) was one of the first scholars to accept the new theory. He took Harvey's ideas a step further when he argued that the heart was like a pump or, better yet, a combustion engine. Yet, he also noted that Harvey had not actually explained the heartbeat.

What made the heartbeat? He wondered.

"We imagine some faculty which causes the movement, the nature of which is much more difficult to conceive than what it is invoked to explain," he said. He believed that the heart had an innate heat, but the true answer would lie far ahead. Meanwhile, Harvey's findings became widely accepted in the decades after his death.

The Heart as Metaphor

We have romanticized the heart perhaps sometime after our species began linking it to love and other emotions. The heart had been romantically characterized throughout the Middle Ages by poets, kings, lords, and their subjects.

"If indeed from the heart alone rise anger or passion, fear, terror, and sadness; if from it alone spring shame, delight, and joy, why should I say more?" wrote Andrés Laguna de Segovia (1499–1559), a Spanish physician to popes and kings and a pharmacologist and botanist.

Just as we know that stars are infernos, yet, they enchant us twinkling in the night, and though we know that the moon is a barren rock, it charms us in the sky, and so it is with the heart. It is associated with love and other emotions as in the phrase "give your heart to" and in ads and stickers as "I ♥ New York," and the heart remains the symbol for Valentine's Day. Pearl Buck (1892–1973) wrote: "The person who tries to live alone will not succeed as a human being. His heart withers if it does not answer another heart."

The heart is our center—a "heart's desire" is an inmost yearning. It is kindness, as "A Good Heart," while a cruel person "doesn't have a heart." It is also an expression of compassion, as in "Have A Heart," the title of my recently published novel, and a "Heart of Gold." It is commitment—we can "no longer have the heart" to perform a task, and we can have a "change of heart." It is intuition, as in *The Little Prince*, Antoine de Saint-Exupéry (1900–1944) wrote, "It is only with the heart that one can see rightly; what is essential is invisible to the eye." It can express an inner truth, when we express feelings "in our hearts." In *The Unbearable Lightness of Being*, Milan Kundera wrote: "When the heart speaks, the mind finds it indecent to object." Poet Ted Hughes (1930–1998) wrote: "The only thing people regret is that they didn't live boldly enough, that they didn't invest enough heart, didn't love enough. Nothing else really counts at all."

In the Old Testament, King David states: "the sacrifices of God are a broken spirit; a broken and contrite heart." Deuteronomy 6:5 instructs to love the Lord your

God with all your heart. The Sacred Heart of Jesus is a Catholic devotion in which the heart of Jesus stands for his love of everyone, while the devotion of the Immaculate Heart of Mary focuses more on her love of Jesus and God. In her image, seven swords typically pierce her heart, for her Seven Sorrows.

These metaphoric expressions give the heart immediacy—symbolizing life.

♥

Chapter 2
The Mysteries of the Age-Old Pulse

Very often conditions are recorded as observable "under thy fingers"… Among such observations it is important to notice that the pulsations of the human heart are observed.

—James Henry Breasted (1865–1935), archeologist, on the Edwin Smith Surgical Papyrus, c. 1600 BCE

I love yoga… I also see an Ayurvedic doctor, which is an ancient Indian thing. I go and see the doctor to balance my system twice a year; it's preventative. They take my pulse, give me some herbs, and tell me what I should eat and what I should avoid.

—Jerry Hall

Since antiquity, the pulse has had a lofty and mysterious position in medical practice. Physicians viewed it not only as a surrogate for the heart but also as evidence of the health of other organs. This was likely because the pulse was the most accessible organ. The liver, kidneys, and lungs are largely silent, but the pulse can always be felt in the neck, the wrist, the feet, and elsewhere. As a result, physicians in antiquity and medieval times used it to diagnose illness, yet they misunderstood its very generation. Some falsely believed that the heart and the arteries each had separate pulses, which contracted at about the same time. Furthermore, they made highly exaggerated claims in diagnosing diseases of a host of organs by feeling the pulse, but there is no evidence that they actually measured its rate (with the exceptions of the Greek Herophilus, the "father of anatomy," and the Ayurveda healers of India). Overall, the pulse was a mystery that became a magnet for some of the best age-old minds.

© The Author(s), under exclusive license to Springer Nature Switzerland AG 2021
J. A. Gomes, *Rhythms of Broken Hearts*,
https://doi.org/10.1007/978-3-030-77382-3_2

The Rosetta Stone of Ancient Egyptian Medicine

In 1872, German Egyptologist George Ebers was investigating sites in Thebes when a prosperous Egyptian approached him with an offer of antiquities. Inside a box, Ebers saw a statue of Osiris carved perhaps in the past year and a papyrus of no value. He politely spurned the offer but said he would pay well for items of value. The next day the man returned and showed him a metal box. Inside were mummy cloths. When Ebers unwrapped them, he found another papyrus. This one was different. It had been discovered 10 years earlier between a mummy's legs in a tomb at Thebes. It was marvelously preserved, with text easy to read, and it seemed to date from at least a millennium before Christ. Ebers was elated, but the seller, perhaps sensing a windfall, asked a price he could hardly afford. Fortunately, a wealthy friend materialized, the deal took place, and Ebers brought the papyrus back to the University of Leipzig.

We now know the Ebers Papyrus (Fig. 2.1) dates back to around 1550 BC, over a thousand years before Hippocrates, and it is one of the most important writings in ancient medicine. It is a 68-foot scroll, replete with archaic phrases and magic chants, but it also has a chapter on the heart and the pulse, for it says: "In the Heart are the vessels to the whole of the body. As to these, every physician, every *sexet*-priest, every magician, will feel them when he lays his finger on the head, on the back of the head, on the hands, on the stomach region, on the arms, on the legs. Everywhere he feels his Heart because its vessels run to all his limbs." In other words, physicians place their hands all over the body, but they are really examining the heart, because it beats before they feel the pulse elsewhere.

It remains unclear whether the Egyptian physicians counted the pulse rate with the help of the clepsydra, the water clock possibly invented under Thutmosis III (18th Dynasty, fifteenth century BCE). It also remains unknown whether they were able to recognize the differences in pulse rate and quality.

Classifying the Pulse: Ancient Asian Medicine

As far back as 600 BCE, Chinese physician Pien Ts'Io asserted the importance of the pulse both for the diagnosis and prognosis of disease. He viewed the human body as a string instrument with a wide array of pulses corresponding to the different strings and their tones. Much later, Wang Shuhe (c. 180–c. 270 CE) wrote a highly influential treatise called *The Pulse Classic*. Born into a noble family and later a physician to royalty, Wang described 24 kinds of pulses, such as slippery, knotted, and scattered, and subdivided each by location, speed, strength, and "feeling," such as "hollow." All told, there were more than 100 variations of the pulse, assessed on both hands in the morning hours when the yin and yang were in balance. "It may be easy to understand the difference among pulse types theoretically," he observed, "but it is difficult to distinguish them with the fingers." And whether right or wrong or highly speculative, ancient Chinese physicians must have

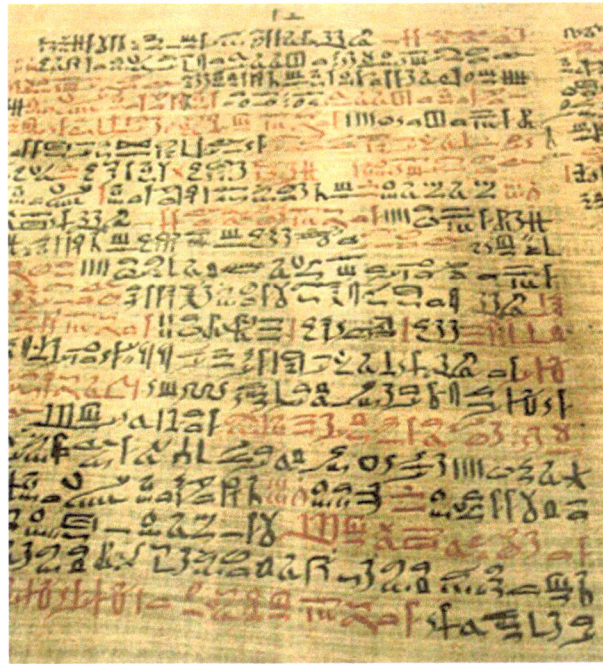

Fig. 2.1 The Ebers Papyrus. Legend: The Ebers Papyrus, also known as Papyrus Ebers, is an Egyptian medical papyrus dating to circa 1550 BC. It was purchased at Luxor (Thebes) by Georg Ebers and is currently kept at the library of the University of Leipzig, in Germany. The papyrus is thought to have been copied from earlier texts, perhaps dating as far back as 3400 BC. It is a 110-page scroll and about 20 meters long and is among the oldest preserved medical documents. The papyrus contains a "treatise on the heart." It notes that the heart is the center of the blood supply, with vessels attached for every member of the body. https://en.wikipedia.org/wiki/Ebers_Papyrus#/media/File:PEbers_c41-bc.jpg

developed outstanding tactile skills. Wang also linked the type of pulse to specific organs, which suggests that these physicians tried to diagnose diseases of other organs such as the liver by taking the pulse. His work dominated Chinese thinking on the pulse for over 1300 years.

Ancient Indian Ayurveda physician Sage Kanád (c. 550 BCE) is best known as a forceful proponent of atomic theory before Democritus (c. 460–c. 370 BCE), and his very name Kanád, bestowed on him later in life, means "atom eater." But he also wrote an important book on the pulse called *Science of Sphygmica*, where he says:

"Immediately after pressing the pulse just below the hand-joint, firstly there is the perception of the beating of *bdyu* (air); secondly . . . there is the perception of *pitta* (bile); thirdly or the last, the perception of the beating of *slesmd* or *kaph* (phlegm), is gained."

As the quote indicates, he theorized that each pulse has three phases, and abnormality in any of them reflects disease in one of the three main humors of the body: air, bile, and phlegm. Perhaps most intriguingly, Ayurveda physicians also counted the pulse rate. They calculated it per "pal," with each pal equaling 24 seconds. It is unclear whether they used a water clock, since one scholar says pulse examination required not only extensive practice but also "trancelike" concentration, so the physician could enter into "the very inside of a patient."

Dissections and Clepsydras: The Ancient Greeks and Romans

Hippocrates (c. 460–c. 375 BCE), the "father of medicine," described the characteristics of the arterial pulse in conditions such as fever and lethargy in his book on humors. But Praxagoras of Kos (c. 340) is the first physician who discovered that pulsations only occur in the arteries, not in the veins. His student Herophilus (c. 335–c. 280 BCE) worked in Alexandria during the few decades when the Ptolemaic rulers allowed dissection of corpses, a practice that would be forbidden for the next 1800 years. He was the first person to measure pulse with an instrument, a portable clepsydra he built for this purpose, which he used on his medical rounds (Fig. 2.2). The clepsydra exploits the principle of the drip—like the regularity of a dripping faucet. He also compared the pulse to musical rhythm, using upbeats and downbeats as units to link the two. Among other phenomena, he described *pulsus caprizans* as similar to the leap of a goat, with two phases, an initial stroke followed by a stronger one, akin to what we call today—*pulsus bisferiens*.

Erasistratus (c. 304–c. 250 BCE) was a Greek anatomist and royal physician under Seleucus I Nicator (or "victor") of Syria, and together with Herophilus, he founded a school of anatomy in Alexandria. They had erroneous ideas on the circulation of blood, believing that arteries contained *pneuma* (air), while veins contained blood. And indeed, our word "artery" is derived from the Greek "airein." They believed that the arterial pulse arose when arteries contracted, drew *pneuma* from the heart, and moved it forward. Additionally, and also falsely, they believed that the pulse was inherent to the arteries and different from that of the heart.

Galen (c. 129–c. 200/216 CE) laid out his thoughts on the pulse in four books entitled *De Pulsuum Differentiis*. He posited that the genesis of the pulse had to lie in the heart itself. He believed that the pulsations of the arteries were unequal and that a variety of pulses arose based on the degree of dilation on each side. Like Herophilus, he wrongly held the view that the arterial wall itself generated the pulse. He described several types of arterial pulse such as saw-edged pulse, undulating pulse, and worm-like pulse. He felt that the pulse varied according to the temperature and illnesses, and in concert with other ancient physicians, he described hot pulses and cold pulses, the pulse of pain, inflammation, lethargy, convulsions, jaundice, and even elephantiasis.[1] Overall, Galen described 27 characteristics for a single pulse based on its size, speed, and frequency.

---

[1] Also known as filariasis and caused by a tropical parasite, this disease affects the lymphatic system, causing blockage and severe swelling of the legs and scrotum. The appearance of the legs led to the name "elephantiasis."

Fig. 2.2 Clepsydra or Greek water clock. A portable water clock used by Herophilus for the purpose of arterial pulse examination. This water clock contained a specified amount of water for natural pulse beats of every age. Nima Ghasemzadeh, A. Maziar Zafari, "A Brief Journey into the History of the Arterial Pulse", *Cardiology Research and Practice*, vol. 2011, Article ID 164832, 14 pages, 2011. https://doi.org/10.4061/2011/164832

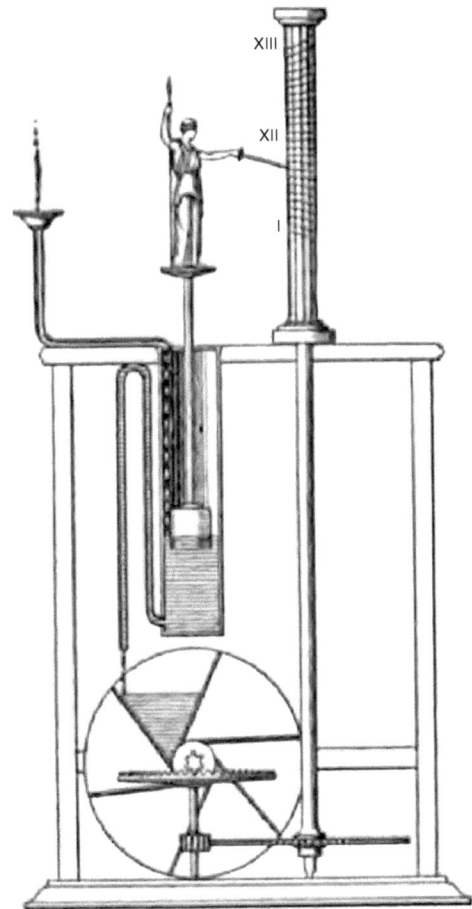

Avicenna and Maimonides

Persian polymath Avicenna (981–1037) helped perpetuate ancient errors about the heart, but he made inroads in our knowledge of the pulse. In his treatise, he described eight different pulse variations depending on dilation, duration, temperature, fullness, compressibility, equality or inequality of consecutive beats, and even regularity or irregularity of rhythm. Thus, in his analysis, we note for the first time an assessment of heart rhythm abnormalities. He was also the first to define resistance and elasticity in the pulse ("compressibility"). His description of the irregularity both in a single pulsation and in a succession of pulses likely reflects premature and dropped heartbeats and atrial fibrillation. He also described several types of pulses in different disease states: the mouse-tail pulse (*pulsus alternans* as it is known today), undulating pulse, dicrotic (M-shaped) pulse, and vermicular pulse (a small, quick pulse that feels like a writhing worm to the finger).

Moses Maimonides (1135–1204) born in Cordoba, Spain, spent much of his early life moving from place to place to avoid persecution. He, together with his family, finally settled in Cairo, then relatively tolerant, but soon after his father and older brother died, his family was in financial straits. He became a physician partly to provide for them. Today, he is best known as a major Jewish philosopher and author of books like the landmark *The Guide for the Perplexed*. He was also a brilliant doctor and eventually became the physician to Saladin, the legendary Muslim general. In his writings, he correlated the pulse with disease severity of a host of organs, as his predecessors had.

The Pulsilogium and the Stopwatch

One day while still a student, Galileo Galilei (1564–1642) was watching a lamp swing back and forth in a cathedral. He began checking its swings with his pulse and found that each swing took the same amount of time, regardless of the distance it covered. He made his findings known and created a few pendulum devices to keep time, known as metronomes.

Venetian physician Santorio Sanctorius (1561–1636) was a friend of Galileo, and he became the first to build a pendulum device explicitly for measuring pulse. Called a "pulsilogium," it consisted of a scale in inches and a cord with a movable weight marked with a crosswise line, and the physician adjusted the length of the pendulum until its swing matched the heartbeat. As a result, he wrote in 1603, "We can monitor at what day and at which hour the pulse deviated in intensity and frequency from its natural state." It has been called "the first man/machine interaction in medicine."

However, it was the English physician Sir John Floyer (1649–1734) who first counted the pulse rate in its current form. There was a clever watchmaker in town, and Floyer had him create a spring-driven watch with two key features: a second hand and a lever to stop it. Thus, Floyer had the first stopwatch with a second hand to enjoy general, practical use. In his book, *The Physician's Pulse Watch* (1707), he wrote in all modesty: "All I pretend is the discovery of a rule whereby we may know the natural pulse and the excesses and defects from this in diseases." He ushered in the modern era of recording the pulse rate in the examination of patients. In fact, his pulse watch gave physicians their first truly effective bedside measuring device of any kind.

The impact was significant. There is a famous painting (Fig. 2.3) of Pablo Picasso done in 1897 in Barcelona when he was just 15 years of age, entitled *Science and Charity*. It is highly realistic, and he executed it just before he began creating his famous semi-representational art. In it, Picasso depicts his own father, José Ruiz Blasco, as a doctor holding the wrist of a bedridden patient and gazing intently at his watch, timing and counting the pulse.

Fig. 2.3 Science and charity by Pablo Picasso. See text for further explanation. https://www.wikiart.org/en/pablo-picasso/science-and-charity-1897

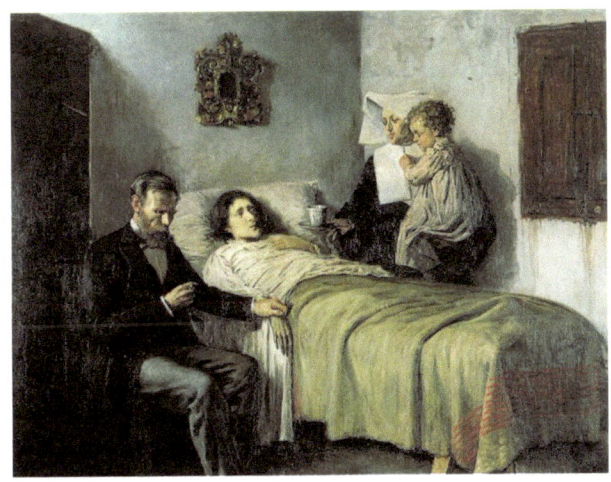

Current Understanding of the Pulse

In modern times, a whole variety of pulses have been described primarily reflecting cardiovascular conditions (Fig. 2.4). The most common and useful include:

1. Pulsus paradoxus (occurs when there is a decrease in blood pressure by more than 10 mm during inspiration). It is seen in a host of cardiac conditions but mostly accessed to determine the presence of significant fluid around the heart what we call pericardial effusion.
2. *Pulsus parvus et tardus* also known as anacrotic pulse (a slow rising pulse seen in severe aortic stenosis, when the aortic valve cannot open adequately).
3. *Pulses bigeminus*: a coupling of the pulse wave in a pair followed by a pause. It is seen in the presence of alternate premature beats and heart block.
4. *Thready pulse*: a very weak pulse seen in shock and in ventricular tachycardia.

Conclusions

When I was a medical student and subsequently a resident in medicine at Mount Sinai's Elmhurst City Hospital, the chairman of medicine, Dr. Stanley Seckler, an old-time clinical professor and a legend in clinical medicine, pressed upon us the need to feel for the pulse and its characteristics. As Wang Shuhe observed long ago, appreciation of pulses requires considerable patience and practice, even though it is highly subjective. It is doubtful that most young doctors and today's medical students can distinguish different types of pulses. Undoubtedly, the pulse has gradually declined in importance from its elevated position in ancient times, the Middle Ages, and even more recently. Although one laments the spiraling fall of the pulse from the altar of worship, the advent of more sophisticated tests and technologies—such

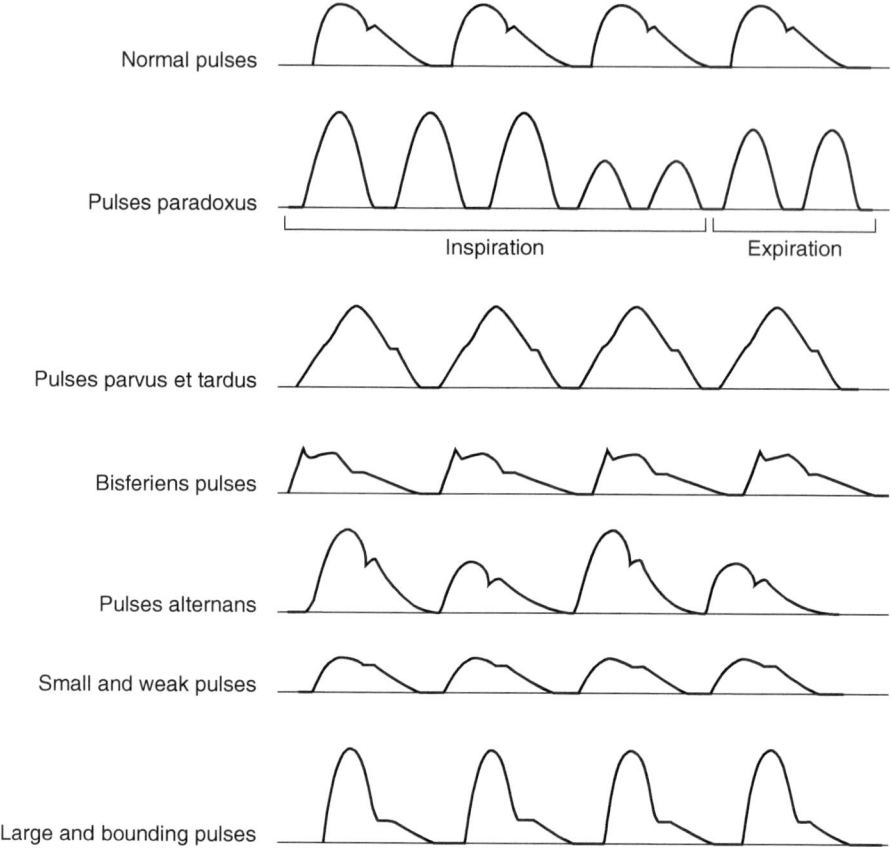

Fig. 2.4 Different types of pulses. A normal and different types of pulses seen in various diseases are shown from top to bottom

as the ECG and echocardiography—provides detailed information on the anatomy and function of the heart. These tests are objective and not subjective. For example, if a patient develops significant fluid around the heart, the decision to insert a needle into the sac surrounding the heart will depend on the echo findings rather than the pulse alone. Furthermore, it has no real value in assessing the condition of other organs beyond the heart.

In today's day and age, the pulse is mostly examined by nurses and medical assistants to determine the heart rate. Pulse quality mainly consists in assessing the weakness or strength of the pulse, identifying a regular or an irregular pulse, and importantly determining response to exercise. During a cardiac arrest, however, one can hear a physician utter aloud, "There is no pulse" or "I feel a weak pulse" and when the patient is revived "I feel a pulse!"—often with great elation and relief that the patient has been saved.

♥

Part II
The Renaissance Period in Heart Rhythm Disorders

Chapter 3
Demystifying the Heart

*Explore, Dream & Discover are three secrets of which the time
traveler is unaware. They demystify as the journey advances!*

—Vishwanath S. J.

*The real voyage of discovery consists not in seeking new
landscapes, but in having new eyes*

—Marcel Proust

Ancient maps showed the world variously as a circular plate, a rectangle, and a
ragged irregular shape. Today with satellites we map it down to dots in the sidewalk.
Similarly, the modern understanding of the anatomy, cellular physiology, and
mechanics of the intact human heart has mostly debunked myths of old discussed in
previous chapters. The heart is very much a dynamic electrical cum mechanical
organ, and engineers have modeled artificial hearts using these properties.

It is undoubtedly a remarkable organ. Just slightly larger than a fist, it beats
incessantly, about 2,759,400,000 times over the average life span, assuming 70
beats per minute for 75 years. Just imagine contracting and relaxing your biceps or
even clenching and unclenching your fist some 100,000 times a day without rest,
come rain or shine, speeding up during the day when active and excited, slowing
down while at rest, and more so while asleep—and going through the same motion
for a whole lifetime without a break until death, the ultimate electrical quiescence.
The heart is a complex but strong, resilient, and reliable structure with great endurance: a true engineering masterpiece.

This hollow structure has four components:

1. Muscle. This tissue is the motor that pumps blood throughout the body.
2. Valves. These gatekeepers open and close to regulate the flow of blood through
   the heart.
3. Two main coronary arteries. They arise from the aorta and branch out to supply
   the heart with oxygen and nutrients.

© The Author(s), under exclusive license to Springer Nature
Switzerland AG 2021
J. A. Gomes, *Rhythms of Broken Hearts*,
https://doi.org/10.1007/978-3-030-77382-3_3

4. Control system. This efficient electrical network causes each beat.

Any derangement in these components will result in heart disease, with their symptoms, disabilities, and potential death.

Harvey described the first three of these—the fourth left him bewildered. Let's take a look at each of them.

The Cartography of the Heart

The most essential fact about the heart's structure is that it consists of four chambers (Fig. 3.1). The two thin-walled upper ones are the right and left atrium. ("Right" and "left" are from one's own perspective, looking out, like your right and left arms.) Physicians used to call them "auricles," but you rarely hear the term anymore. "Atria" is much more descriptive. Like the atria in buildings, they are open spaces for arrivals. The two lower chambers are thicker and stronger, because they have to pump blood much further. They are the right and left ventricles. "Ventricle" comes from a diminutive of the Latin word *venter* that meant "little belly." And with a little imagination, the slight outswellings of the ventricles can seem like bellies.

Harvey observed that oxygen-poor blood enters the right atrium through two large veins: the superior and inferior vena cava (IVC and SVC, respectively) (Latin for "hollow veins," and they would have looked hollow in dissections). The superior vena cava brings in blood from the head and upper body. The inferior vena cava delivers it from everywhere else.

The right atrium is a collecting receptacle (Fig. 3.1) As it gathers blood, the tricuspid valve between it and the right ventricle below stay closed to keep the blood in. When the right atrium is full, it contracts, opening the tricuspid valve and forcing blood down into the right ventricle.

The right ventricle (Fig. 3.1) is a much stronger pump. About two-tenths of a second later, it squeezes suddenly, and blood shoots up into the pulmonary artery, which carries it to the lungs, where the blood takes in enriched oxygen, which becomes part of the carrier molecule hemoglobin. It also releases waste like carbon dioxide into the lungs, which we exhale. The swap is efficient. Each minute, the blood picks up about three-tenths of a quart of oxygen and discharges the same amount of carbon dioxide.

Now the blood is scarlet, and it looks bright with life. Four pulmonary veins take this freshened blood into the left atrium. It is a collecting chamber like its cousin, the right atrium, and behaves the same way. When full, it contracts and opens the mitral valve at the bottom, so named because of a fancied resemblance to a bishop's *mitre* or hat. Blood then pours down into the left ventricle.

The left ventricle is a stronger pump than the right and generates a higher pressure (Fig. 3.1). When it contracts, it forces blood through the aortic valve into the aorta and outward. Some of it goes quickly back to nourish the heart through the coronary arteries. The rest travels the 60,000 miles of blood vessels in the body.

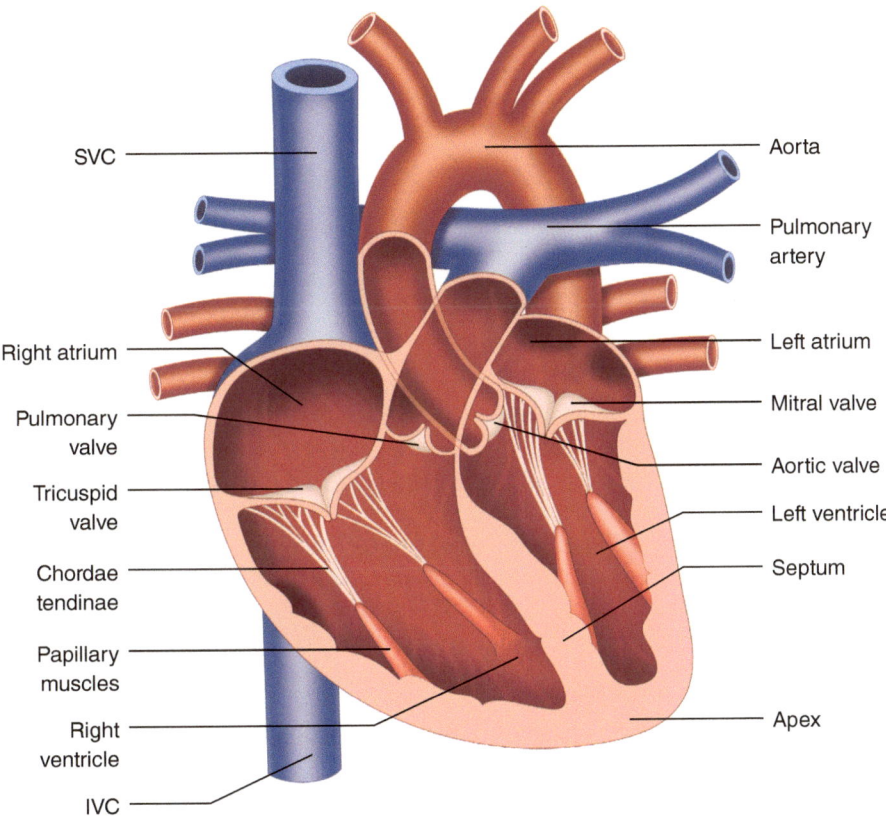

SVC

Aorta

Pulmonary artery

Right atrium

Left atrium

Pulmonary valve

Mitral valve

Aortic valve

Tricuspid valve

Left ventricle

Chordae tendinae

Septum

Papillary muscles

Right ventricle

Apex

IVC

Fig. 3.1 Interior view of the mechanical elements of the heart (*corresponds to B1-Slide 01. pdf...attached*). Legend: Red depicts the arterial blood vessels, heart cavity, and muscle and purple the venous system. The valves appear in white. Note that the right and left ventricles are separated by a muscular structure known as the septum or septal wall of the heart. The tricuspid and the mitral valve are tethered to the heart muscle (papillary muscles) by chords known as chordae tendineae. Abbreviations: SVC superior vena cava, IVC inferior vena cava

The arteries get smaller and smaller, until blood passes through microscopic capillaries, just big enough for red blood cells to come through in single file. There, another exchange occurs. The blood feeds oxygen, glucose, and other nutrients to cells through the thin capillary walls while picking up waste. It darkens, emerges into a vein, and finally spills back into the right atrium again through one of the vena cavae.

This life-sustaining circulation is surprisingly quick. A red blood cell makes a full cycle once every 30 seconds or so.

Heart disease can arise in any aspect of this system. The heart walls can grow too thick. The valves can narrow or leak. The coronary arteries can get blocked, causing myocardial infarction ("muscle-heart-stuffing") and death to part or all of the heart tissue. These maladies were mysteries since antiquity, and now we understand them rather well.

But French philosopher Rene Descartes, who was the first to accept Harvey's theory on the circulation of blood, asserted that an important question still remained: What makes the heartbeat? Where is the control system?

The command system of the heart continued a mystery even to well-informed doctors of yester years. Yet, it's the essence of the heartbeat, the secret to that thump you feel and hear in your chest. It is the most fascinating aspect of all.

The Search for the Command Center

In the 1770s, physician Luigi Galvani (1737–1798) grew interested in nerves. During one experiment, he saw a frog's muscles twitch when he touched them with scissors during a thunderstorm and stared at them in wonder. In another, he accidentally touched a dead frog's leg with a scalpel that gained an electrical charge, a spark flew, and the leg kicked as if alive. He eventually showed that electricity passed through nerves to muscles, making them jump. This finding did more than upend ancient notions about "animal spirits." The observations gave birth to the relationship between electricity and physiology.

Simply put, without electrical activation, there can be no muscle contraction. Every time you snap your fingers or lift your eyebrows or throw a ball, an electric current has stimulated muscle fibers and made them contract. An electrical current makes the heart beat too. But where does this signal originate and how does it get to all the muscle fibers of the heart?

Galen had observed that an excised heart whose nerves had been cut continued beating for some time after its removal. He wrote: "The heart, removed from the thorax, can be seen to move for a considerable time... a definite indication that it does not need the nerves to perform its function." Leonardo da Vinci, who drew anatomic details of the organs of the body with unsurpassed draftsmanship and who dissected corpses, said: *Del core. Questo si muove da se`, e non si ferma, se non eternalmente.* ("As to the heart: it moves itself, and doth never stop, except it be for eternity.")

The origin of the heartbeat remained the subject of much interest and research in the nineteenth century. Ultimately, the debate was settled by anatomists who discovered the site of origin of the electrical impulse and its conducting pathways.

The first advance toward mapping the cardiac electrical system came from Czech experimental physiologist Jan Evangelista Purkyně, commonly known as Johannes Purkinje ("per-KIN-jee," 1787–1869). In 1839, he described a mesh of gray, gelatinlike fibers across the ventricless. He didn't know what they were: at first, he thought they were cartilage, but his name became attached to them—Purkinje fibers (Fig. 3.2). As it turns out, there are millions of them, and they carry electrical current to the heart muscle.

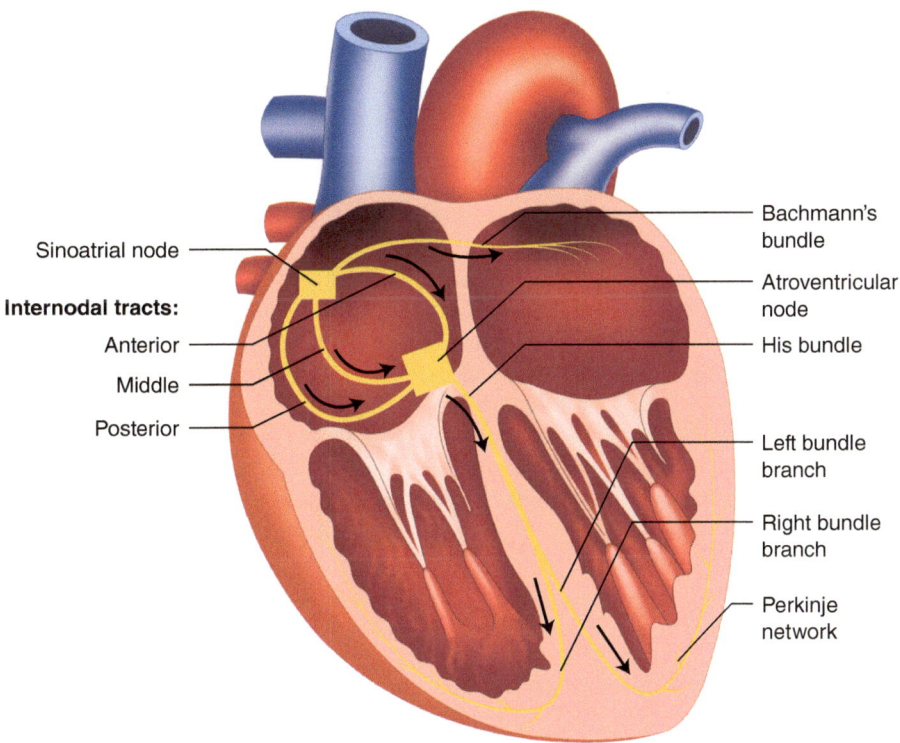

Fig. 3.2 The electrical system of the heart (*corresponds to figure B1-Slider 09.pdf...attached*). Legend: Current starts at the sinus or sinoatrial node and ends in the Purkinje system. The cable network of the heart is shown in yellow. The dark arrows show the direction of electrical activation. The sinus node has the fastest rate of spontaneous firing, followed by the A-V node, while the Purkinje fibers have the slowest rate

By the late nineteenth century, the search for the origin of the heartbeat had become intense, almost like the search for the source of the Nile.

In 1893, Swiss anatomist Wilhelm His, Jr. (1863–1934) discovered that tract at the University of Leipzig. It was a bundle of tissue leading away from the base of the atrium and down into the septal wall. This formation became known as the bundle of His (Fig. 3.2). It is a very important structure and a landmark to distinguish rhythm disorders that arise in the upper chambers of the heart from those in the lower.

Pioneering Japanese pathologist Dr. Sunao Tawara (1873–1953) in 1906 working at the Philipps University of Marburg, Germany, traced the bundle of His up to the base of the atrium, where he found the tight knot of fibers that caused the pause in the current flow. This is the atrioventricular node, usually called the A-V node (Fig. 3.2).

The capstone came next year. Scottish anatomist and anthropologist Dr. Arthur Keith had been looking for an assistant, and his grocer suggested his own son, Martin Flack, then a medical student at Oxford. One summer day in 1906, Flack was working in a laboratory in a cottage in the English countryside. Once, a drawing room, it had been converted into a lab by its owner, Dr. Arthur Keith. The cottage itself was a fine, two-story, multi-bedroom, red-gabled building with creepers climbing up the front, a broad lawn, a lush garden, and a horse plodding in circles around a well. On this day, Flack was hunched over his microscope examining sections of the mole heart.

At the same time, his mentor, Dr. Keith, was taking a well-earned break, bicycling with his wife through the pretty cherry orchards nearby. One of Keith's medical students said of him, "He was a great favorite with everyone there… He won you to learning anatomy in that he never seemed to deal out information, but rather to accompany you in the search for an understanding of it." He and Flack were searching intensely for *the source of the heartbeat*.

When Dr. Keith and his wife returned that evening, they found Flack highly agitated. He greeted them with "Eureka!" and showed Keith a "wonderful structure he had discovered in the right auricle (atrium) of the mole, just where the superior vena cava enters that chamber."

Keith realized that the structure resembled the A-V node, which Dr. Sunao Tawara had described earlier that year. Dr. Tawara had aptly said the entire system "resembles a tree, having a beginning, or root, and branches," and Keith and Flack had found that beginning. They named it the sinoauricular node, abbreviated to sinus node (Fig. 3.2). It lay atop the right atrium and had its own blood supply. It was a breathtaking discovery. In 1907, they wrote that "the dominating rhythm of the heart is believed to normally arise" in it. They were right. They had found the source of the heartbeat.

The Org Chart of Control

The heart's electrical system is all about distributing orders. It's about sparking an electric current and sending it to the muscle fibers to make them contract. In a way, it resembles the top-down command structure in the army, from general to myriad privates, or in a corporation, from CEO down to entry-level employees. And so, I'll recapitulate in this direction too, from sinus node to Purkinje fibers (Fig. 3.2).

The sinus node—or sinoatrial node or SA node—is the heart's dominant pacemaker. It triggers every beat and controls beat frequency. I like to call it the "maestro" of the conducting system and what a maestro it is! It can go from *larghissimo* to *adagio* to *prestissimo*[1] in a moment, and likewise, it can change its tempo to

---

[1] As slowly as possible, to slowly, to very quickly.

rallentando.[2] It fires independently, but it is heavily influenced by the autonomic nervous system, which regulates the myriad inner processes that occur without our awareness, such as breathing, digestion, and body temperature. The sympathetic or stimulating part of that system can speed up the heart rate and the force of muscle contraction, while the parasympathetic or inhibiting part can slow it down. As a result, the heart reacts rapidly to fear, sexual, and other forms of excitement, increasing its rate in an instant. On the other hand, the sinus node can slow down its rate when a person is at rest and during sleep. Long-distance athletes and marathon runners have rates less than 60 beats per minute during the day; and five-time Tour de France winner Miguel Indurain reportedly had a resting heart rate of 28. Their bigger, stronger hearts pump blood more efficiently with each beat.

When the sinus node discharges, it activates the right atrial muscle, or myocardium ("myo" = muscle), and almost simultaneously the left atrium through a special pathway known as the Bachman's bundle, discovered in 1916 by Dr. Jean George Bachmann (1877–1959), who unusual for a cardiologist was also a landscape artist, linguist, and professional chef. Because of Bachmann's bundle, both atria contract at about the same time.

From the right atrium, the electrical impulse spreads through internodal tracts to Tawara's A-V node, where it pauses. The A-V node, like the sinus node, is unique in form and function. It acts like a railway station except that normally electrical conduction doesn't quite stop there but moves more slowly. The effect is the same: delay. After the A-V node fires, current races down the bundle of His. Then it reaches a branching point. The right bundle branch carries it to a right ventricle, the left bundle branch to the left. Both branches finally ramify into the mesh of Purkinje fibers, which spread it out all over the ventricles. The Purkinje network activates both, making them pump at the same time.

The cable system of the heart is prey to other problems as well. It can fire spontaneously and produce abnormal and runaway heart rhythms, via a host of mechanisms. In addition, a person can be born with extra muscle bands and connections that provide an alternate and additional pathway for conduction. Such extra connections can wreak havoc, resulting in a host of abnormal runaway rhythms (see Chap. 4).

Meanwhile, there is one more question: Exactly how do these electrical impulses reach the heart muscle at all?

This is the final mystery, a question the ancients could not have even fantasized.

---

[2] Becoming slower.

Inside the Command Fibers

In 1952, Hodgkin and Huxley (1) reported their findings on the channel theory and the gating system in the squid axon, by demonstrating how channels open and close and how ions pass through open channels. Their pioneering work won them a share of the 1963 Nobel Prize in Physiology of Medicine.

Thus, at the cellular level, electrical activation of the heart occurs through a special system, which consists of opening and closing of "gates" or "channels." These gates let electrically charged ions, positive or negative, flow in or out of the cell. Because they are electrically charged, their inward and outward flow can change the voltage of the cell. Hence, their movement generates the electrical waveform known as the "action potential."

The action potential consists of five phases, shown in Fig. 3.3, with their respective inward and outward flow of sodium (Na^+), potassium (K^+), calcium (Ca^+), and chloride (CL^-) ions. The phases of the action potential are labeled 0–4 by convention. The resting membrane potential is phase 4. Then depolarization (phase 0) occurs. That is, as ions move back and forth, the charge in the cell quickly becomes positive compared to the outside. On the ECG, phase 0 corresponds to the QRS

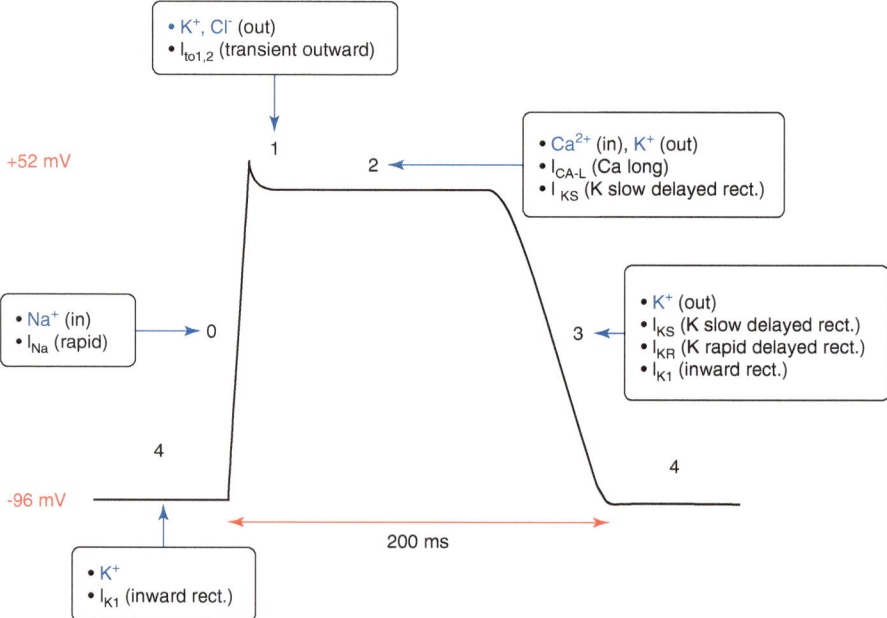

Fig. 3.3 Cardiac action potential (*corresponds to Figure 4.1 jpeg…same figure used in the book Heart Rhythm Disorders*). Legend: Phase 4 is the resting state (at −96 mV), 0 is depolarization, 1 and 2 are the plateau, 3 is repolarization, and 4 is the resting state again. "I" stands for movement into the cell, "out" for movement out of it. "Na" is the symbol for sodium, Ca for calcium, CL for chloride, and "K" for potassium

complex. Since the whole heart is much larger than a single cell, the QRS complex is much wider than the sharp upstroke (phase 0) of the single cell. During the plateau phase (1–2), the cell remains depolarized. Repolarization or change back to resting membrane potential occurs in (phase 3), and the T wave of the ECG reflects this reverse shift in electrical charge. At the end of the T wave, the single cell is back in phase 4—the resting membrane potential.

It is noteworthy that unequal distribution of ions produces electrochemical gradients across the cell membrane. The large differences in sodium and potassium concentration are made possible by the energy-dependent Na/K pump that requires adenosine triphosphate (ATP) for energy. The Na/K pump works like a shape-shifting machine (for animation, see Sodium-Potassium Exchange Pump Animated Lecture-YouTube: *https://www.youtube.com/watch?v=xweYA-IJTqs*). It actually changes its form, over and over, to control the level of these ions in the cell. It first opens up inside the cell, pulls sodium into it, and then closes. Once it has trapped the sodium, it opens at the end outside the cell, expels the sodium, and draws potassium ions in. It closes outside, opens inside, and releases the potassium. Then it pulls in sodium again, and it repeats this cycle over and over. Critically, it moves three positive sodium ions out of the cell for every two positive potassium ions it pulls in. All this work has the effect of creating a higher positive charge outside the cell than inside.

However, drugs and genetic abnormalities (inherited or mutated) can cause blocks in the gating system (see Chap. 10) and result in heart rhythm abnormalities. Failure in conduction at the level of the A-V node or the bundle of His can result in heart block, for instance. And in some cases of tachycardia, excess stimuli strike outside the shield of the plateau. Certain drugs will block or slow the potassium channels, so these ions take longer to reenter the cell. They expand the plateau phase and can be helpful in both preventing and terminating rapid heart rhythms.

What triggers an action potential? A cell generates one when it receives a sufficient stimulus from a neighbor cell, across a synapse. It needs a prod. But that doesn't explain how a heart can beat when it is detached from the body. The ultimate secret of the heartbeat lies in one final fact: pacemaker cells like those in the sinus node don't need a prod. They have no true resting state. On their own, they open the gates regularly to start the action potential. And so, when the sinus node fires, say, 75 times per minute, each time it generates an action potential which spreads cell to cell down to the A-V node, the bundle of His, and eventually the Purkinje fibers and the muscle.

Deep facts like these were as unimaginable to Galen as pulsars. And as we came to understand the physiology of impulse generation and transmission, it opened doors to the treatment of heart rhythm disorders.

♥

Chapter 4
Understanding Heart Rhythm Disorders: The Birth of the ECG and Clinical Cardiac Electrophysiology

I am one of those who think like Nobel, that humanity will draw more good than evil from new discoveries.

—Marie Curie

There is not a discovery in science, however revolutionary, however sparkling with insight, that does not arise out of what went before. 'If I have seen further than other men,' said Isaac Newton, 'it is because I have stood on the shoulders of giants.'

—Isaac Asimov, Adding a Dimension: Seventeen Essays on the History of Science

At the outset of my career as a heart rhythm expert, few cardiologists understood our specialty of clinical cardiac electrophysiology. They were a visual breed, and they saw cardiac electrophysiology as esoteric, mathematical, mechanistic, abstract, and cerebral. It was a realm of electrical waves, signals, and numbers, all beyond the scope of the clinician. Indeed, to the doctors unfamiliar with the field, and that was almost everyone outside the field itself, the waveforms of the heart's electrical system seemed a *helter-skelter*—a ride into oblivion much like the lyrics in the Beatles song: "When I get to the bottom I go back to the top of the slide. Where I stop and I turn and I go for a ride."

But the discovery of the electrical activation of the heart and the waves it produced in the electrocardiogram and from inside the heart itself would prove vastly different and important. It would open up the central mysteries of the heart's electrical activation and give us profound healing powers. And the road to it began with a mere hunch, long ago.

The Code of the Electrocardiogram (ECG)

In 1887, British physiologist Augustus D. Waller (1856–1922) became interested in a novel device called a capillary electrometer. The device could measure small bursts of electricity, and he wondered what would happen if he tried to record the electrical activity of the heart with it. His hunch paid off. His instrument was, arguably, the first electrocardiograph, but it was hard to use and yielded little detail. He seemed rather unimpressed by his own achievement and in 1911 made one of those ill-fated utterances that trail after one in posterity: "I do not imagine the electrocardiography is likely to find any extensive use in the hospital."

Dutch physician Willem Einthoven (1860–1927, Fig. 4.1) was born in Java, Indonesia, then called the Dutch East Indies. He returned to Holland at the age of ten, and as a college student, he was an ardent gymnast, fencer, and rower. In 1889, he attended the First International Congress of Physiology in Basel, Switzerland, and this visit changed his life's trajectory and the course of medicine. There, Einthoven saw Waller record electrical waves from the heart. He was fascinated by its possibilities.

Through much of the 1890s, he worked to improve the capillary electrometer but eventually gave up on it, unable to break through to the kind of precision he wanted. He switched to a different machine, called a string galvanometer. It comprised of a thin, silver-coated quartz filament that passed between two electromagnets. An electric current passing through the filament produced a movement that projected a shadow, which was magnified and registered. It provided readings of higher quality than its precursor, the capillary electrometer due to the thinness and minimal mass

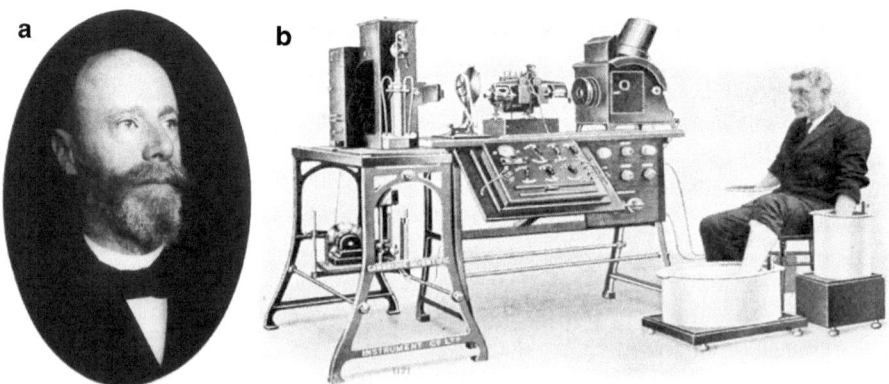

Fig. 4.1 Willem Einthoven and the string galvanometer. Panel A: Willem Einthoven. (Reprinted from Moises Rivera-Ruiz, Christian Cajavilca, Joseph Varon. Einthoven's String Galvanometer: The First Electrocardiograph *Tex Heart Inst J*. 2008; 35(2): 174–178. Panel B: An early commercial ECG machine, built in 1911 by the Cambridge Scientific Instrument Company showing the manner in which the electrodes are attached to the patient. In this case, the hands and one foot are immersed in jars containing salt solution. (Reprinted from: https://en.wikipedia.org/wiki/String_galvanometer)

of the string and the ability to adjust tension to regulate sensitivity and response time. He refined it endlessly, and in 1901, he described a different and far more sensitive electrocardiograph.

The procedure could be used on anyone with minimal discomfort, and it used just three leads,[1] a more economical approach. In 1905, Einthoven began sending ECGs or electrocardiograms via telephone wires from the hospital to his lab about a mile away—an early example of telemedicine. By 1906, he demonstrated the extraordinary usefulness of the device, showing how it detected such problems as hypertrophy (excess thickness) of the heart chambers, heart block, an atrial arrhythmia (atrial flutter), and premature (extra) beats. By all accounts, he was a kind and thoughtful man. When he received the Nobel Prize in Medicine in 1924, he split the $40,000 award with the impoverished heirs of his assistant.

The first ECG machine—the Edelman string electrocardiograph—was introduced in the United States in 1909 by Dr. Alfred Cohn, at the Mount Sinai Hospital in New York City.

Most inventions go through cycles of improvement, and Einthoven's was no different. His electrocardiograph weighed 600 pounds. Japanese physician Taro Takemi (1904–1983) developed the first portable one in 1937. Today, it is highly mobile and computerized. It takes 5–10 minutes in a doctor's office to obtain a 12-lead ECG.

The ECG is a treasure chest of data compared to the pulse. It records the heart's electrical activity in some detail, capturing each phase from many sites at once, and the information it provides is about the critical command system. The electrical waves go out in certain directions, so some leads naturally yield different shapes. Individual hearts and their position in the chest also vary somewhat. A physician can quickly gain crucial insights from the length of the waves, their distance apart from each other, their strength (voltage), and their overall pattern. Einthoven named its waves PQRST (Fig. 4.2).

There is an interesting story of Einthoven's labeling of the ECG waves as PQRST. During my final medical oral examination in medicine in 1969, at Goa Medical College of the University of Bombay, I was to rapidly examine a young man and provide a diagnosis, what was called a "short case." I took a quick history and went about palpating, percussing, and listening to his heart with the stethoscope, after which I looked at his ECG.

My clinical diagnosis: mitral stenosis—narrowing and thickening of the mitral valve between the left atrium and ventricle—due to rheumatic heart disease. I rather confidently awaited the visiting examiner from Bombay, who was in the process of questioning my colleague a few feet away. He was a rather famous consultant in cardiology, Dr. Ivan Pinto, a British-trained member of the Royal College of

---

[1] Leads are not the same as electrodes. Electrodes are the pads placed on your body. A lead is the connector attached to the pads, and two pads can have one connector. A specific lead is also the number of angles you can record the heart's electrical activity from, that is, the number of comparisons of electrical activity, and the number of voltages you can record. Today a technician will normally put 10 electrodes on you, but there are 12 leads.

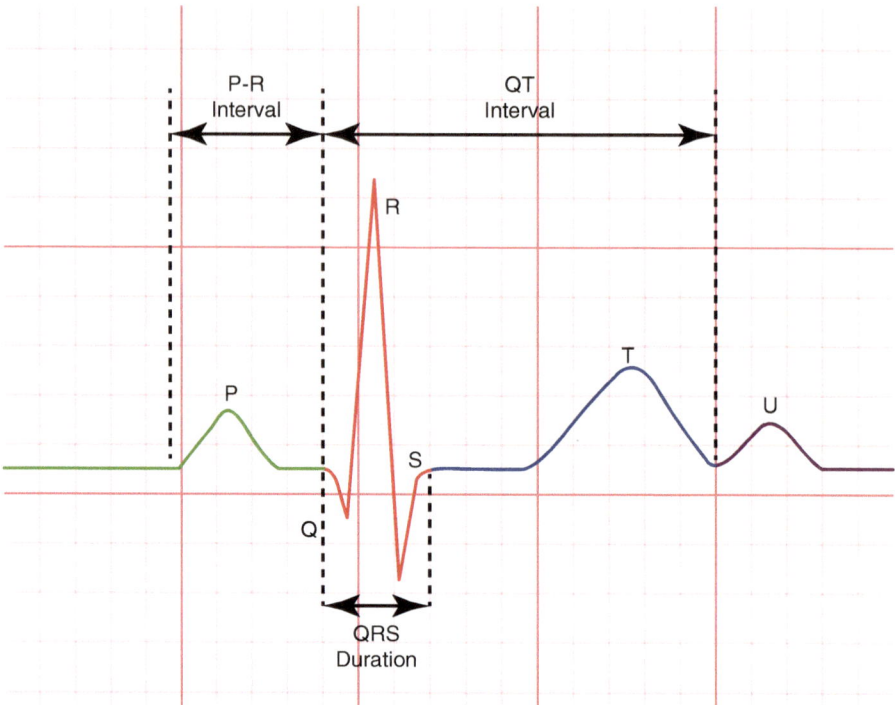

Fig. 4.2 PQRST corresponding to different waves of the ECG. Legend: Shows the five waves of the ECG shown in different colors. The P wave (green) is due to electrical activation of the atria. The PR interval that follows, before the Q wave, represents the signal flowing down the A-V node, the His bundle, and the bundle branches, into the Purkinje fibers. The QRS wave (shown in red) is due to activation of the ventricles; here, the heart pumps blood to the lungs and the rest of the body. Notice the stable line that follows, between the S and T waves, known as the ST segment. Finally, there is the half-moon near the end, the T wave (shown in blue), followed by the U wave (shown in grey). It shows the repolarization of the ventricles, with a rising and declining waveform. The entire QT interval shows the cycle of the ventricles, i.e., depolarization and repolarization. The genesis of the U wave which is variable in its presence or absence and its duration and voltage as well as its continuation or separation from the T-wave has been controversial. It is hypothesized that it represents (1) the repolarization of the Purkinje fibers, (2) the prolonged repolarization of the M-cells in the midmyocardium, and (3) afterpotentials, possibly caused by mechanical forces in the ventricular wall

Physicians, the type one finds on Harley Street in London. He asked me a few questions about rheumatic disease, which I answered, after which came the bombshell. He asked me to identify the waves of the electrocardiogram, which I did promptly as "PQRST." The next question took me entirely by surprise:

"Why are they named PQRST and not ABCDE?" he asked.

I was dumbfounded and overtaken by nervousness. I didn't know the answer. After a long silence, I said: "I don't know…perhaps, it's just nomenclature!"

He shook his head and abruptly left. I was certain he would fail me. On second thought, I wondered whether he was just kidding along after a heavy lunch and gulps of beer plentiful in wet Goa, unlike in prohibition-weary Bombay of those days. Dr. Pinto was related to my brother-in-law, and I wondered whether he knew who I was. This occurred to me only after I left the hospital ward, where the exam had taken place rather downcast and depressed. He did not fail me; after all it had nothing to do with my correct diagnosis, but neither did he give me a high mark. Subsequently, I tried to find the answer to his question but to no avail. Even after I came to the United States, I asked my attending cardiologists, but was met with blank stares, rather surprised at the question as I was. Almost 30 years later, I read an article by Dr. J. Willis Hurst from Emory University entitled: "Naming of the Waves in the ECG, With a Brief Account of Their Genesis." And I finally found the answer, long after I became a cardiologist and a heart rhythm expert to whom the ECG is a way of life, so to speak, the very imprint of the heart's rhythm that tells a spectrum of different stories.

According to Willem Einthoven's official biographer, he chose the letters PQRST because they were near the middle of the alphabet. He wanted other letters to be available for waves that might be discovered later, and indeed he later discovered a wave he named "U." He was also probably influenced by the work of French philosopher René Descartes, who had used P and Q to label successive points on a curve. He invented analytical geometry and was the first scientist to state the law of refraction. There is also another likely possibility. At first when Einthoven was using the capillary electrometer, he recorded raw, inaccurate data and labeled them ABCD. Then he corrected for inertia and friction, got a much better curve, and chose the letters PQRST that we use today, and the ECG has retained the letters for over a century.

For curiosity's sake, I recently searched the genesis of the PQRST of the ECG on Google, and not surprisingly found a trove of information. We have come a long way in the dissemination of knowledge and access to the history of medicine.

Most discoveries in medical science has occurred like Einthoven's, by careful, methodical, scientific investigation, often stimulated by intuition. But not uncommonly, there is a stroke of serendipity. In cardiovascular medicine, we have a wonderful example of this accidental good fortune in the discovery of coronary angiography ("angio" = "blood vessel"; "graphy" = "writing"), penicillin, quinine, streptokinase, and other drugs. However, the renaissance in heart rhythm disorders had an entirely different take: one of step-by-step, careful scientific investigation.

Starting and Stopping Heartbeats

Over 60 years from the discovery of the ECG, in 1967, a milestone occurred. Two European groups—one in Holland led by Drs. Dirk Durrer ("the godfather of Dutch cardiology") and his coworkers and the other in France led by Drs. Philippe Coumel and his associates—reported almost simultaneously and independently that they had started and stopped cardiac rhythm disorders in patients by introducing extra beats through a catheter in the right atrium. For the first time, they had invaded the heart chamber with an electrode catheter passed through a vein and by introducing electrical current through an external stimulator could induce and terminate the rather elusive, sporadic rhythm abnormalities such as supraventricular ("supra" = "above," hence above the ventricles) and ventricular tachycardia in the laboratory. This new approach was called programmed electrical stimulation (PES) of the heart, which is used to this day to initiate and treat heart rhythm disorders.

And if these artificially introduced beats could induce arrhythmias, the implication was that most heart arrhythmias we see in patients arise from reentry of current. I'll give reentry the space it deserves in the next chapter, but briefly, some current gets sidetracked, circles back, and enters the electrical system again, causing rapid heart beating.

This discovery was a key undertaking. With this kind of control over the electrical system of the heart, we could—among other things better assess the effects of medications and other treatment modalities for these rhythm disorders. "We were able to initiate and terminate tachycardia by appropriately timed stimuli," wrote the late Dr. Hein J.J. Wellens (personal communication). "This was the birth of programmed stimulation of the heart, over 50 years ago, and we danced in the catheterization lab!"

Tapping the Signals From Within the Heart

Coronary artery angiography lets us peer right into the heart arteries. The ECG was unable to do the same. It had revolutionized cardiology and it remained a vital tool. Yet, it couldn't record information from discrete sections of the electrical system, and by the 1960s, physicians often considered ideas based on its data to be conjecture or hypothesis. No new methods had appeared to access the heart's electrical activity since 1901.

Enter Dr. Benjamin Scherlag, Ph.D.

> In some strange way, any new fact or insight that I may have found has not seemed to me as a "discovery" of mine, but rather something that had always been there and that I had chanced to pick up.—Subrahmanijan Chandrasekhar, Indian-American astrophysicist

In 1965, Dr. Benjamin Scherlag (Fig. 4.3) was approaching the end of his postdoctoral tenure. Much later he confessed, "My initial career objective was to teach high school biology," but then he landed a technician job with one of the top researchers in basic electrophysiology and expanded his goals dramatically. In 1965, he was working in the laboratory of Dr. Brian Hoffman (1925–2013) in the Department of Pharmacology of Columbia University. He was given a project to

Fig. 4.3 Dr. Benjamin Scherlag. (Courtesy of Dr. Benjamin Scherlag)

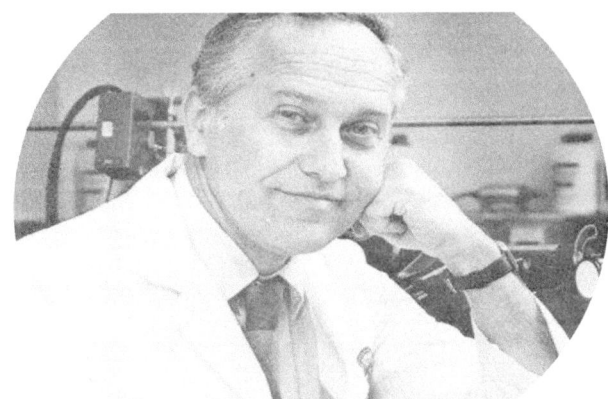

create heart block by interrupting current between the upper and lower chambers of the heart in the anesthetized dog.

He focused on His bundle, that keystone structure in the cardiac conducting system, which sits in the septum between the upper and lower chambers of the heart at about the level of the tricuspid valve (see Chap. 3, Fig. 3.2). It was a challenging target. The bundle is about 1.5 mm across or 1/17 of an inch. It also lies in the depths of the heart itself. Recording its electrical activity seemed an insurmountable task. After many trials and errors, Scherlag finally developed a procedure for injecting formaldehyde through the atrial wall into the dog's His bundle. Using this method, he shut down the current and achieved permanent heart block.

After Scherlag obtained his doctorate, he joined Dr. Anthony N. Damato at the Staten Island Public Health Service Hospital (part of the US Public Health Service (USPHS) system). Dr. Damato was keenly interested in setting up an experimental laboratory. In a short time, he set one up in a single room, complete with a catheterization table, an X-ray unit, a recorder, and a stimulator. It was called the "dog lab." It was here that Scherlag improved his technique and ultimately would use a special catheter in the dog to record electrical activity of His bundle. Soon thereafter, his clinician coworkers at the USPHS Hospital at the time, which included Drs. Sun Lau, Anthony Damato, Richard Helfant, and others, were anxious to move on to human studies.

Drs. Scherlag and Lau were the first to attempt to record an electrical deflection from the bundle of His in a human being. In 1969, they, together with his colleagues wrote an account of the novel technique (Fig. 4.4).

They sent the manuscript to Dr. Howard Burchell, chief editor of *Circulation*, one of the world's most prestigious heart research journals. The reviewers were harsh, expressing disbelief in the accomplishment. Dr. Burchell ultimately published the paper and predicted that it would become a "standard reference," and it did for years to come.

This was a groundbreaking achievement in cardiovascular medicine, since for the first time we could systematically explore the conducting system of the human

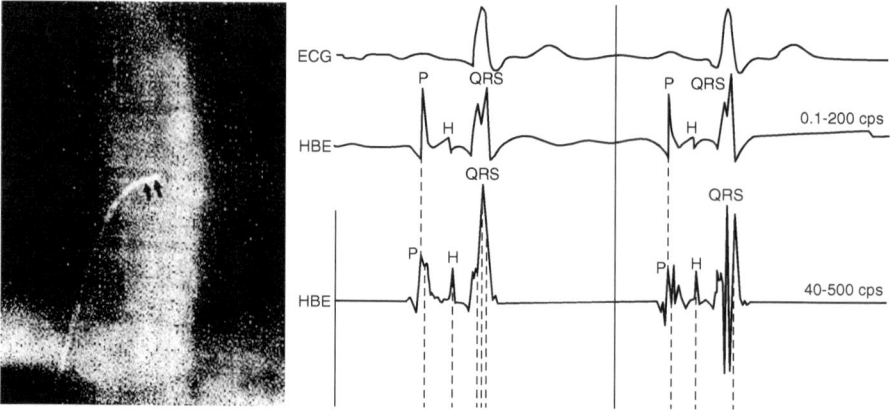

Fig. 4.4 Catheter recording of electrical activity of the bundle of His. Left panel: chest X-ray showing an anteroposterior view of a multipolar catheter across the tricuspid valve for His bundle recording. (Reprinted with permission from Scherlag B, Lau SH, Helfant RH et al. Catheter techniques for recording His bundle activity in man: *Circulation,169;39:*13–18.) Right panel shows an ECG lead and bipolar recordings from the various poles of the catheter. The lower two show a His spike (H) sandwiched between a P wave from the atria and a QRS wave from the ventricles. (Modified from Scherlag B, Lau SH, Helfant RH et al. Catheter techniques for recording His bundle activity in man.: *Circulation,169;39:*13–18)

heart from inside its chambers without open heart surgery. It was akin to the discovery of coronary angiography by Mason Sones.

As soon as the Staten Island group discovered the ease of recording His bundle activity in humans, several studies were launched to study the electrical properties of the human conduction system.

The USPHS Hospital and Its Electrophysiology Laboratory

The USPHS Hospital—where I worked from 1975 to 1979—had a remarkable history. It nurtured two giants in medical research: Dr. Joseph James Kinyoun and Dr. Anthony N. Damato. Previously known as the Marine Hospital, it was constructed in 1831 in Staten Island, New York, for retired naval and commercial sailors. The neighborhood mood toward newly arrived immigrants was hostile at the time, and history seems to have repeated itself. On May 6, 1857, a local mob attacked the nearby Port of New York Quarantine Hospital in Tompkinsville, Staten Island, fearful of immigrant detainees with communicable diseases. On the night of September 1, 1858, a mob again attacked the hospital, burning it down while three local fire companies stood nearby and watched.

In 1874, many of its quarantine resources for newly arrived immigrants were transferred to the Marine Hospital. By the latter half of the century, physicians were realizing that microbes caused many dreaded illnesses like smallpox and yellow fever. For instance, in 1883, Robert Koch (1843–1910) showed that a tiny bacillus caused tuberculosis. Thus, the study of communicable diseases assumed great urgency. Soon after, in 1887, a 27-year-old doctor named Joseph James Kinyoun (1860–1919) established a single-room bacteriology lab on the top floor of the Marine Hospital. The Laboratory of Hygiene for Bacteriological Investigation remained in the attic from 1887 to 1891, supporting quarantine activities against the four epidemic diseases: cholera, plague, smallpox, and yellow fever. In 1891, the surgeon general moved the laboratory from Staten Island to Washington, DC, and placed Dr. Joseph J. Kinyoun in charge of the nation's first federal bacteriology laboratory. In 1897, Dr. Kinyoun advised that the government should create a broad-based research agency to explore "the nature, origin, and prevention of contagious epidemics, and other diseases affecting the people, and should also make investigations into other matters relating to public health." In 1930, the Ransdell Act renamed it the National Institute of Health (NIH). *Thus, what is now the National Institutes of Health began as a single room Laboratory of Hygiene for Bacteriological Investigation established by the US Marine Hospital at Stapleton, Staten Island, New York, in 1887.* Drs. David M. Morens and renowned Anthony S. Fauci, the current director of the National Institute of Allergy and Infectious Diseases and a member of the Task Force for COVID-19, called Dr. Joseph James Kinyoun, the forgotten forefather of the NIH. The NIH budget for 2020 was 42 billion.

The USPHS Hospital itself remained in Staten Island, and it was highly unusual even when I worked there. It served only people from the merchant marine (thus the name Marine Hospital) and had no university affiliation. Many of its staff doctors were commissioned naval uniformed officers. Moreover, most of us were there to do research, supported by grants from the Bureau of Health services of the US Public Health.

At the USPHS Electrophysiology Laboratory, the first of its kind in the United States, under the tutelage of Dr. Anthony N. Damato, we embarked on projects deciphering the mysteries of the cardiac electrical system and the genesis of abnormal and rapid heart rhythms. We did these studies by introducing catheters into the heart advanced through a vein in the groin under fluoroscopic guidance that had electrical poles at the tip. At the time, these catheters were custom designed for our use. The catheters were connected to a recording system (also custom designed), and the tracings of these electrical signals were recorded on rolls of photographic paper. The rolls, which were in metal boxes, were carried to a dark room where the paper was developed. Subsequently, we spent days, evenings, and even many late nights reading reams and reams of photographic paper, since in those times anything we discovered was a novelty and therefore publishable. After long reading sessions, our hands had an alkaline vinegary smell, and not uncommonly some even developed palmer rashes. At the time, nobody fantasized that cardiac electrophysiology would become a clinical specialty and would assume such importance in medicine.

The modus operandi at the USPHS Electrophysiology Laboratory was rather unconventional. I did not meet Dr. Anthony Damato for a couple of months after joining the place. I roamed around the clinical and animal laboratories observing what others were doing, somewhat lost and wondering when I would start a project of my own. Most often I kept the company of Dr. Masood Akhtar, a highly intelligent man with a mercurial personality and with whom I developed a close friendship. I also interacted with Dr. Sun H. Lau, a pleasant and perfect gentleman with a chortle, who was instrumental in teaching the technique to fellows in training and national and international visitors and scholars to the laboratory.

Finally, one day, Dr. Damato called me to his office and asked me what I wanted to do. I discussed with him several projects, both in electrophysiology and echocardiography. I was surprised when he gave me free reign to pursue my interests.

Human research was done under guided principles, and the physicians maintained a high standard and thoroughness in the investigative process. *Primum non nocere*, which means, "first, do no harm," was always uppermost in our minds. However, the guidelines, institutional review boards, and HIPA regulations that are current today did not exist then.

Initially, whenever I had questions, I approached Dr. Masood Akhtar or Dr. Sun Lau, but subsequently, when Dr. Damato familiarized with me and greatly appreciated my scientific productivity, we became good friends, and I was at leisure to approach him at any time. During most of the 4.5 years I spent at this institution, I shared an office with Drs. Pratap Reddy and Masood Akhtar. Often, we read and reread rolls and rolls of photographic paper—the Torah's of electrophysiology—and not only discussed heart rhythms but also talked about life and politics. We developed a close lifelong friendship that continued to this day; however, Dr. Masood Akhtar passed away in 2019.

Besides research, we also saw patients in our offices or in the clinics and had responsibilities for rounding in the coronary care unit and in the medical wards. Career wise, we did not know where we were going. We had no idea whether the field of cardiac electrophysiology would take off clinically or had any clinical value for that matter. We made very little money; the salary was in the ballpark of $19,000 a year for the first 2 years, and then it went up to $24,000. Undoubtedly, we did not think much about money in those days. Our quest was knowledge. Seminal work was done in the laboratory in deciphering the physiology of the conduction system of the human heart, the mechanism of heart rhythm disorders, and the effects of drugs on the human conducting system. Studies done in this laboratory laid the groundwork for the future.

Many of the bright young Americans (except for the immigrants and foreigners) joined the institution for exemption from the draft to fight in Vietnam. However, their contributions to the advancement of medical science, their teaching of future heart rhythm specialists, and their dissemination of cardiac electrophysiology provided a great service to humanity—and far outweighed the contribution they might have made fighting a doomed, unpopular war in a distant land. Young physicians who opposed the Vietnam War also joined the National Cancer Institute (NCI), since, as with the USPHS, enrollment in a federal research program exempted them from the draft. These were brilliant and energetic young doctors ready to embark into new frontiers in cancer treatment at the NCI and into cardiac rhythm disorders at the USPHS Hospital.

Dr. Anthony N. Damato: The Grandfather of Clinical Electrophysiology

One of the greatest values of mentors is the ability to see ahead what others cannot see and to help them navigate a course to their destination.—John C. Maxwell

After Dr. Scherlag moved to Miami, Dr. Anthony N. Damato (Fig. 4.5) and Dr. Sun H. Lau spearheaded all research activities in the Cardiac Electrophysiology Lab at the USPHS Hospital. I came to know him as a fine-looking American academician of average height and weight with an interesting personality and a rather conservative political outlook. He had assumed the position of chief of the Cardiovascular Program and director of the Cardiac Fellowships Program at the Hospital in 1962. Several of his coworkers and fellows in training described him as an honest and conscientious clinician-scientist, a brilliant mind, and a dedicated mentor.

Despite his creative investigative mind, he remained shy, unassuming, often withdrawn, and fearful of celebrity status. He mostly remained sequestered in his office reading scientific journals and reviewing manuscripts.

He was passionate about medicine, and although his focus was research in understanding heart rhythm disorders, patient care was uppermost in his mind. When he walked around the corridors, we immediately picked up his raspy cough from a distance, which he had from heavy smoking. He had a very genteel manner and usually kept to himself; however, once he became familiar and relaxed with an associate, he was a good and trusted friend. He avoided brash and aggressive individuals, however. He was not fond of the limelight and never sought high-powered university chairmanships even at the peak of his career. Most of the time, he did not go to

Fig. 4.5 Dr. Anthony N. Damato. (Courtesy of the Heart Rhythm Society)

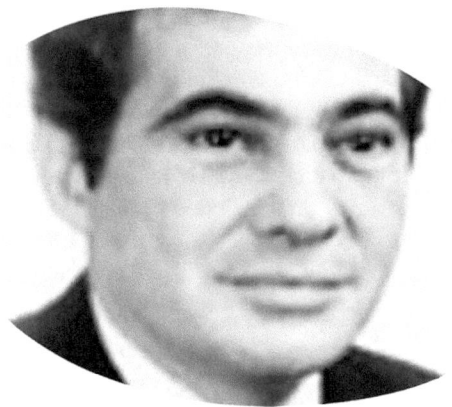

accept any of the awards he received. Usually, he sent one of his current or ex-associates in his place, with one exception: he attended an award ceremony at the New York Academy of Medicine, where Dr. Brian Hoffman, the David Hosack professor and chair of Pharmacology at Columbia University, College of Physicians and Surgeons, presented the award.

When I assumed the position of director of Cardiac Electrophysiology and Electrocardiography at the Mount Sinai Medical Center in New York City, I had invited my two friends and colleagues at the USPHS Hospital—Dr. Jeremy Ruskin, the director of the Arrhythmia Service at the Massachusetts General Hospital in Boston of Harvard University, and Dr. Masood Akhtar, the director of Electrophysiology at the Mount Sinai Hospital in Milwaukee—as guest speakers for the Consultants Course in Cardiology held at our medical center. I also invited Dr. Damato to dine with us at the Riverboat Café in Manhattan. I was not entirely sure he would show up, until he actually made his appearance. Both Drs. Ruskin and Akhtar were surprised and thrilled when he appeared. To pull Dr. Damato out of his seclusion was a tall order, somewhat akin to pulling out Howard Hughes out of his isolation. But he came because he was among friends—a great fondness for the three of us. We had a wonderful time reminiscing the past and anticipating a bright future for the field we were at the forefront at the time. And rather unabashedly, we smoked almost two packs of cigarettes among ourselves and drank a couple of bottles of wine.

After the Reagan Administration closed the USPHS Hospital in 1981, Dr. Damato became chairman of Medicine at the Misericordia Hospital in the Bronx and soon after joined the Jersey City Medical Center as chairman of Medicine, where he remained until his retirement. During these years, he dedicated himself to the training of medical house staff, interns, and residents and even took his boards in geriatric medicine after the age of 60. He came to work at 5:30 AM and conducted morning rounds with his residents and chief residents at 6 o'clock. It seemed that chairmanship of medicine gave him a second wind. He was entirely dedicated to teaching and gave himself to an inner-city hospital when he could have easily sought and obtained a university hospital position. He often invited me to lecture at his institution and referred patients to my service at Mount Sinai Medical Center for electrophysiological studies.

Dr. Damato trained a cadre of electrophysiologists many of whom opened laboratories and arrhythmia units in the major university medical centers, passing their expertise on to the young fellows in training, the future heart rhythm experts. He created a continuum of excellence that translated into the creation of a new specialty for the benefit of patient care. He joins the ranks of heart electrophysiology luminaries of those times that included Drs. Dirk Durrer and Hein J. J. Wellens of the Netherlands, Dr. Phillip Coumel of France, and Drs. Gordon Moe and Brian Hoffman of the United States. These extraordinary men not only trained a whole generation of young doctors but also inculcated a sense of excitement to expand the frontier they had opened up.

In his grayer years, Dr. Damato continued his mission of education, training house staff in internal medicine with equal vigor. Only recently I learned from his wife that he had taken a course in advanced gardening at Rutgers University and became an avid flower gardener in his retirement years. He passed away in 2001.

The combination of His bundle recording and the ability to start and stop heart rhythm disorders was a revolutionary undertaking—it ushered the modern era of clinical cardiac electrophysiology. In the late 1970s and early 1980s, clinical cardiac electrophysiology and its associated electrophysiological studies or EPS[2] were poorly grasped by general cardiologists, whether academic or in clinical practice. It took a lot of time, patience, and education to create a measure of understanding of the field. Even at a prestigious institution like Mount Sinai Hospital, I had my work cut out not only explaining the indications for a procedure, but more so in discussing a patient's electrical tracings, I had obtained from inside the heart. What I found encouraging, however, was the interest and enthusiasm not only from the fellows and residents in training but also from the full-time and voluntary faculty.

Indeed, when the medical community realized that the "heart rhythm expert" could totally cure an arrhythmia and instantly terminate a cardiac arrest, the specialty shot up in prominence like a spectacular stock offering.

Over the last several decades, we have made great strides in heart rhythm disorders, not only in understanding the mechanisms but also in technological advancement for mapping and treatment of cardiac rhythm disorders with catheter ablation, in the development and use of specialized pacemakers and defibrillators, and in the genetics of heart rhythm disorders. A host of pioneering individuals and their groups laid the foundation stones in these important endeavors. Unlike when I started in cardiac electrophysiology 45 years ago, the control room in the electrophysiological laboratory abounding in technology looks more like in the movie *Star Wars*.

Today, clinical cardiac electrophysiology is one of the most crucial and exciting fields in cardiovascular medicine. There are many reasons why, and I'll start with Maria.

♥

[2] An EPS is commonly a test, hence "studies," but it can also do more. It involves introducing catheters via a vein or artery in the patient's groin and advancing them to the heart. These catheters have sensitive poles at the tip that record its electrical conducting system and its impulse generation and transmission. Cardiologists use EPS to examine a host of abnormal rhythms of the patient's heart, to determine their circuits and sites of origin, and to assess the effects of drugs. But the catheter can also stimulate the heart and destroy malfunctioning tissue.

Part III
Galloping Away in the Atrium

Chapter 5
Living with a Galloping Heart

Among my stillness was a pounding heart.

—Shannon A. Thomson, Seconds before Sunrise

Having this thing totally wrecked my life. I felt so scared and helpless because I never knew when I'd have another episode, how bad that episode would be, if this new drug would work ... because many of them didn't... or if it never stopped racing... would I die?

—Kathryn A. Wood, Supraventricular Tachycardia and the Struggle to Be Believed

Paroxysmal supraventricular tachycardia (PSVT) as the name implies is a rapid regular heartbeat in the range of 150–240 beats/min, arising in the upper chambers of the heart, above the bundle of His that occurs sporadically and often unexpectedly. These tachycardias are seen in patients with and without the so-called Wolff-Parkinson-White syndrome. At other times, but less often, the tachycardia can occur due to rapid firing in the atria, referred to as atrial tachycardia. In the majority of patients, the mechanism of tachycardia is reentry or a circulating electric wave front.

George Ralph Mines and the Circles of PSVT

On November 7, 1914, a man was found mysteriously unconscious in the physiology laboratory at McGill University. He died later around midnight, and the postmortem failed to show a cause of death. He was just 28 years old. His name was George Ralph Mines (Fig. 5.1), and he is probably cardiac electrophysiology's only martyr.

He seemed to have endless energy, a deep enjoyment of life, and a creativity that brightened everything he touched. He married an aspiring poet, and he seriously

© The Author(s), under exclusive license to Springer Nature
Switzerland AG 2021
J. A. Gomes, *Rhythms of Broken Hearts*,
https://doi.org/10.1007/978-3-030-77382-3_5

Fig. 5.1 George Ralph
Mines. (Source: Regis A.
DeSilvaMB, FRCP(C),
FACCA: *Journal of the
American College of
Cardiology* 1997;
29:1397–1402)

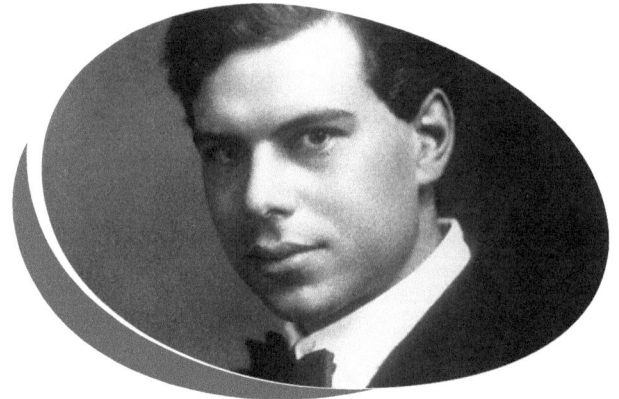

considered a career as a concert pianist before turning to physiology. There, his rise
in academia was meteoric for the times. He graduated from Sidney Sussex College,
Cambridge University, at the age of 22, and at 24, he was elected to the Physiological
Society. A year later, he received the Gedge Prize, bestowed by Cambridge for the
best original observations in physiology. In 1914, at 28, he was offered the position
of professor and chair of the McGill University Department of Physiology.

His death came soon after. In an address to the McGill faculty, he had spoken of
researchers who experimented on themselves. He had likely immersed himself in
the same adventure, since when found unconscious he was attached to his physiological monitoring devices. We will, of course, never know all this brilliant man
could have contributed to the field of cardiac physiology.

But in 1913, he first conceptualized the true mechanism of PSVT.

He observed that in PSVT, the atrium seemed to cause the beats of the ventricle,
and the ventricle seemed to cause the beats of the atrium. "The rhythm of each
chamber was directly dependent on that of the other," he wrote and called it "reciprocating rhythm."

What could cause such a pattern?

He noted that the electrical link between the atrium and ventricle was never just
one muscle fiber, but always a bundle of them. So perhaps they could become separated into two pathways like two parallel streets. He also noted that just after the
excitation of the ventricle, a signal immediately went back to the atrium and caused
it to contract. It was unlikely that the returning signal used the same path, he said.
The return was just too fast. Hence, one path took it forward and the other right
back. There was a circulating excitation, with current going round-and-round like a
dog chasing its tail. "I venture to suggest," he concluded, "that a circulating excitation of this type may be responsible for some cases of paroxysmal tachycardia."
And indeed, most PSVTs are due to "reentrant excitation."

Maria's PSVT

I first met Maria when my associate Dr. Winters and I were called to the ER to manage her runaway rhythm. She was a 26-year-old rather attractive woman, but episodes of palpitations and fainting spells had plagued her since the age of 10. The first time she felt her heart racing, she was biking. Her heart wouldn't stop galloping away and she had to be rushed to the ER. As she arrived there, the episode stopped on its own.

These attacks were entirely unpredictable, and they kept on recurring when least expected. Sometimes she was able to stop them by taking deep breaths and straining. Initially, the doctors didn't know what she had, and some believed it was an anxiety disorder. Often when she went out with her friends, the rapid rhythm suddenly afflicted her, and instead of socializing, she landed in the ER. On several occasions, her heart rate was clocked at 200–240 beats per minute, resulting in a blackout spell. During one instance, an electrical shock was applied to her chest to terminate an irregular tachycardia of 220–280 beats per minute. She stopped venturing out with friends. She felt ashamed and insecure. When she was 16, she had had enough.

"I ran away from home. I just wanted to die," she said. "But suddenly while walking the Brooklyn streets the tachycardia started and I blacked out. I was rushed to the ER in an ambulance."

When we saw her at the Mount Sinai Hospital ER, she was sweating profusely with a weak and erratic pulse and low blood pressure. The ECG showed an irregular heart rhythm—atrial fibrillation at rates of 200–250 beats per minute. We couldn't record a blood pressure. We ended the tachycardia by delivering an electrical shock to her chest.

Maria had paroxysmal supraventricular tachycardia (PSVT) and atrial fibrillation. PSVT results in a rapid heartbeat of usually over 150 beats per minute and arises in the upper chambers of the heart, "supra" the ventricles. It is "paroxysmal" because the galloping starts at intervals of days, months, or even years and stops suddenly or has to be stopped with drugs or electrical shock to the chest. Cases like Maria's had long puzzled doctors. Not uncommonly, the malady was misdiagnosed particularly in women and labeled as panic attacks or an anxiety disorder. Currently there are long-term monitoring systems such as event recorder used externally for a 3–4-week period or an internal recorder that has a battery life of 3 years. These recording systems have the capability of transmitting the event tachycardia to the physician. More recently, iPhone apps are available that can record an ECG during the episode, which can be messaged to the physician.

Identifying Maria's Syndrome

Maria had a distinctive kind of PSVT due to the Wolff-Parkinson-White syndrome.
The mechanism of the tachycardia remained baffling and controversial for centuries.

On April 2, 1928, Dr. Paul Dudley White (1886–1973) was working at Massachusetts General Hospital in Boston. He was an energetic advocate of optimism, work, and physical activity at a time when some cardiologists thought exercise harmed the heart. In 1924, he founded the American Heart Association. On that very day, he saw a patient, an 18-year-old freshman on the Harvard swim team who suffered from sudden attacks of rapid heartbeat that lasted about 15 minutes. Dr. White examined him and found nothing unusual. The response to exercise was normal. A few days later, as it happened, his colleague Dr. Louis Wolff (1898–1972) referred a similar case to him, that of a 35-year-old gymnast who had experienced palpitations for several years. Both men were in good health and examination revealed no clue to their problem. After a careful search, they found only two more cases, in their own hospital. They were stumped.

In those days, before World War II, scientific advances occurred mostly in Europe, and it was not uncommon for American academicians in medicine and in other disciplines to visit and even specialize in Europe. And so Dr. White went on a trip to Europe, with information about these four cases. He found little interest in Vienna or at first among doctors in London. However, there he came across Dr. John Parkinson (1885–1976) who was a gracious host; a connoisseur of wine, food, and art; and a man of renowned punctuality. One colleague said of him: "He had a passion for truth. He relied on facts; he was never given to imagination, for the truth to him was what he saw. Indeed, he seemed a tyrant for truth, and through his diligent search for it, he often presaged it." The cases intrigued him and he provided White with seven more such cases.

In 1930, the three men (Fig. 5.2) described the phenomenon in the *American Heart Journal*. They stated that none of the patients had disease of the heart structure. However, all had similarities in their ECGs "of bundle branch block and a short PR interval," as well as PVST and/or atrial fibrillation. They also credited Drs. F.N Wilson and A.M. Wedd who had described such symptoms in a single patient as far back as 1915 and 1921, respectively. Since 1930, this disease entity has become known as the Wolff-Parkinson-White or WPW syndrome. It has held the interest of internists, cardiologists, anatomists, heart surgeons, and above all heart rhythm specialists.

All three of these eminent men would go on to further achievements. Dr. White would become one of the best-known cardiologists in the United States, treating prominent patients, among them Pablo Casals, Albert Schweitzer, and President Dwight Eisenhower. He would also record the ECGs of a living elephant and beluga whale. When he died, *Time* called him "Dr. Cardiology." Dr. Parkinson would help found cardiology as an independent discipline in Britain, and he and White coordinated the field across the Atlantic, at a time when communication was much harder.

Fig. 5.2 Wolff, Parkinson, and White (from left to right). (Source: https://en. ecgpedia.org/wiki/ Ventricular_pre-excitation_ (Wolff-Parkinson-White_ pattern))

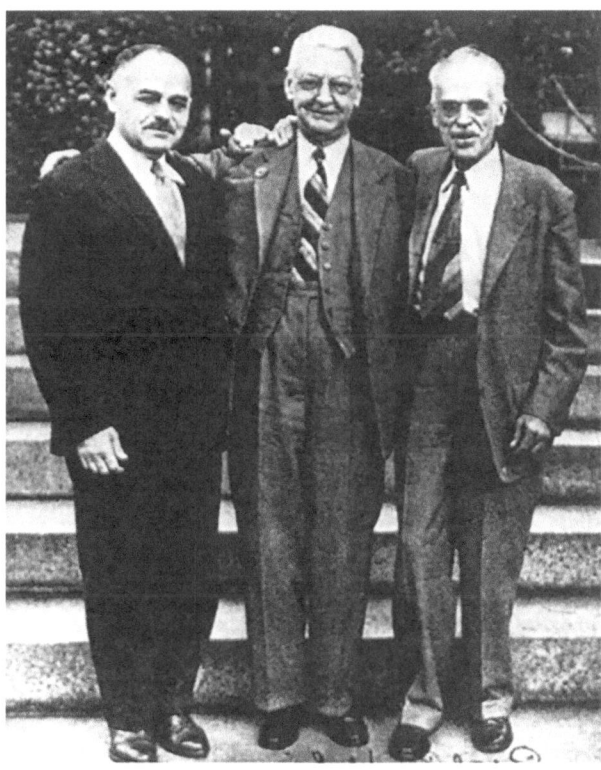

As mentioned, Maria had WPW syndrome.[1] In the past, the syndrome was often misdiagnosed as a panic attack or anxiety disorder, as it had initially with Maria. However, the abnormality has a recognizable signature on the ECG (Fig. 5.3). There is a short PR interval—the time between when the atria start pumping followed by the ventricles. There is also a widened, slurred QRS complex (which Wolff, Parkinson, and White erroneously called bundle branch block). The QRS begins early, cutting into the normal PR interval with a rising line called a "delta wave" (so named because of a resemblance to the capitalized Greek letter delta, a triangle). In the past, clinicians sometimes misread this ECG as indicating bundle branch block and heart damage (the "pseudo-infarct pattern"); as a consequence, the armed forces barred some young men with WPW ECG pattern from serving in World War II, on the grounds that they had a previous heart attack.

With better knowledge, we readily diagnosed Maria's condition.

---

[1] The prevalence of preexcitation (WPW pattern) on ECG is estimated to be between 0.1% and 0.3%.

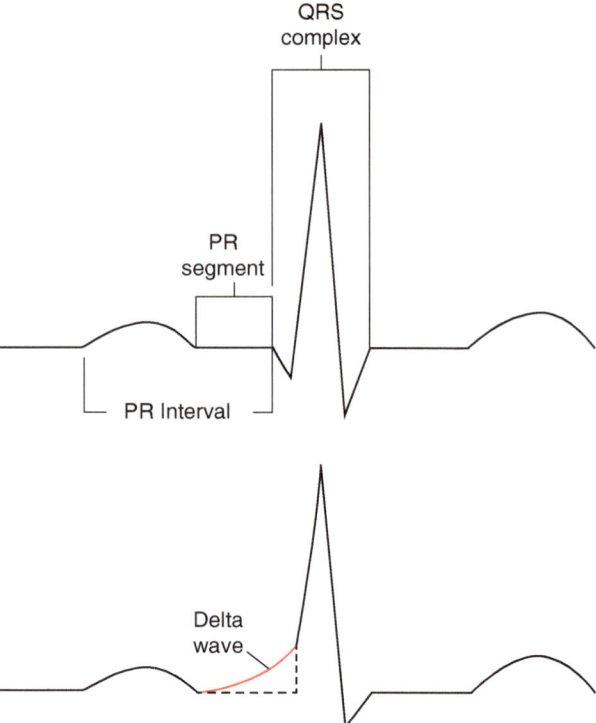

Fig. 5.3 ECG of the normal heart and the WPW syndrome. Legend: The top panel shows a normal ECG. The lower one shows an ECG from a person with Wolff-Parkinson-White syndrome. Note the shortened PR interval, cut off by the delta wave, and the initial slur of the QRS complex shown in red. This makes the QRS duration longer than normal. The delta wave is due to muscle activation via the bypass tract, whereas the remaining part of the QRS complex is due to activation via the normal conducting pathway; thus, the QRS complex is a "fusion." There are instances when the heart activation can occur entirely over the accessory pathway, in which case the QRS complex is very broad and bizarre looking. (Reprinted with permission from *Heart Rhythm Disorders: History, Mechanisms, and Management Perspectives*, by J. Anthony Gomes; Springer, Switzerland, 2020)

What Causes WPW Syndrome?

As far back as 1932, Holzman and Scherf hypothesized that there were two insulated pathways in WPW syndrome: the normal cable system, described earlier, and a second, accessory connection, shown in Fig. 5.4 that one is born with and could be related to a genetic mutation. (You might think of "accessory" as a partner in crime, though here it is more of a saboteur.) Subsequently, in 1943, Drs. Francis Clark Wood, Charles C. Wolferth, and George D. Geckeler, after examining the heart of a young man who had died of this condition, found three muscle connections between the right atrium and right ventricle, each of which could carry an

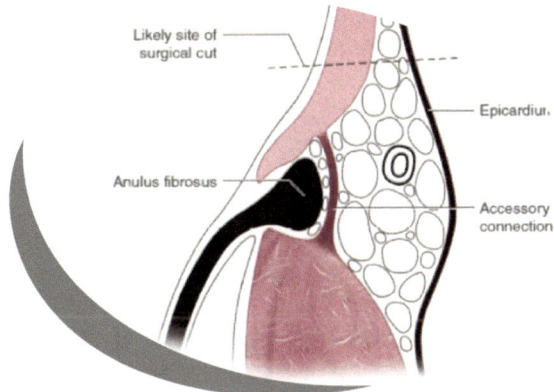

Fig. 5.4 Accessory muscle connection in WPW syndrome. Legend: Diagrammatic representation of left-sided accessory pathway(depicted in brown color) connecting the atrium (light pink) to the ventricular muscle (darker pink). (Modified from Anton E. Becker, Robert H. Anderson, MD; MRC Path; Dirk Durrer, MD; and Hein J.J. Wellems, MD. The Anatomical Substrates of Wolff-Parkinson-White Syndrome: A Clinicopathologic Correlation in Seven Patients. *Circulation* 1978; 57: 870–879, with permission)

electric current. Microscopic examination showed the existence of such accessory pathways.

In the mid-1960s, Dr. Dirk Durrer, a giant of Dutch cardiology, was discussing the WPW syndrome with Dr. Howard Burchell (1907–2009) from the Mayo Clinic, when the latter was a visiting professor at the University of Amsterdam. These men were aware of the two-pathway hypothesis functioning at the same time in WPW syndrome and that the electrical impulses moving along them in two different directions might be responsible for the syndrome. Then a unique opportunity came along. In 1966, a patient needed an operation to close a hole in the upper chambers of the heart (known as an "atrial septal defect"). He also had WPW syndrome on the ECG. Since they had to open his chest and expose the heart, Durrer decided to map the epicardium or outer surface of the heart muscle, by placing electrodes on it. These electrodes would record electric current and show him the activation pattern of the heart in the patient. He found early activation on the side of the patient's right ventricle, where it should not have occurred. He thus proved that there were, indeed, two pathways—a normal cable system and an accessory connection—that is also conducting in the WPW syndrome. This second route was commonly called the bundle of Kent, eponymously named for British physiologist Albert Frank Stanley Kent (1863–1958), who described lateral branches in the A-V groove of the monkey heart.

Durrer's thinking went even further. Since the two pathways would have different electrical properties, maybe one could alter the conduction pattern by artificially introducing an extra beat. Instead of the impulse going down both pathways at the same time, it might make it circulate. But how?

It comes down to timing. The two pathways have different refractory periods, those plateaus of the nerve or muscle cells when they don't respond to stimuli. Think of the pathways as roads with stoplights with different timing that alternate from red to green to red to green. Every time a car moves through, if the stop light is green, the road is available, while the other is red and unavailable. Now suppose an electrical signal arrives when the normal channel has a green stoplight and the *accessory bundle* a red one. The regular path will carry it down to the ventricle. But there, if the *accessory bundle* has recovered, its stoplight will be green. The signal will split. It will go to the ventricle, but also into the *accessory bundle* and right back to the atrium where it started. If the normal path has recovered by then, it will be green, respond to the impulse coming via the *accessory bundle*, and send another bolt of current down to the ventricle. And that in turn will go back up the *accessory bundle*. The current will move round and round, in Mines' "reciprocating rhythm." If the stimulus hits a red stoplight, the current will die, but otherwise the ventricles will keep responding and beat at a rapid rate.

Circulation of the electrical impulse in the two pathways would produce the phenomenon that is known as "reentry" and result in PSVT.

When Durrer and his coworkers applied an extra beat at the right time, its activation went down only though the normal pathway from the atrium to the ventricle but blocked in the *accessory bundle*. When the electrical wave front approached the end of the *accessory bundle* in the ventricular muscle (Fig. 5.5), it turned around to flow backward over the *accessory bundle*. The current returned again to the atrium, completed the circuit, and flowed back down again. The continuous electrical circulation resulted in a sustained tachycardia.

Moreover, they could use an extra beat to stop it. That sounds highly counterintuitive. How could an extra beat actually stop a racing heart? Timing is the secret again. That extra beat would disrupt the stoplight pattern. It could trigger an extra impulse in the normal pathway, and the pathway could be blocked when the signal arrived from the *accessory bundle*. The stoplight would be red, and the current would stop dead. And the endless circuit would cease. The heart would resume its normal pace.

That's how, as I mentioned earlier, one could start and stop PSVT in the laboratory. By introducing extra beats, Durrer's group demonstrated not only that the mechanism of the tachycardia in WPW syndrome was reentry but also that it could be controlled.

This was a spectacular accomplishment. The method is used today to initiate the tachycardia in the laboratory, to map the activation sequence, and to locate the extra cable so we can destroy it, what is referred to as ablation which will be discussed in the next chapter.

Maria's Life-Threatening Complication

It was disconcerting that Maria had atrial fibrillation in addition to a regular rapid tachycardia. Normally, a very rapid beating in the atrium is not as dangerous as ventricular fibrillation. A barrier of nonconducting collagen separates the two chambers, and the only way through is the A-V node, which slows down conduction like a railway station will slow a train. But Maria's case was different. During the atrial fibrillation, most of her impulses were moving through the accessory pathway and bypassing the normal conducting system, the A-V node. Since they were skipping the A-V node and its delay mechanism, they were making the ventricles beat much faster (Fig. 5.5, panel C). This situation increased Maria's risk of sudden cardiac death.

However, an accessory pathway isn't always available. Again, it has a recharging period, when the red stoplight is up. The shorter this red light period (known as the refractory period), the more of the rapid atrial impulses the pathway can send along.

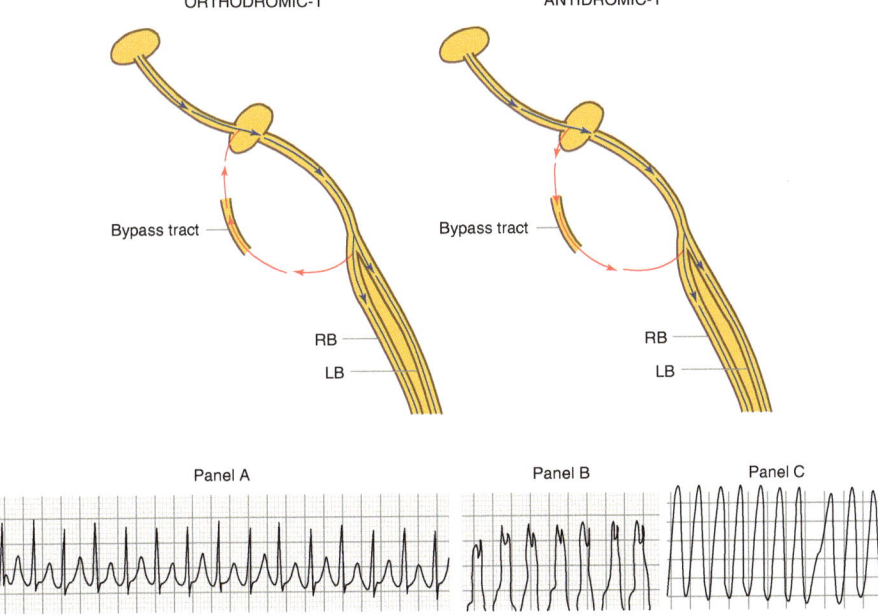

Fig. 5.5 Reentrant circuit in the WPW syndrome. Legend: Top left hand panel shows a reentrant circuit going down the A-V node and coming up the bypass tract (the reentrant circuit is shown in red. This is known as an orthodromic tachycardia and corresponds to the tachycardia in panel A which shows a narrow complex tachycardia. Top right hand panel shows the reverse: the electrical activation goes down the bypass tract and comes up over the normal pathway. This is known as an antidromic tachycardia and has a broad QRS complex (panel B). Panel C shows atrial fibrillation at a rate of 300 beats per minute due to conduction going entirely through the bypass tract

And if it is brief enough, WPW can be abruptly fatal. A refractory period of less than 240 milliseconds lets a swift series of signals race through. If that period is equal to or less than 200 milliseconds, say, the heart will beat 300 or more times per minute. Such fast rates cannot sustain the blood pressure to keep the heart muscle supplied with enough oxygen, and if not terminated promptly, it will result in ventricular fibrillation and sudden death.

Fortunately, this event is indeed rare, occurring in about 1 percent of patients with WPW syndrome.

How could we treat Maria? We managed her with one drug after another and even inserted a pacemaker. Unfortunately, these didn't help. I will revisit Maria in the next chapter when I relate breathtaking advances for conquering PSVT permanently.

The Commonest Supraventricular Tachycardia

WPW is not the only malfunction that causes PSVT. Indeed, the kind most often seen in clinical practice is known as atrioventricular nodal reentrant tachycardia or (AVNRT) (Fig. 5.6). The name is a mouthful, and the acronym itself can take getting used to, but the key to the latter is AVN, for A-V node. The A-V node is the focal point for this arrhythmia.

AVNRT can make the heart suddenly start beating over 150 times a minute. Like WPW, it is usually congenital, and women are about three times more likely to suffer from it than men. It is usually not life-threatening. Sir Thomas Lewis (1881–1945), the great British cardiologist of the early twentieth century (and one who smoked 70 cigarettes a day until a heart attack at 45 convinced him of their danger), rightly held that the rhythm arose in the A-V node. With some exceptions, most physicians of the time felt that PSVT arose in the A-V node or near it and that the tachycardia had "nervous origins."

The mechanism of the tachycardia remained controversial since the animal studies of Dr. Gordon Kenneth Moe (1915–1989), "the grandfather of basic cardiac

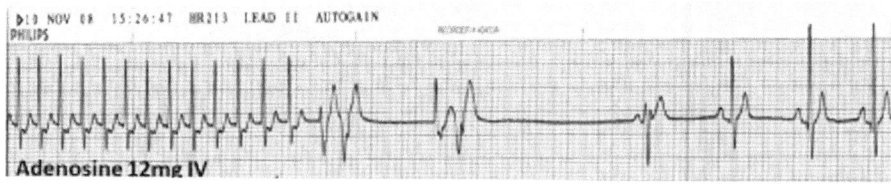

Fig. 5.6 AVNRT terminated by injecting adenosine. Legend: The left side of this ECG shows a rapid, regular, narrow complex tachycardia, at approximately 210 beats per minute. The AVNRT ceases with the injection of adenosine, a medication that induces block of conduction in the A-V node. Immediately afterward, there are seen ventricular extra beats (VPCs) and pauses, and then normal sinus activity resumes (extreme right)

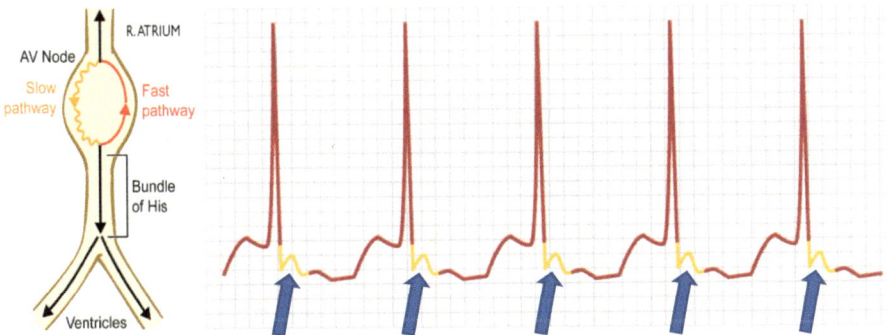

Fig. 5.7 Dual pathways within the A-V node. Legend: The left side panel (A) shows the A-V node separating into two pathways, a slow one conducting forward (serrated lines) and a fast one conducting backward (arrow). An impulse comes down the slow pathway and meets a fork. Part of it goes to the backward fast conducting pathway producing a retrograde atrial deflection shown in yellow and blue arrows in the right hand panel, and part of it goes forward to the ventricles. According to this concept as shown, both pathways are within the A-V node consisting of a proximal and distal meeting of the two pathways according to the concept of dual-pathway physiology. However, it has been shown that the proximal common pathway is not intranodal, but rather atrial in location (see Fig. 5.8)

electrophysiology" and a man who could deliver a deadpan joke. He and his associates demonstrated in 1956 that electrical conduction in the A-V node of the dog can dissociate into two pathways, one slow and one fast. According to this concept, when an atrial premature complex (APC) occurs at a critical timing, it blocks in the fast antegrade pathway and so conducts through the antegrade slow pathway. When the impulse enters the distal common pathway in the A-V node, it finds the fast pathway no longer refractory and conducts back to the atrium via the fast pathway to re-engage the slow pathway (Fig. 5.7). Reciprocation within the antegrade slow pathway and the retrograde fast pathway results in tachycardia. This reasoning was labeled the "dual-pathway concept." Subsequently, Dr. Kenneth Rosen, another alumnus of the USPHS Laboratory, and his associates demonstrated the "dual-pathway" phenomenon in the human A-V node. In 1979, I showed that in some patients, specialized fibers with properties unlike those of the A-V node were partly responsible for AVNRT. My observations were confirmed by Japanese investigators almost 30 years later. Needless to say, our understanding of this tachycardia has evolved over time. We now believe that one of the pathways (the slow pathway) is located in the atrium and conducts the impulse down the A-V node that then links with the fast pathway in the lower aspect of the A-V node (Fig. 5.8, top panel), while in some patients, there is an accessory pathway (the fast pathway) that is connected to His bundle (Fig. 5.8, bottom panel).

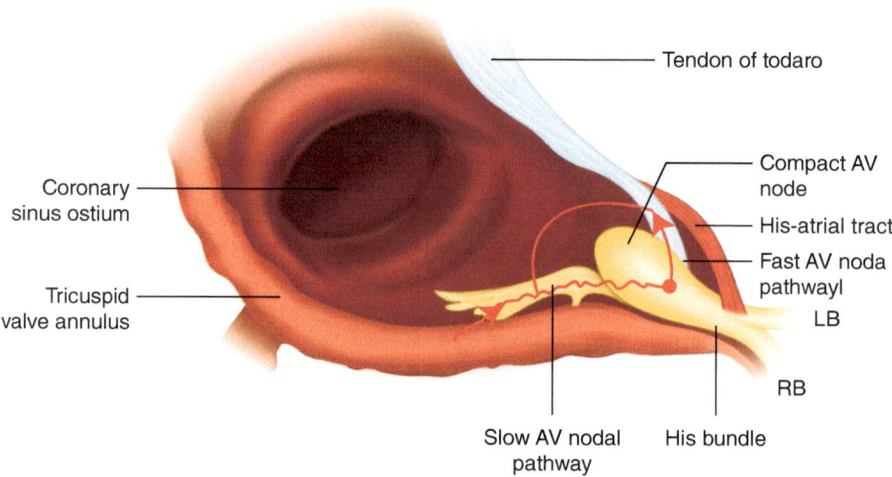

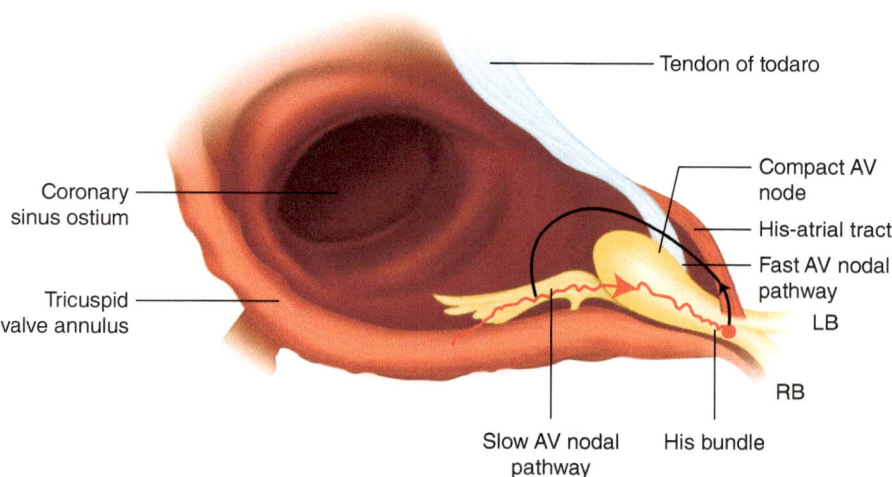

Fig. 5.8 Schematic conceptualization of slow/fast AVNRT. Legend: Schematic reconstruction of the triangle of Koch depicting the coronary sinus, the tricuspid annulus, the tendon of Todaro, the A-V node, the His bundle and the right (RB) and left bundles (LB), the slow A-V nodal pathway, and retrograde fast A-V nodal pathways consisting of an A-V nodal fast pathway and His atrial tract. *Although the latter and former are shown in both panels, it does not mean the His atrial tract is present in all patients with AVNRT.* Top panel shows activation of the slow pathway entering the A-V node and turning around (distal common pathway) into the retrograde fast pathway with activation near the tendon of Todaro. Bottom panel shows the activation of the slow pathway with turnaround near His bundle to activate the fast pathway which is depicted as a His atrial tract. In either case, the backward conducting pathway is fast enough to activate the atrium even before forward activation of the ventricles. It results in the ECG pattern called a "retrograde P wave," a P wave backed up toward the QRS wave, shown in yellow in Fig. 5.7, right hand panel. It is reasonable to conclude that AVNRT is due to the presence of two or more congenital accessory connections (atrial A-V node) and His atrial. In some patients, these tracts can be located on the left rather than the right side of the septum

The Case of Antoinette

In the late 1990s, I encountered a young woman in her late 20s, a lawyer by profession, who while defending a case in court felt palpitations, a dense fog in front of her eyes, and then briefly passed out. Obviously, there was a lot of commotion in the court room. She was taken by ambulance to the ER of a neighboring hospital, where she was found to be in normal rhythm. She was however admitted and an extensive workup revealed no cardiac abnormalities. She was referred to me for an opinion. She gave a history of recent onset of palpitations when excited (had several episodes during sexual activity) and recently during stress (like in court). I surmised that she could well have a PSVT of the A-V nodal variety. I submitted her to an EPS, but after introducing extrabeats through a catheter in the right cardiac chamber, the atrium, though an electrical stimulator, I could not initiate any tachycardia. Previously, in the 1980s, we had shown that in some patients an adrenergic surge was necessary to initiate tachycardia. And so, after infusing a drug known as isoproterenol, which is like introducing adrenaline in the system, I could easily as predicted induce a rapid tachycardia due to A-V nodal reentry. Antoinette's treatment and cure of the tachycardia will be discussed in the next chapter when I present advances in treatment of PSVT.

♥

Chapter 6
Radical Ideas: The Road to Conquering Supraventricular Tachycardia

Over every mountain there is a path, although it may not be seen from the valley.

—Theodore Roethke

First comes thought; then organization of that thought, into ideas and plans; then transformation of those plans into reality. The beginning, as you will observe, is in your imagination.

—Napoleon Hill

In the distant past, management of recurrent paroxysmal supraventricular tachycardia (PSVT) with or without WPW syndrome consisted of lifelong drug therapy, much of which was ineffective or associated with side effects. Doctors had to simply watch patients suffer despite their best efforts. Ideally, it would be best to get rid of the troubling *accessory pathway* or bypass tract altogether. But how?

The Road to Ending PSVT

The first surgical attempt at getting rid of a bypass tract occurred in 1968 at Duke University. A team consisting of Drs. Frederick Cobb, Sarah Blumenschein, Will Sealy, and their associates operated on a 32-year-old man with heart failure thought to be related to recurrent rapid heart palpitations. They had tried a host of drugs and even implanted a pacemaker but to no avail. They finally decided to place the patient on cardiopulmonary bypass, and after opening his heart, they cut the abnormal bypass tract. When the heart began beating again, the abnormal delta wave had vanished from the ECG, and he was cured of the tachycardia.

This team was the first to successfully destroy the *accessory pathway* in a patient with WPW syndrome with open heart surgery. We call these destructions "surgical ablation," and subsequently many techniques were utilized for it: surgical interruption, as here, as well as freezing at −60 °C, lasering, and using radiofrequency current. The team's subsequent results showed that the vast majority of WPW patients could be cured by surgical ablation. Although the procedure had a high success rate, it required open heart surgery with its attendant risks. Moreover, it was not possible to locate the camouflaged bypass tracts by sight, and the surgeon depended completely on the heart rhythm expert and his mapping prowess to localize the bypass tract so that he could tell the surgeon where to cut or freeze. This was one of a few times I saw a heart surgeon show a degree of humility in the operating room, where he or she is usually the lion king or queen of the realm. Thus, surgery for WPW syndrome remained a complex undertaking, and very few major centers in North America and in Europe performed it. Therefore, most patients with WPW syndrome suffered from ineffective lifelong drug regimens.

At the age of 27, Maria underwent surgery at Mount Sinai Medical Center. We opened her chest and under cardiopulmonary bypass destroyed her accessory pathway connecting the left atrium to the left ventricle by cutting it. The operation was successful and afterward Maria's quality of life gradually improved. Permanently cured, on no medications, she developed a relationship, got married in her 30s, and had a child.

The Attempt to Save Diane

No patient I've ever seen illustrates the progress in our treatment of PSVT better than the 74-year-old woman I shall call Diane, who was emergently transferred to my service for treatment in the late 1980s. She was a medium-sized woman somewhat rounded at the waist and of average height. After a hip replacement at the Hospital for Joint Diseases, in New York City, her recovery was complicated by a heart rate of 200 beats per minute that caused repeated fainting spells. She received several electrical shocks to her chest to halt the rapid heartbeat, only to have it recur soon after. A host of medications were tried, unsuccessfully.

I diagnosed her condition as PSVT due to a circulating electrical wave involving an *accessory pathway* in the heart, which she was born with. This extra cable, unlike that in the classic WPW syndrome, conducted electricity solely from the ventricle back to the atrium, like a one-way street. Consequently, its presence could not be identified on the surface ECG. It was commonly referred to as a *concealed bypass tract*, first identified by Drs. Roworth Spurrell, Dennis Krikler, and Edgar Sowton in England and Dr. Douglas P. Zipes and his associates in the United States.

We immediately ended Diane's rapid heartbeat by injecting intravenously a powerful drug—amiodarone. Its intravenous form was still experimental then, and only a few investigators in the country had access to it. The medication having done the job, I started her on the oral form of the drug.

Amiodarone was originally developed in Belgium in the late 1950s and used as a coronary dilator for treating angina. It quickly became a rather popular anti-angina drug in Europe and South America, but the drug company did not seek release in the United States likely because of tough US regulations. Subsequently, it was seren-dipitously found that it abolished heart rhythm abnormalities by Argentinian cardi-ologist Dr. Mauricio Rosenbaum. The drug's reputation as a highly effective agent in controlling heart rhythm disorders spread far and wide. It took many years for the oral form of the drug to be approved in the United States with many caveats after a host of studies found a plethora of long-term side effects mostly discovered by US investigators. It is an unusual drug with multiple and diverse properties used com-monly in clinical practice. It remains an effective drug, popular even today. However, its long-term use can lead to serious side effects in 1–3% of patients, including lung, liver, thyroid, central nervous system, and eye toxicity. The drug is replete with paradoxes: concurrently, some fear it, yet some love it!

Diane was thoroughly pleased with the outcome and baked me her favorite choc-olate cake when she came to see me in the clinic. When I asked her how long she had had the rapid heartbeat, she said, "Oh, on and off since the age of six." I was not at all surprised. I believed she was born with an *accessory pathway* about which our medical forefathers in the early twentieth century where entirely unaware.

I saw her regularly, every 3 months, and she always embraced me, saying, "Doc, you cured me, you saved my life." The truth of the matter is that I hadn't cured her yet—the extra cable was still there, perhaps blocked by the drug I had placed her on or by preventing the extra beats, which were like the sparks for a forest fire that initi-ated the tachycardia.

A couple of years later, she called me saying that she was getting winded and could barely walk a block. I immediately saw her in the clinic and ordered a chest X-ray and an echocardiogram to access the pumping action of the heart. The dark side of amiodarone had appeared, and I made a diagnosis of lung toxicity related to it. This problem, if not recognized and treated immediately, can result in severe dis-ability and even death. I stopped the drug and placed her on steroids to reduce the inflammation in her lungs. She recovered completely. However, her palpitations, dizzy spells, and rapid heartbeat reappeared about 6 weeks later. There were no medications left to try. They either didn't help or brought on side effects.

But since we operated on Maria, major advances had occurred.

Catheters and Radio Waves

In the early 1980s, electrical shocks via a catheter were used to ablate the A-V junc-tion pioneered by Drs. Melvin N. Scheinman at Moffitt Hospital in San Francisco and Dr. John J. Gallagher at Duke University, both alumni of the Staten Island elec-trophysiology laboratory. The tissue damage as a result of the procedure stemmed from the *blast effect* of the shock, akin to a *bomb going off inside the heart*, a rather barbaric undertaking. Heart rhythm experts used the technique mostly to ablate the

A-V junction, between the upper and lower chambers of the heart on patients with atrial fibrillation who had a rapid heart rate along with symptoms of shortness of breath, exercise intolerance, and heart failure and who did not respond to drug treatment. However, not uncommonly, the technique only produced numbing of the tissue and conduction resumed after 20–30 minutes, and the shock had to be readministered. Additionally, the partly damaged cardiac tissue also had the disturbing potential to create a new rhythm abnormality.

In 1987, Stephen Huang and Frank Marcus took a completely new tack. They performed ablation experiments in the dog heart using radiofrequency energy, that is, high-frequency alternating current, and reported its first use in patients. This is the same energy we use for radios, televisions, and microwave ovens. Shortly thereafter, after conducting similar animal experiments, Dr. Martin Borggrefe and his associates in Germany had a 40-year-old patient with WPW and a galloping heart. They blasted the extra-cable with electrical shocks and managed to stop the tachycardia. However, 8 hours later, the tachycardia resumed again. They then turned to a different current, namely, radiofrequency waves. Three days later, they brought the patient back to the laboratory and used radiofrequency current, and the tachycardia stopped. Moreover, the tachycardia did not recur in the next 5 months.

They had successfully destroyed the accessory pathway without open heart surgery.

Ultimately, the use of radiofrequency current for catheter ablation was a paradigm shift in medical practice. The technique eliminated the need for general anesthesia, limited the desiccation of tissue to a few millimeters, and cut cost and shortened convalescence (Figs. 6.1 and 6.2).

Soon after, in 1991, Dr. Warren Jackman together with his associates at the University of Oklahoma Health Science Center reported their findings in a large number of patients in *The New England Journal of Medicine.* Using radiofrequency current, they eliminated accessory pathways in 164 of 166 WPW patients, or 99%, without any major complications. In the same issue, Dr. Hugh Calkins and his associates from Johns Hopkins Hospital reported success in 93% of patients, and Dr. Karl-Heinz Kuck and coworkers in Germany reported successful ablation in 89% of patients.

These were transformative observations.

For AVNRT, Jackman used the recording of an electrical deflection of the "slow pathway" at the atrial site (Fig. 6.3) to ablate the slow pathway in this tachycardia and largely prevented heart block. This was another spectacular accomplishment, since it resulted in a cure rate of almost 96–99% with a less than 3% chance of heart block in patients plagued by this tachycardia.

Jackman's elegant studies established his laboratory as one of the prime US centers for cardiac ablative therapy of WPW syndrome particularly for patients with multiple accessory pathways whose ablation had failed at other facilities.

In addition to reentrant tachycardia, focal and micro-reentrant tachycardia can occur anywhere in the upper chambers of the heart. The development of a three-dimensional electro-anatomic cardiac mapping system in the late 1990s based on

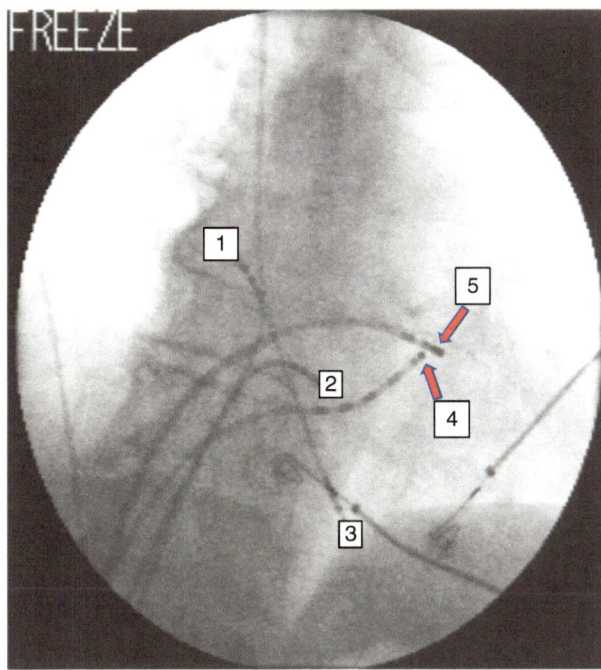

Fig. 6.1 X-ray showing catheter positioning in the heart chambers for ablation. Legend: X-ray showing position of five catheters inserted into the cardiac chambers, four through the veins in the groin, and one the ablation catheter inserted through the groin vein into the right atrium and then through a puncture in the wall that separated the right from the left atrium inserted in the distal left atrium to ablate the accessory pathway connecting the left atrium to the left ventricle. The catheter positions are shown in numbers: 1, right atrium; 2, His bundle; 3, right ventricle; 4, coronary sinus; and 5, ablation catheter that delivers radiofrequency current

electromagnetic technology that enabled more accurate mapping of rhythm disorders facilitated the ablative therapy of a host of atrial arrhythmias (Fig. 6.4) and substantially shortened the mapping time. The method is also useful in identifying and marking the location of the His bundle and assists in positioning of the ablation catheter to avoid and prevent heart block.

Radiofrequency catheter ablation was a paradigm shift in medical practice that afforded complete cure and high cost-effectiveness for patients with PSVT, with or without WPW syndrome. Indeed, some of my patients fearful of recurrent PSVT and fainting episodes expanded their lives dramatically after a successful ablation. One of my young patients wrote to me: "I can't believe I'm on no medications and that I haven't been to the ER since the procedure. Now I feel like a new person. I can have a drink or two, and I have been living a normal life. I went on vacation abroad for the first time." The advent of radiofrequency catheter ablation sounded the death knell of open heart arrhythmia surgery.

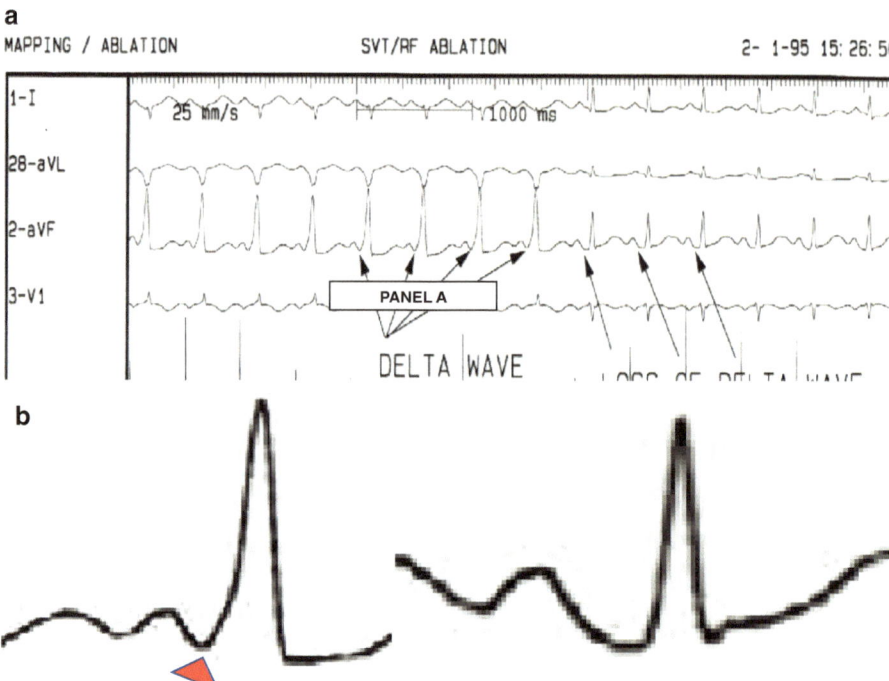

Fig. 6.2 ECG showing disappearance of the delta wave within 8 beats of radiofrequency current. Legend: Panel A, from top to bottom are four ECG leads. Note the presence of a delta wave best marked in lead aVF, which disappears within seconds after delivering current implying successful ablation of a left sided bypass tract. Panel B, enlarged lead aVF showing the delta wave (shown in red) before ablation and absence of the delta wave post-ablation

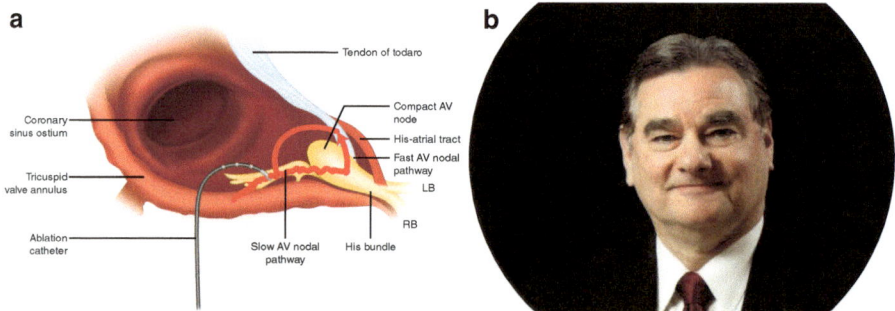

Fig. 6.3 Schematic representation of the circuit of AVNRT and ablation of slow pathway and photo of Dr. Warren Jackman. Legend: Panel A shows a cartoon of the reentrant circuit in AVNRT according to current understanding and catheter position for ablating the slow pathway. (Photo of Dr. Warren Jackman, courtesy of Dr. Jackman)

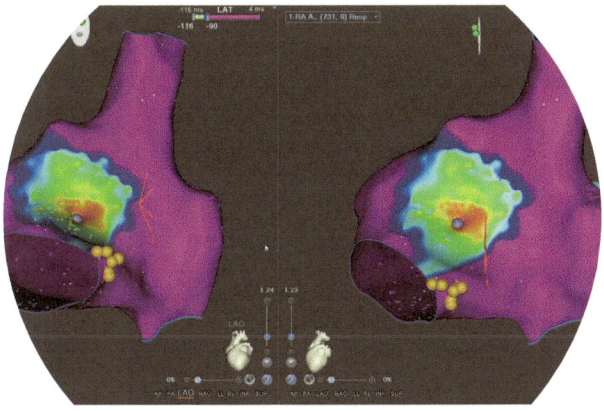

Fig. 6.4 Three-dimensional map of a right atrial septal tachycardia. Legend: Three-dimensional electro-anatomic activation map in two views (left anterior oblique and left lateral) with CARTO mapping system. Note that activation proceeds from the red area to the yellow and then the green area. This suggests that the red area is the focal point where an atrial tachycardia arises in the septum (shown in red). The successful ablation site is shown with a green dot in the red area. The yellow dots show the location of the His bundle. (Courtesy of Dr. William Wang)

Diane and Her Secret Companion

I explained the ablative procedure to Diane, the patient I referred to before who had developed side effects to amiodarone and who developed recurrence of palpitations and fainting spells after stopping the drug. "We will insert catheters into your heart through the veins in your groin, locate the accessory cable, and with radiofrequency current 'zap' it and destroy it for good," I said.

On the day of the procedure, a sense of doom was visible on her features. "Doctor," she said. "I've lived with this problem my entire life. The tachycardia has been my secret companion: my foe—I learned to live with for nearly all my life. I don't want to die on the table."

Hearing these ominous sentiments made my hair stand on end, but I recollected myself and reassured her. I remained optimistic even though we were about to perform a complex procedure that had just come into the armamentarium of the heart rhythm expert, and ours was the prime center in New York City that offered it at the time. Nonetheless, her words were unsettling and gave me pause as I scrubbed for the procedure. I had, however, explained to her all the possible complications including puncture of the wall of the heart, a stroke, and even death.

A couple of months before, I was supposed to do a diagnostic procedure on a Holocaust survivor. I had spent a lot of time explaining the procedure, and it carried few minor risks, if any. One can quote statistics and percentages. However, often, for the patient in question, he or she is the only statistic. On the evening of the procedure, she called me and said, "Doctor, I survived the Holocaust. I don't want to die from the procedure." I immediately cancelled it and asked her to see me in the clinic at her convenience. Ultimately, she had the procedure, and all went well.

Coming back to Diane, I held her hand and reassured her that I would be extra careful and diligent and wouldn't expose her to a lengthy procedure with its attendant risks. In those early days of ablative treatment, the procedure could take longer than 6 hours. We spent most of the time seeking the location of the hidden pathway to be destroyed within a 5-millimeter range. Undoubtedly, the recording of a pathway deflection which Drs. Jackman, Borggrefe, and our group pioneered implied that one was right at the site of the pathway; however, recording of pathway electrical activation was time-consuming.

After injecting her groin area with an anesthetic and puncturing her veins four times, I navigated catheters into her heart. With a special stimulator, extra beats were introduced. Easily and effortlessly, a rapid heartbeat of almost 200 beats per minute was initiated. We located the extra cable after carefully "mapping" the electrical activation. We delivered radiofrequency current, and within 10 seconds or so, the rapid heartbeat abruptly stopped. We continued for another 50 seconds, after which I could no longer initiate the tachycardia. After an additional two 1-minute lesions and several "electrophysiological maneuvers," we determined that the extra cable was destroyed for good.

Just a few years back, this woman would have to be subjected to open heart surgery like Maria, with all its attendant risks and prolonged hospitalization. Now, she left the hospital the following day.

The most interesting part of this narrative is the story of her life she related to me after I saw her almost a year after the procedure. By then she was entirely reassured that the rapid heartbeat she suffered intermittently for most of her life had finally left her.

"It's miraculous Doc, you cured me with the *Zap*," she said, accompanied by a hearty embrace. "I am 78 now, but I had 6 months to live in 1917. You stopped my racing heart, those palpitations that pounded in my head and made me oozy, foggy, and blackout. Radio…abb..lation, right? I've to write that big name down."

"Radiofrequency catheter ablation," I said.

"You stopped my racing heart. I love you, doc, 'cause of you I'm alive today."

"That's very kind of you," I said. "But what happened in 1917?"

"I was at The Mount Sinai Hospital for several months with rapid heartbeat and dizzy spells. I was only allowed to be in bed. I heard the doctor tell my sobbing mother: "'It's no good. The poor kid is going to die in 6 months. We have no treatment for her condition.'" His words befitted those of the Anglo-French writer and historian Hilaire Belloc:

Physicians of the Utmost Fame
Were called at once; but when they came
They answered, as they took their fees,
There is no cure for this Disease.

"'If she's a burden take her to the Hospital of the Incurables,'" he said to my mother.

"What's the Hospital of the Incurables?" I asked.

"St. Barnabas Hospital in the Bronx founded in the late 1800s, where people with strokes or crippling heart disease went to die," she said.

"Wow! I never knew such a hospital existed."

"But my mother took me home and put me to bed. I lay there with a rapid heart-beat, staring at the wall, staring at the ceiling, and they stared back at me. To hear the children play and hear the trains by day—a poor little kid of six—as the clock ticked by, I waited for the big day."

"You were waiting for your death!" I said. "How horrible!"

"Yes. One fine day the rapid heartbeat stopped, as I gave a loud cough. But they came back to haunt me now and then. I coughed and strained, and they stopped and came. A year passed by, I was still around. Why hadn't I died? Well the docs' in those days probably didn't know much anyway."

"That's right! That's some story there. Please continue," I said.

"Then came Christmas and they stopped—a gift from Santa Claus! The next year I went to regular school and hopped and jumped and ran. Oh boy, what a day, but on and off they came. I learned—with a cough or a good solid strain these damn palpitations would go away. I went on living, I became a woman. I beat them palpitations. I licked death! Was I a super woman or something like that? But they never left me; on and off they would come, and I'd rush to the ER. In my 74th year while having a knee replacement, they came back very strong. My orthopedic doctor in sheer panic transferred me here—back to the *Mount* after 67 years. You did it, doc'! I'm finally cured!" she said.

"Yes, indeed," I said.

"Oops, my other knee hurts! After 71 years. I'm still here, 78 and all."

This was a great story, one to reckon with. This woman had lived with her heart condition for almost all her life! And at the age of 77, she was finally cured. Wow!

Death had taunted her all along and she had won. As she told me her story, I could see a sudden tremor in her voice, as if even today, 71 years after her encounter with death, the memory still haunted her.

"Do you have any regrets?" I asked.

"It had a profound effect on my psyche. Imagine being 6 years old and hearing that you were going to die in 6 months. It stayed with me my entire life. The idea that the rapid heartbeat would one day kill me would never leave."

Her face grew serious. Her eyes flooded with tears. I left my desk and embraced her.

Antoinette's Curative Ablation of AVNRT

The reader will recall the case of Antoinette, a lawyer by profession who was plagued by palpitations, dizziness, and blackout spells when stressed and when excited (had episodes in court and several episodes during sexual activity). After inducing the tachycardia in the laboratory, I proceeded to ablate the slow pathway

(Fig. 6.3, panel A). After a 60-second ablative lesion, no tachycardia was inducible. A year later, she wrote to me: "I can't believe I'm on no medications and that I haven't been to the ER since the procedure. Now I feel like a new person. I can argue my cases in court, have a drink or two, and climax without fear of fainting. I have been living a normal life. I went on vacation abroad to Paris for the first time." She would remain free of tachycardia for the rest of her life on no medications.

The Management of AVNRT

The management of PSVT can be divided into acute, chronic preventive treatment with drugs and curative treatment with ablation. For acute termination of AVNRT, adenosine triphosphate in a dose of 12–18 mg will result in termination in over 93% of patients.

Chronic preventive management for recurrent episodes includes drugs such as beta-adrenergic blockers, calcium channel blockers, and type IC antiarrhythmic drugs such as flecainide or propafenone and type III drugs such as sotalol or amiodarone. *However, the introduction of ablative curative therapy has made the use of chronic drug therapy obsolete.* The 2015 guidelines from major cardiac American and European societies listed catheter ablation as a class I indication in patients with recurrent episodes of tachycardia.

♥

Chapter 7
Atrial Fibrillation: The Heart's Tap Dance

Don't let anyone, especially your doctor, tell you that A-Fib isn't that serious, or you should just learn to live with it.

—Steve S. Ryan, Beat Your A-Fib: The Essential Guide to Finding Your Cure

"Beginning with the first few months of my sudden and strangely tumbling heart, my life changed," said my patient, Marjorie Robinson. She was a lifelong professional actress, both in movies and in the theater. A tall striking woman of exquisite features with high cheekbones, an upright slim noble posture, and piercing yet sedate blue eyes, she carried herself in a dignified manner and, not surprisingly, spoke with an eloquent timbre.

Her worst incident occurred on Christmas day 2012. She was with her partner and her son at home, and they'd planned to visit neighbors and relatives and later have a dinner at her home. She woke up early for a jog before breakfast, and since her nose was a little runny, she grabbed a sinutab and downed it with coffee.

"When I returned, I felt dizzy as I walked through the kitchen door," she said. "I headed straight to the shower, hot and welcome. As I stood in it, suddenly my heart popped off and started racing; my legs went limp, I shut off the water, opened the glass door of the shower, pulled down a large bath towel from the rack as I fell out of the shower onto the bathroom floor. I crawled out to the bedroom, which is a corner room with windows on three sides and open drapes. All I could see was an opaque golden shield; nothing outside was visible. I couldn't get up to lie on the bed, and so I lay on the carpeted floor. It was as if death was dancing all around me!"

Her family heard her call and came in. "My partner wanted to call an ambulance, but I said no. I wasn't going to any hospital on Christmas day.

"After about 6 hours, I came out of it," she recalled. "My heart started to slow and eventually I was able to stand. But I was as weak as a kitten. It was the worst Christmas of my life, except that it could have been so much worse if I had a stroke or a heart attack. I attributed the incident to the over-the-counter medicine for a

J. A. Gomes, *Rhythms of Broken Hearts*, https://doi.org/10.1007/978-3-030-77382-3_7

runny nose. But when I put two and two together, I began to believe something much worse was wrong with me.

"As time went by, I could hardly get up a flight of stairs. Truthfully, I became an old woman inside of 1–2 years. My quality of life went from 100% to 25%, and I saw no way to continue my career. I welcomed any chance to get my old life back."

Marjorie was referred to me by her general practitioner of 25 years, Dr. Frank Weiser of New York City. He had placed her on a heart monitor for 24 hours and found that she had frequent rapid episodes of 170–200 heartbeats per minute.

She had no history of heart disease. She was well aware of the importance of healthy eating, and she wasn't overweight. The rapid heartbeat was often triggered by sinus medication, but not by wine, martinis, or coffee, unlike another patient of mine, an art dealer who owns a gallery in New York City, and many homes, and in whom it occurs only when she drinks a half-glass of wine. The petty curse despite the affluence—her inability to enjoy the nectar of Bacchus—the elixir of life!

Marjorie's episodes occurred during the day, sometimes at night, and they would last for 2 days at a time. She had no risk factors such as high blood pressure, obesity, obstructive sleep apnea, and other ailments like diabetes and heart valve diseases. And yet, her condition was truly frightening for her job, with all the lines to learn and all the energy required to perform eight shows a week or to spend the day on a film set or location.

Marjorie had atrial fibrillation (AF) that stops on its own of the "lone," variety (i.e., no cause for the rhythm abnormality). She revealed the psychological as well as physical burdens of AF, and I'll come back to her story later.

Before 2000, AF was the lowest figure on the totem pole of heart arrhythmias. However, its incidence has shot up dramatically in recent years, and today it is the most common heart rhythm disorder seen in the clinic, the hospital setting, and the emergency room afflicting between 2.7 and 6.1 million people in the United States and increasing to 12.1 million in 2030. It's hard to be more precise since people can have mild symptoms and either ignore them or not feel them at all.

The chaotic irregularity of the pulse was likely known since antiquity. Its earliest description probably dates back to the Chinese, in *The Yellow Emperor's Classic of Internal Medicine*, while William Harvey was presumably the first to describe "fibrillation of the auricles" in animals in 1628. The first ECG recording of AF was made by William Einthoven in 1906. He named it *pulsus inadequalis et irregularis* without speculating on the mechanism that caused irregular QRS complexes and chaotic undulating baseline, whereas it was Sir Thomas Lewis in London and Rothberger and Winterberg in Vienna in 1909 and 1910, respectively, who independently established AF as a clinical entity.

We now classify AF into three varieties: paroxysmal when the AF terminates on its own without intervention, persistent when it lasts for days and weeks and needs to be terminated with the administration of drugs or electrical shock, and permanent or chronic when it lasts for a year or more and cannot be terminated.

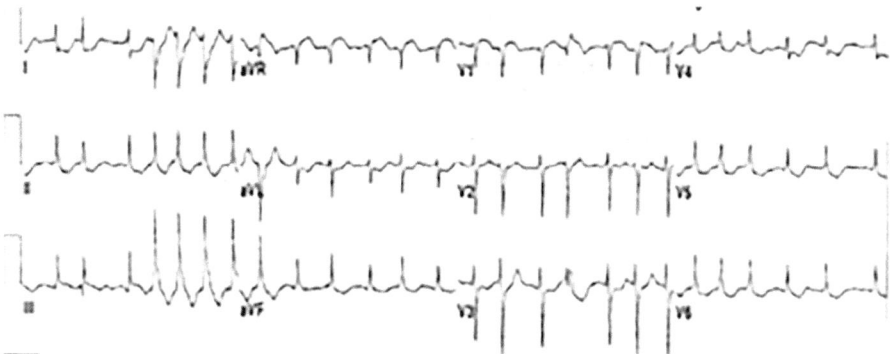

Fig. 7.1 Atrial fibrillation. Legend: From top to bottom, the ECG leads I, II, and III show an irregularly irregular rhythm. Note the variable height (amplitude), shape, and timing of the QRS complexes. Some of the fast and broad ones conduct aberrantly (intermittent abnormal conduction) down the ventricles

The AF heartbeat is "irregularly irregular" (Fig. 7.1)—a macabre sort of heart dance without a pattern. What does that mean? If your heart skips every fourth beat, it is regularly irregular. But in AF, the irregularity itself is unpredictable. There is no pattern, just chaos.

It usually arises in the left atrium—not the right, as you might expect—which starts quivering at 300–600 times per minute or 5–10 times *per second*. These impulses spread to the right atrium, and if they went straight down to the ventricles, death would quickly follow. Luckily in the majority, the A-V node blocks many of them. The result can be a heart rate (commonly called a "ventricular response") of 150–220 beats per minute. However, in patients with WPW syndrome like Maria, who had the bypass of the A-V node, the ventricles can in fact exceed 300 beats per minute, and sudden cardiac death can follow.

For much of the twentieth century, the prevailing mechanism of AF was thought to be reentry, initially conceptualized in 1962 by Gordon Moe and his colleagues in their "multiple wavelet hypothesis" and subsequently elegantly demonstrated in the animal model by the compelling studies of Dutch investigator Professor Maurits Alessie and his coworkers. But it was the groundbreaking work in the late 1990s of the brilliant French electrophysiologist Michel Haïssaguerre (Fig. 7.2) who revised this thinking.

Haïssaguerre was born and brought up in a small village in the Basque country, in Bayonne, France. During his childhood, he was so fascinated by the caves and ruined chateaus in the Pyrenees that he wanted to be an archeologist. Later, in his teens, he was inclined toward psychology, and as a medical student in Paris, his intention was to become a psychiatrist. But all that changed. When doing his training in cardiology in Bordeaux, he became interested in electrophysiology encouraged by his then mentor Professor Warin. After completing his cardiology training, Professor Warin recommended him to one of Europe's preeminent electrophysiologist, Dr. Philippe Coumel, professor of Cardiology at Lariboisière Hospital in Paris.

Fig. 7.2 Dr. Michel
Haïssaguerre. (Source:
https://alchetron.com/
Michel-Haïssaguerre)

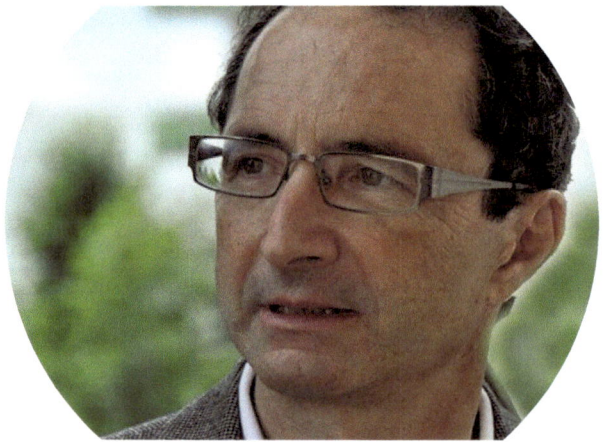

This was at the very down of interventional electrophysiology when the field was gradually transitioning from a diagnostic and mechanistic domain to curative treatment. Haïssaguerre became enamored with the advances of Scheinman and Gallagher in catheter ablation. "Their results were magic to me," he said. In 1982, he moved back to Bordeaux, but after Professor Warin passed away, he moved to Hôpital Cardiologique du Haut-Lévêque and worked under Professor Jacques Clementy, who gave him total freedom to pursue his interests.

When he and his team were attempting a procedure in a patient, they happened to see sudden, new atrial premature complexes (APCs). They recognized them on the ECG. They turned out to be the initiating beats of AF, and the atria began their characteristic quiver. He with his team then spent long days tracking the source of these extra beats finally discovering that paroxysmal AF arose in the pulmonary veins, which carry blood from the lungs to the left atrium (see Fig. 3.1, Chap. 3). The finding surprised not only Dr. Haïssaguerre but also heart doctors all over the world, since most physicians believed these veins were irrelevant to the conducting system. And of course, the veins themselves cannot initiate firing, because they're blood vessels. But a sleeve of the left atrial muscle extends up into them, and they are the source of rapid firing like machine guns. Finding the source of AF, they targeted it with catheter ablation.

Triggers and Genes

The common triggers of AF episodes include alcohol (particularly wine), chocolates, and psychological or exercise-related stress. In some cases, the cause is genetic and it can run in families. In some people, attacks occur after eating or at night or in the early morning hours, when the activity of the vagal nerve is high.

One rare trigger is weekend or holiday alcoholic binging, and it's called "holiday heart syndrome." After a heavy weekend of intoxication, these individuals usually present with rapid AF on Monday or Tuesday complaining of shortness of breath and palpitations. In such cases, the delay in the occurrence of AF is related to an excessive outpouring of adrenaline in response to acetaldehyde, a metabolite of alcohol.

The Cost of Atrial Fibrillation

AF substantially affects quality of life due to symptoms of recurrent palpitations, shortness of breath, heart failure, chest pain, dizziness, increased frequency of urination, blackout spells, and worst of all debilitating strokes. Its major impact is on the elderly since its prevalence increases as the population ages—and the developed world is graying. As a result, it is estimated that the number of sufferers will double in the next 25 years.

The Insidious Upshots of Atrial Fibrillation

AF is linked to diseases most people fear. For instance, it clearly increases the risk of dementia. Many years ago, in 1990, I was consulted on a prominent New Yorker with chronic long standing AF and dementia. At that time, we did not know that AF can result in dementia. Looking back, it is possible that this elderly gentleman's dementia was partly related to the AF.

AF can also cause heart failure. For example, I was referred a patient many years ago, a prominent financier, Andrew, for management of heart failure and consideration for a heart transplant. Andrew gave a history of AF for over a year. More recently, he was getting winded on just minimal exertion. He was a man in his 50s who showed all the signs of heart failure. Indeed, his heart function had hit the ground. We have a measure called the "ejection fraction," which is simply the percentage of the blood already in the ventricles that gets pumped out with each beat. Normal is around 55–70%, but his was 15%. His body was receiving less than half the blood it normally receives with every throb. When I looked at a portable monitor he brought from his primary doctor, I noticed that he was in AF all the time and that his heart rate was not under control, ranging from 110 to 150 beats per minute. Indeed, it's not uncommon for an otherwise healthy individual to present in heart failure because of AF. Since AF can reduce the heart's ability to pump, over time, it can strain and weaken the organ. This failure, known as "AF-induced cardiomyopathy," is becoming more prevalent.

When I saw Andrew, AF-related cardiomyopathy was not yet a solidly established entity. Nonetheless, I felt it was a distinct possibility. I told Andrew that I wanted him back into normal rhythm, and since he was already on warfarin, a blood thinner to prevent strokes, I started him on amiodarone. If he did not convert to normal rhythm within 3–4 weeks, I said, I would use electrical shock.

When Andrew came to see me 3 weeks later, I was surprised to see that the drug had done its job. Andrew was in normal rhythm. A month later, his echocardiogram showed that his ejection fraction was normal at 56%, and he was out of heart failure. I was simply overjoyed. Andrew was elated, in seventh heaven, happier than after any of the big deals he had made in his hedge fund. He continued seeing me for another year. He maintained normal rhythm on the amiodarone, had an active lifestyle, and ultimately continued following up with his primary doctor. But Andrew was not home yet.

Evolution of Clot Prevention in AF Treatment

In addition to dementia and heart failure, AF is a serious risk factor for stroke. If you suffer from AF, you are five times more likely to have a stroke. Indeed, around 50% of patients who experience a debilitating stroke already suffer from AF. Yet, many people with a stroke are unaware of AF. Thus, in AF, anticlotting drugs are used. They come in two kinds: anticoagulants and antiplatelets. Each addresses a different key element in the formation of clots.

The Story of Warfarin

Until recently and since its commercialization, warfarin was the most used anticoagulant in the United States and in the world. The story of warfarin is as interesting and fascinating as the discovery of penicillin.

In the late 1920s, previously healthy livestock began dying of internal bleeding on the prairies of North America and Canada. For one reason or another, it seemed clots were not forming to block tears in these animals' blood vessels. It was found that the cattle and sheep had grazed on sweet clover hay, but the bleeding only occurred when they ingested damp hay. Normally, farmers would have discarded this feed, but during the Depression years that followed, few could afford extra fodder for their cattle, so they used it. However, the moisture allowed the harmful molds *Penicillium nigricans* and *Penicillium jensi* to thrive. They caused the ailment that became known as sweet clover disease, which appeared within 15 days and killed the animal within 30–50 days.

About 10 years after the outbreak of sweet clover disease, a young Wisconsin farmer named Ed Carlson, who had lost many cattle from internal bleeding, took it upon himself one winter day to travel 200 miles with a dead cow in the back of his truck to the local agricultural station. There he met Karl Link and his senior student

Wilhelm Schoeffel. He handed them a milk can of un-clotted blood. As it happened, Link had gotten interested in the problem just a month back. He was sympathetic and suggested that Carlson avoid moldy hay, since two veterinary surgeons had shown animals might recover without such feed or with transfusions.

Then, together with his colleagues, Link went to work finding the active substance from the spoiled hay. After nearly 6 years, his laboratory was able to crystallize a substance that proved to be 3,3′-methylene-bis(4-hydroxycoumarin). It was a natural coumarin—the chemical that gives freshly mowed hay its scent. But when oxidized in moldy, infested hay, it formed a substance called dicoumarol, which, in turn, disabled the cows' ability to form clots and thus caused their hemorrhaging. Graduate student Mark Stahman achieved large-scale isolation of it, and he ultimately became professor of Biochemistry at the University of Wisconsin. Since the Wisconsin Alumni Research Foundation (WARF) had funded this research, it received the patent rights for dicoumarol in 1941.

In 1945, when Link was recovering in a sanatorium from wet pleurisy—a disease in which too much fluid collects between two layers of the lungs—he got the idea of using a coumarin derivative as a rat poison (Fig. 7.3). After all, if it could make cows bleed to death, it should do the same to rats. Of all the coumarin variants on his list, one seemed an especially effective rat killer, and it got the name warfarin after the patron foundation. It was marketed as a rodenticide in 1948, but soon its value as an anticoagulant for humans became clearer, for in the right doses it could disrupt clots that were harmful. It was approved for human use in 1954 and marketed as Coumadin. That was just in time for President Dwight Eisenhower, who received Coumadin in 1955 after suffering a heart attack. As two observers pointed out, "What was good for a war hero and the President of the United States must be good for all despite being a rat poison." *And so, it was: rat poison was given to humans to prevent blood from clotting until recently!*

In the early 1990s, several major studies performed in the United States, Europe, and Canada established the important role of warfarin in stroke prevention in

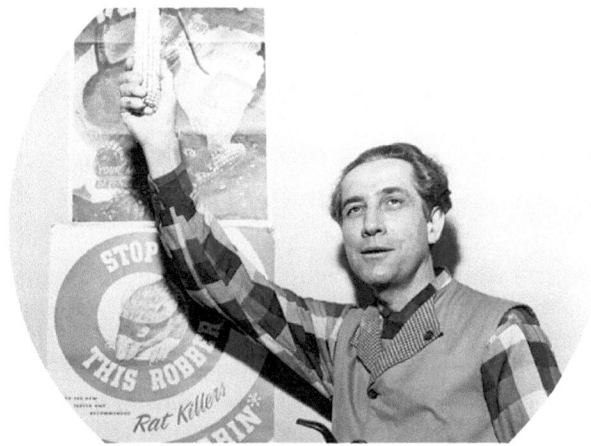

Fig. 7.3 Karl Link promoting warfarin as a rodenticide. (Source: https://www.sciencehistory. org/ distillations/a-study-in-scarlet)

patients with AF. In the United States, many of these studies were spearheaded by Dr. Jonathan Halperin at the Mount Sinai Medical Center in New York City.

Warfarin poses difficulties in dosing. It produces wild swings in "prothrombin time," a measure of how long it takes the blood to clot expressed as INR (international normalized ratio) that requires constant dose adjustment. It interacts with a host of drugs as well as leafy green vegetables. Despite all these disadvantages and the risk of bleeding, Coumadin continued being used for stroke prevention in AF, and in patients with artificial valves, and in those with blood clots, throughout the world. In 2010, pharmacists filled over 25 million prescriptions for the drug in the United States alone.

Bleeding remains a hazard, just as it was for the livestock eating the damp hay. In 2010, warfarin caused a third of all US emergency hospitalizations due to adverse drug events in patients 65 and older. Major warfarin-related bleeding is often fatal.

Andrew the financier had remained on warfarin and amiodarone watched by his general practitioner to keep him on the right dose of warfarin. But dose adjustment is hard, and one day I received a call from a family member. Andrew bled in his brain and died. Today, he might have survived.

The New Anticoagulants

We are no longer chained to warfarin. Several pharmaceutical companies were hard at work in the development and marketing of novel and more specific anticoagulants. In 2010, the FDA approved dabigatran (Pradaxa). Soon after, it approved two more anticoagulants: rivaroxaban (Xarelto) in 2011 and apixaban (Eliquis) in 2012. Unlike warfarin, these three don't require monitoring or have widespread interaction with other drugs and leafy vegetables. Xarelto and Eliquis are the new anticoagulants most often used to prevent strokes. All three go by the acronym NOACS ("novel oral anticoagulants") and are indicated for patients with no valve disease ("non-valvular AF"). In patients with valve disease, warfarin remains the drug of choice.

All anticoagulants increase the risk of bleeding, and this is true for the NOACS. Even so, the risk from bleeding seems less for the NOACS than warfarin.

Preventing Strokes in Patients with AF

Which AF patients are most at risk of stroke? Currently most American medical societies including the Heart Rhythm Society recommend using the CHA$_2$DS$_2$VASc ("chads-vasc") point scale, recommended in 2010 by the Task Force for the Management of Atrial Fibrillation of the European Society of Cardiology. In this scoring system, each capital letter stands for a factor with 1 point, unless it has a 2 after it, in which case it has 2 points. Here is the rundown:

C = congestive heart failure (1 point)
H = hypertension (1 point)
A = age greater than 74 (2 points)
D = diabetes (1 point)
S = prior stroke or "transient ischemic attack" (a mini-stroke that clears on its own, 2 points)
V = vascular disease (1 point)
A = age of 65 through 74 (1 point)
S = sex category, with female gender conferring higher risk (1 point)

If the score is zero, no anticlotting drugs are recommended. We call such medications "antithrombotic," since a "thrombus" is a clot. But the higher the score, the greater the risk. For example, if the total is 1, the risk of stroke is 1.3% per year, and baby aspirin (81 mg) usually suffices. If the score is 2 or higher, therapy with antithrombotic is preferred. The midway score of 5 carries a 6.7% risk, and with the maximum, 9, the risk is 15.2%.

New Devices for Stroke Prevention

The standard treatment for stroke prevention remains anticoagulation with warfarin and the new anticoagulants. However, there are patients who are prone to bleed on anticoagulation therapy through the gastrointestinal system and unfortunately into the brain. Moreover, they are at increased risk for repeated bleeding if left on anticoagulation therapy, and at the same time, they are at a high risk of stroke if left without anticoagulants. It is well established that the left atrial appendage (LAA) is the major source of clots in patients with AF. Therefore, the obvious solution to this problem is to insert a device that can close the LAA. Currently, there are two devices, the Watchman and the Amulet, which are most commonly implanted through a catheter for occlusion of the appendage. The Watchman device (Fig. 7.4)

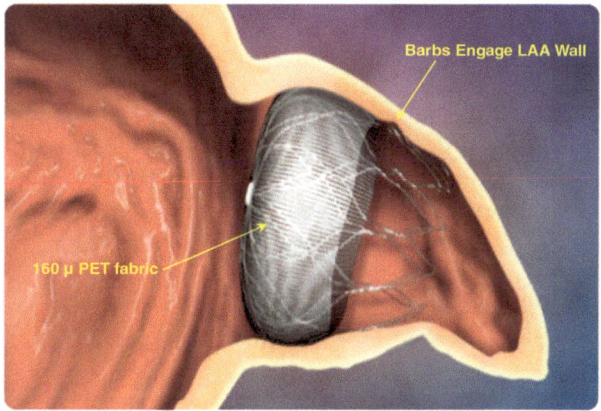

Fig. 7.4 The Watchman device. Legend: A schematic of the Watchman and its position in the left atrial appendage. (Modified from J. Anthony Gomes, *Heart Rhythm Disorders: History, Mechanisms and Management Perspectives*, Chap. 34, Fig. 34.2; Springer 2020, with permission)

Barbs Engage LAA Wall

160 μ PET fabric

is mostly used in the United States, while the Amulet device has a higher penetration in Europe. The device is mostly indicated to reduce the risk of stroke and systemic embolism in patients who are candidates for anticoagulation therapy and are at risk of bleeding. It has also been shown to be more cost-effective than warfarin and the new anticoagulants over the long term.

Evolution of Rhythm and Rate Control in AF

In the majority of AF patients, treatment usually involves drugs and/or ablation, and it has three overall goals: rate control, rhythm control, and stroke prevention.

Rate control is a more modest goal. It brings the heartbeat down to less than 110 beats per minute, without trying to control the rhythm itself. It can be a better option in elderly patients, those with chronic AF, and even those who are relatively young but asymptomatic if the AF is longstanding. In a large multicenter study called the *Atrial Fibrillation Follow-up Investigation of Rhythm Management* (AFFIRM), no difference was found in survival between rate and rhythm control. However, in many patients, rhythm control was not actually achieved. It is noteworthy that some "asymptomatic" patients feel much better and have a superior quality of life when in normal rhythm. Therefore, in most patients, I prefer at least one shot at rhythm rather than rate control.

For rate control, drugs such as the beta-adrenergic blockers (propranolol, atenolol, metoprolol, pindolol, nadolol), calcium channel blockers (diltiazem, verapamil), and digitalis are used. When these drugs do not work and the patient experiences exercise-induced shortness of breath or develops low heart function or heart failure, ablation of the A-V junction and a pacemaker is usually recommended.

Through most of the twentieth century, good treatments for rhythm control of AF (i.e., prevention of recurrence of AF) had been lacking. Rhythm control seeks to end AF and return complete control to the sinus node.

Cardioversion

For immediate conversion of AF to normal rhythm, called "cardioversion," electrical shock or drugs are used. The first electrical shock cardioversion of AF was performed in the Soviet Union in February 1959 by Vishnevskii and Tsukerman during open heart surgery. In 1960, they reported the first successful transthoracic cardioversion of atrial arrhythmias in 20 patients using electrical shock. In the United States, it was Dr. Bernard Lown who reported the use of shock to convert AF in a large cohort of patients in 1963 after which cardioversion of AF gained momentum and the method began to be used worldwide.

Chemical cardioversion with a drug such as intravenously administered Ibutilide (Covert) is less often used because of its lower success rate and the 3–4% risk of *torsade de pointes*[1] ventricular tachycardia.

To keep AF from recurring, a host of drugs, flecainide, propafenone, sotalol, dofetilide, dronedarone, and amiodarone, are used. However, these drugs have differing efficacies (50–75%) as well as side effects on the long run. Of these drugs, amiodarone is most effective in rhythm control. Flecainide and propafenone should not be used in patients with coronary disease and in those with enlarged hearts and heart failure.

The Story of Maze

As AF assumed a commanding presence in heart rhythm disorders, doctors and clinician scientists began a concerted search to cure AF. Then in the early 1980s, erudite surgeon Dr. James Cox and his team, after performing animal experimentation, developed a technique for cutting and sewing a mazelike pattern of incisions in the atrium. These had the effect of redirecting the current harmlessly.

In September 1987, he performed the operation on a human being, a pilot from Cyprus. It was the first procedure to reliably free people from AF. In 1990, before the advent of catheter ablation, we invited Dr. Cox as a visiting professor, and he along with our heart surgeon Dr. Arisan Ergin performed the maze procedure on a young patient of mine, Ms. Swope, plagued by AF episodes resulting in blackouts. She was recalcitrant to all drugs including amiodarone. She was completely cured after the procedure with no need for drug therapy. She remains free of AF for the last 30 years. However, in view of the complexity of the open heart surgery, the maze procedure was performed only in a handful of major academic centers. Besides, most patients were unwilling to undergo such major heart surgery unless they were highly symptomatic with recurrent episodes of AF recalcitrant to drug therapy.

Currently, the Cox maze is abandoned in favor of catheter ablation, enabled by the findings of Dr. Haïssaguerre. However, in patients undergoing valve surgery, surgeons use several variations of it, called "mini-maze."

---

[1] <Footnote ID="Fn1"><Para ID="Par5800">From the French "twisting of the points," used in ballet when the dancer twists around the tips of her shoes</Para></Footnote>

Medical Societies and Their Guidelines

There are well-established treatment guidelines, initially spearheaded by Dr. Valentin Fuster in 2006, on behalf of the American Heart Societies. These societies revise the guidelines periodically to keep up with recent advances. Nonetheless, often one needs to tailor therapy to the patient's symptoms and the type of AF.

Regardless, it is important to treat AF early, because as mentioned previously, it can be associated with grave consequences.

Ablation: Fire and Ice

Ablation of AF ushered in by the pioneering work of Michel Haïssaguerre is a complex procedure that has evolved over the last two decades and is still evolving. Moreover, it is becoming clearer that ablation for rhythm control is better done when the condition is paroxysmal rather than persistent or chronic. The success rate of the procedure is around 80% in the paroxysmal variety but around 60% in the persistent. The latter variety usually requires a second procedure and in some cases a third—not to mention the need for drug therapy and repeated cardioversion. Evidence is accumulating that ablation is associated with a lower incidence of stroke than drug therapy, amelioration of heart failure, as well as better long-term survival.

If you ever experience AF ablation, first, the electrophysiologist will obtain a CAT scan to get an image of your left atrium and pulmonary veins. When you come in for the procedure, you will be put under general anesthesia. The heart rhythm experts will introduce one or more catheters into your right atrium. Next, using a long-shielded needle, they will usually make two punctures in the septal wall of your heart, to slip the catheters into your left atrium. In most institutions, including our own, physicians perform this procedure with the aid of ultrasound that enables online identification of cardiovascular structures. Furthermore, if there is perforation of the heart, resulting in cardiac tamponade—that pooling of blood in the pericardial sac that encloses the organ—it can be immediately spotted and drained.

Once the catheter is in the left atrium, the CAT scan will be merged on a computer screen with the anatomic details of the left atrium and pulmonary veins obtained through a 3D mapping system. Radiofrequency lesions are then given around the four pulmonary veins to isolate them electrically (Fig. 7.5). We break the currents path. It's like turning off the switch of a rapidly firing flickering light.

The procedure takes around 4 hours, and you might stay a night or two in the hospital afterward. There is a low incidence of serious complications including perforation of the heart resulting in cardiac tamponade ($\leq 3\%$); stroke ($<1\%$); atrioesophageal fistula, a communication between the left atrium and the esophagus which can be fatal ($<1\%$); and death ($\leq 0.1\%$).

Fig. 7.5 Pulmonary vein isolation procedure for AF. Legend: 3D computer map of the left atrium and pulmonary veins. Note the radiofrequency lesions (red) encircling the pulmonary veins, from two different views. (Courtesy of Dr. Srinivas Dukkipati)

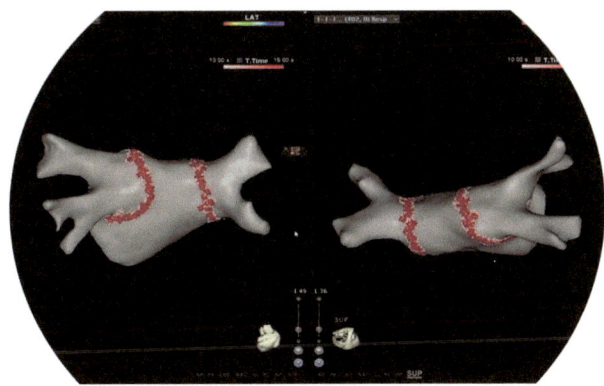

Other sources of ablation are available. Radiofrequency requires point-by-point searing, but in cryoablation using a balloon, the doctor inserts the catheter, expands the balloon with coolant, and touches it to the vein. The chill ablates a single, wide circle. The technique is easier to learn and can be done without general anesthesia. Laser ablation, also with a balloon, lets the operator actually see the targets, so they can spot overheating or gaps between the ablation lines. It was pioneered in our institution by Drs. Vivek Reddy and Srinivas Dukkipati.

A recent German study entitled *FIRE AND ICE* compared radiofrequency and cryoablation and found similar success rates. However, radiofrequency allows more flexible targeting and can ablate atrial flutter as well as the extra beats that can arise elsewhere in the atria besides the pulmonary veins.

It is noteworthy that the technology in the area of AF ablation is advancing at a rapid pace (e.g., pulsed field ablation), which has the potential of shortening the length of the procedure and a higher success rate.

Treating Marjorie

My choices for treating Marjorie were drugs and ablation. Though she worried about medications, I told her I would prefer to begin with the drug flecainide in combination with a beta-adrenergic blocker like metoprolol. I started her on flecainide with a low dose of metoprolol in October of 2013. She proved intolerant of the drugs, which caused her considerable fatigue. The dose of metoprolol was halved, and she took the flecainide on "a pill in the pocket approach," that is, only if she developed AF.

But by November of 2013, she was having more and more AF attacks. I reiterated my belief that ablation was ultimately the best solution for her. Since her AF hadn't gone beyond paroxysmal, she was a better candidate for it. However, she was already committed to doing a play out of town, so I decided to keep her on flecainide and revisit ablation when she came back to New York. Before she left, this approach was working pretty well for her, and it kept her from being completely wiped out both physically and mentally.

On her return, I asked her if she had AF during any of her performances, and if so, how she had handled it.

"While I was performing out of town," she said, "one of my entrances was down a long staircase. Standing at the top of the stairs, I felt my heart rate jump precipitously, at the same moment my legs felt as if they were limp and full of warm water. My vision started to blur, my mouth became dry, and I had to sit down on the top step. I immediately began a conversation with myself and with God. I'm not a religious person, nor am I a churchgoer, but I do believe in the power of prayer, and in that moment, I made a solemn promise that if I could just get through that performance, I would donate to Doctors Without Borders, my charity, and do something nice for someone else for the rest of my life.

"My cue was coming. I pulled myself up by the banister and started to move down the stairs with my heart pounding in my ears. I momentarily decided to act the way I felt in the performance. Thus, my character appeared slightly drunk. I wobbled and held onto the banister as I came down the stairs. Instead of standing for my tirade at 'my sister' in the cast, I sat on the arm of the couch. I simply put one word in front of the other by rote, and somehow, they came out in the right order. I only know that because I was so told, later. I couldn't remember anything during that 15-minute scene. I made my exit directly to the dressing room for a tablet of flecainide.

"By the time the interval was over, I took another flecainide and went backstage to await my entrance in Act 2. Fortunately, by the time I was back in front of the audience, I could feel my heart slow, my persona began to open up again from its closed and terrified state, and the air around my nose felt cooler, and the feeling of floating subsided."

We decided to go forward with ablation. I placed her on the blood thinner Xarelto for 8 days before the procedure (and she stayed on it for 2 months afterward). I introduced her to my colleague, Dr. Srinivas Dukkipati, the director of our EPS laboratories who would perform the ablation. She liked him immediately and admired his modesty and straightforwardness. The procedure was set for March 7, 2014.

She is now just past the 5-year mark. She has returned to her previous lifestyle including working out at a gym, yoga, speed walking, eating healthy food and drinking some wine, making a movie, and performing in a play in New York City.

"I am the most grateful person you'll ever meet," she wrote. "My quality of life was severely compromised. I feared I would not be able to continue my career, my activities, my way of life which is usually pretty high energy, and indeed, whether or not I would have a stroke and die or worse, live as a vegetable—a dreadful expression but one that says it like it is."

We gave our very best to Marjorie, and deeply appreciate her gratitude, and hope we can be as successful with other patients.

♥

Chapter 8
The Sawtooth Rhythm: Atrial Flutter

The gloom encroaches upon my mind, and my heart flutters like a bird held fast in a fist.

—Hannah Kent

Barney was a famous 70-year-old saxophonist who played for a jazz band. Suddenly, one night when he was blowing his horn in a nightclub, he felt his heart racing when he hit a few high notes, followed by shortness of breath and a dizzy spell so bad he almost fell. Luckily, he was at the end of his number, and he managed to walk off the stage and rest. His musician friend who was my patient called me the following day, and I saw him on that evening. Barney's heart was racing at 150 beats per minute. The ECG showed that he was in atrial flutter (AFL). After questioning him, it was clear that he had been having palpitations and near dizzy spells on and off for a couple of weeks. I admitted him to the hospital and started a blood thinner and an intravenous drug to slow his heart rate. The next day, after an echo showed no clots, I applied the paddles and shocked his heart back to normal rhythm. I told him that the odds were high that he would go back into the abnormal rhythm and perhaps even in atrial fibrillation (AF) and to continue the blood thinner for 4 weeks. I asked him to see me in the clinic in 2 weeks. I will revisit Barney a bit later in this narrative.

AFL is less common rhythm than AF, but sometimes it goes hand-in-hand with AF, often preceding it or even occurring interchangeably with it. You might consider AFL a close cousin of AF. In the elderly, there is at least a 30% chance that patients with AFL will develop AF in the future.

And just like in AF, AFL carries a risk of stroke and heart failure, as well as "AFL-related cardiomyopathy." The guidelines for stroke prevention described for AF apply to AFL as well.

The characteristic sawtooth flutter waves (Fig. 8.1) in the inferior ECG leads, which are seen in what is referred to as "typical flutter," were originally reported by Jollie and Rittche as far back as 1911, although Einthoven was the first to record AFL on an ECG in 1906. However, when these typical sawtooth waves are absent,

J. A. Gomes, *Rhythms of Broken Hearts*,
https://doi.org/10.1007/978-3-030-77382-3_8

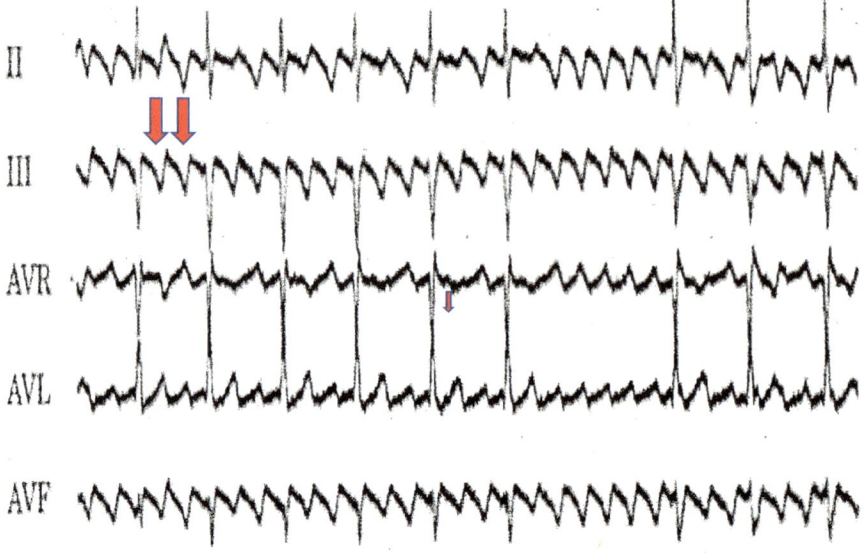

Fig. 8.1 The sawtooth waves in typical atrial flutter. Legend: From top to bottom, ECG leads II and III, AVR, AVL, AVF. Note the classical sawtooth serrated pattern of the P waves (flutter waves) in ECG leads II and III (red arrows) and AVF

the AF is referred to as "atypical flutter" and in contrast to the typical variety arises in the left atrium.

In contrast to AF, AFL occurs less than one-tenth as often. However, with more people living longer with heart disease and after complex heart surgery, as well as the advent of ablative therapy for AF, the incidence of atypical AF has gone up considerably, and the figure reported in the past probably doesn't hold true today.

Elderly subjects, those with heart failure, lung disease, and congenital heart disease, are at the highest risk of developing this arrhythmia. It can also occur in young subjects and in those without heart disease as well. More recently a genetic link has been found like in AF.

Commonly, the atria in AFL beat at 300 beats per minute (range = 280–320 beats per minute), while the ventricles beat at 150 beats per minute (a ratio of 2:1). However, as shown in Fig. 8.1, in elderly patients with diseases of the A-V node, it can be associated with varying degrees of block. Furthermore, any exertion can drive the ventricular rate even faster to 200–300 beats per minute (a 1:1 ratio) resulting in syncope. And as with AF, AFL is a dangerous rhythm in WPW syndrome in association with a short refractory period of the accessory pathway.

The rhythm is often paroxysmal like in AF but can be persistent and even chronic. It often results in palpitations, shortness of breath, and sometimes even blackout spells when the heart rate is fast. And like in AF, it can cause heart failure and heart enlargement.

It has been difficult to treat AFL since its description. Before the advent of beta-adrenergic blockers, calcium channel blockers, and other drugs to block conduction in the A-V node, the only drug available came from a plant with flowers of purple splendid bells.

The Story of the Purple Foxglove (Digitalis)

The foxglove, with its stately bells Of purple, shall adorn thy dells.—David Macbeth Moir

O Solitude! if I must with thee dwell, Let it not be among the jumbled heap Of murky build-ings: climb with me the steep, Nature's observatory whence the dell, In flowery slopes, its river's crystal swell, May seem a span; let me thy vigils keep 'Mongst boughs pavilion'd, where the deer's swift leap Startles the wild bee from the foxglove bell. —John Keats

The story of digitalis goes back to the Scottish doctor William Withering. In 1775, one of his patients developed dropsy. Withering had no treatment for the man and thought he was going to die. The patient went in search of a local healer, by some accounts a gypsy woman, who gave him a secret herbal remedy, and lo and behold, the man got better. When Withering heard of it, he searched for the gypsy woman throughout the back roads of Shropshire. After he found her, he urged her to tell him what was in the secret remedy. After much bargaining, she handed him the concoction, which was made up of over 20 ingredients. He ultimately found that the main ingredient was the plant purple foxglove (*Digitalis purpurea*) (Fig. 8.2). Withering tried a host of formulations of the digitalis plant extract on 163 patients and found that the dried and powdered leaf had the best results. He officially intro-duced its use in 1785. Thanks to the gypsy healer and Withering's dogged efforts, he became the richest doctor outside of London at the young age of 46.

For centuries, drugs based on digitalis extract, such as digitoxin and digoxin, were the only ones available to block the A-V node. Doctors often used large dos-ages of the drug that resulted in serious side effects and even death. The powerful effect of the drug was known in the Dark Ages when it was used as a poison for the "trial by ordeal." Indeed, people used digitalis glycosides to commit suicide, more so in France than in England or the United States. Killers used it in the novels of Mary Webb, Dorothy Sayers, and Agatha Christie. In the 1970s, I personally attended to two cases of suicide poisoning and several cases of toxicity resulting in heart block and ventricular tachycardia. However, digitalis in regular dosages was not highly effective in blocking the A-V node conduction in AFL, usually because of its fixed 2:1 response, unlike in AF. In 1976, digoxin-specific antibody (Fab) fragments that bind molecules of digoxin were first used successfully to treat patients with digitalis toxicity.

The introduction of beta-adrenergic blockers in the 1970s and later calcium channel blockers such as verapamil was an improvement, but they too were not highly effective in slowing the heart rate or terminating the rhythm unlike in other PSVTs. The only available option was to shock the patient to stop the rhythm or to pace the atrium at rates over 300 beats per minute as Dr. Jacob I. Haft at the Staten

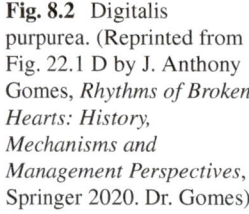

Fig. 8.2 Digitalis purpurea. (Reprinted from Fig. 22.1 D by J. Anthony Gomes, *Rhythms of Broken Hearts: History, Mechanisms and Management Perspectives*, Springer 2020. Dr. Gomes)

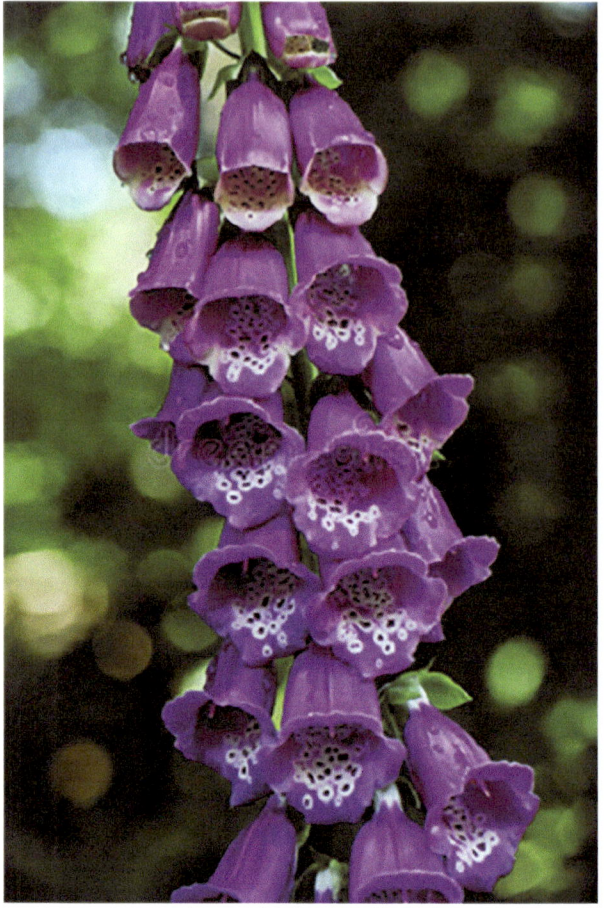

Island Lab in New York first demonstrated in 1967. However, the odds were that the rhythm would recur.

The Road to Definitive Treatment

What is happening in atrial flutter? From the beginning of the twentieth century to the end of the twenty-first century, several investigators[1] studied the mechanism of AFL in the animal model and in man. These investigations pointed to reentry (Fig. 8.3) within the right upper chamber in the great majority of patients. Finally, in 1992 and 1993, Gregory Feld and coworkers in the United States and Francisco

---

[1] Sir Thomas Lewis, Arturo Rosenblueth and Juan Garcia Ramos, Jacob Haft and Anthony Damato, Albert Waldo, George Klein, Hiroshi Inoue, and Nabil El-Sherif

Fig. 8.3 Typical atrial flutter circuit. Legend: Cartoon of the right and left atrium. The solid yellow arrows show the circus movement activation pattern in typical right AFL. IVC, inferior vena cava; CS, coronary sinus. Note that the activation is counterclockwise. This type of flutter is isthmus-dependent, i.e., the area between the IVC and the CS is the area of slow conduction critical for reentrant flutter rhythm. Ablation at this site (with a catheter, shown in black) is usually associated with termination of the rhythm. The activation of the remaining right and left atrium is passive and does not form part of the reentrant circuit

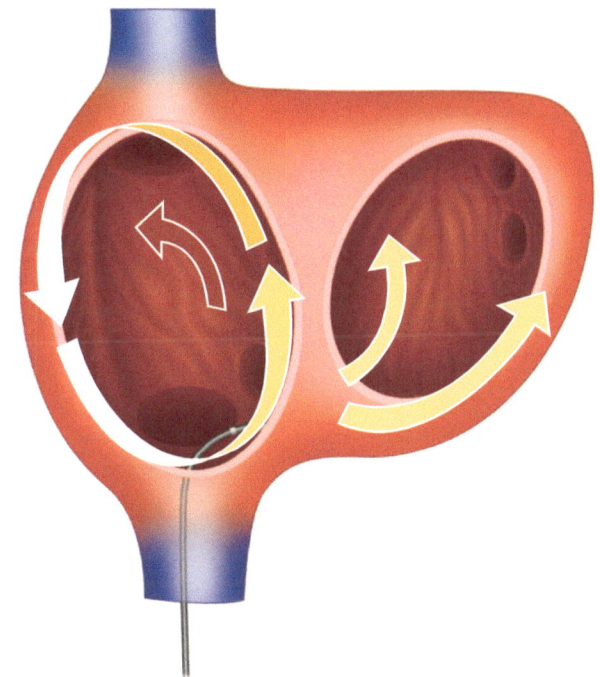

Cosio and his associates in Spain, respectively, reported success in ablating the rhythm abnormality with a catheter by using radiofrequency current (Fig. 8.3). As with PSVT described earlier, catheter ablation was a game-changer in this malady. It is curative in around 90% of patients.

And to Barney—the saxophonist—not surprisingly, he went back into AFL within 3 weeks of the shock therapy. Since catheter ablation with radiofrequency current has a high success rate, the choice was easy. Barney had a successful ablation, and he carries on blowing his sax in the United States and abroad with much gusto and bravado.

♥

Part IV
Abnormal Rhythms Arising from the Ventricles

Chapter 9
The Elusive Ventricular Extra-Beat

lab/dab ------ lab/dab --- dab ------------ lab/dab
My heart skips: the ventricular premature beat¬
the heart tumbles, the chest heaves
pain, dizziness, delirium.
What is it white knight?
An impending infarction, or death?
Out of my lungs, the last breath?
lab/dab ------ lab/dab --- dab ------------ lab/dab

—Modified from Mirrored Reflections, António Gomes

What heart rhythm disorder are you most likely to get? You might already have without knowing about it. However, in some, the symptoms can be unnerving. They usually range from palpitations, chest-thumping, strong or hard beats, and skipped beats. Other symptoms might include chest discomfort, a need to take a deep breath, a sudden cough, dizziness, and shortness of breath. Yet, you may not have any symptoms at all.

The disorder is an extra beat referred to as a premature beat arising in the ventricle that goes by the name of premature ventricular complex or depolarization or beat or contraction or the extrasystole that has had a host of abbreviations: VPC, VPD, VPB, or PVC or PVD—I prefer the abbreviation VPC. And it's normally harmless—but not always.

VPCs go far back in the history of medicine. A thousand years ago, Avicenna (981–1037) likely perceived its presence. Dutchman Dr. Karel Wenckebach ("ven-keh-BAK," 1864–1940) definitely recognized them in 1899. He had begun his career as a zoologist, but color blindness forced him to switch to physiology. Before the ECG was available, to his great credit, he was able to differentiate VPCs from a kind of heart block that now goes by the name Wenckebach block. Though he earned many honors in life, he once wrote: "In medical science there are vast realms of which I have no special knowledge...."

J. A. Gomes, *Rhythms of Broken Hearts*,
https://doi.org/10.1007/978-3-030-77382-3_9

Estimates of its prevalence in the general population have ranged from 1% to 4% on a single-test ECG, such as the one administered in a doctor's office. But the real figure is certainly far higher. As far back as 1992, we measured its incidence in 20 healthy medical interns on call, none of whom were aware of any arrhythmia. We did continuous 24-hour ECG monitoring and found that 12 or 60% of them had VPCs. Again, these were young doctors, and VPCs occur much more frequently in older subjects.

Some of the triggers include anxiety or fatigue, and our interns with VPCs were under greater stress than those without. VPCs are also common after intake of stimulants, such as coffee, tea, chocolates, alcohol, and recreational drugs.

It is noteworthy that the VPC and pause go together. You can see the pattern in the first line of the poem above: *lab/dab* ------ *lab/dab* --- *dab* ------------ *lab/dab*. The chest thumps are actually not the VPCs, but rather the beat *after* the pause. VPC makes the ventricles contract a little too early. This weak extra beat is the VPC (Fig. 9.1 A), and it slightly disrupts the rhythm of the heart. In the pause that follows, more blood than usual fills the ventricles. It is the stretching, which makes the ventricles contract more powerfully for the next beat, a phenomenon known as the Starling Law. You feel your heart pounding, and you are not imagining it. It really is

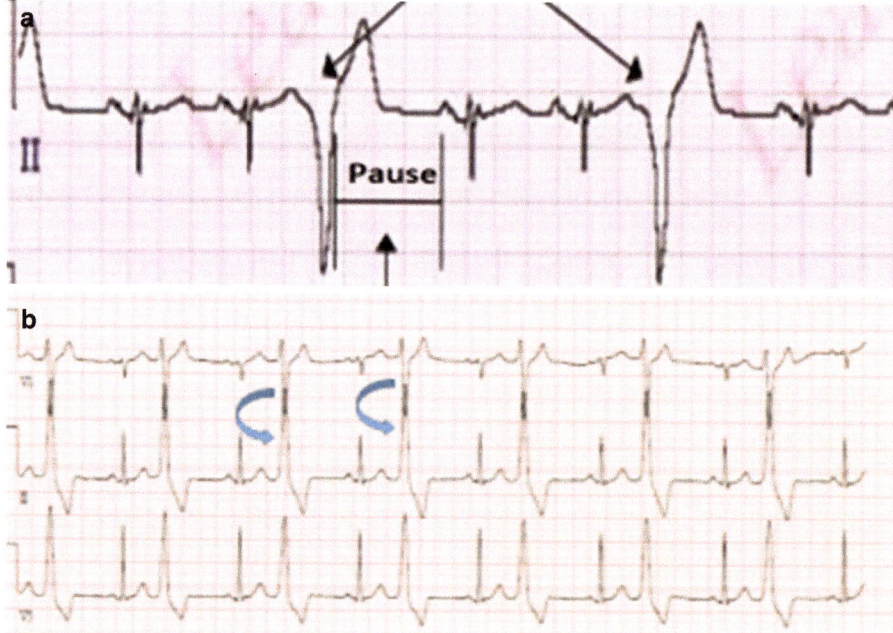

Fig. 9.1 The ventricular premature complex. Legend: **Panel A**. the arrows point to the VPCs. Note the pause after the VPC which occurs early. **Panel B**, the curved arrows point to the VPCs on a three-lead ECG. Note that they occur early—so they're premature—and their configurations differ markedly from normal beats. Note the pause after each VPC, known as the post-extra-systolic pause. The configuration of the VPC in V1 and LII (LBBB + R axis) suggests that it is arising in the right ventricular outflow tract. Note that every other beat is a VPC. This is known as bigeminy

beating harder than normally. Premature beats can also arise in the atria, in which case they are called atrial premature contraction (APCs).

In my experience, people with normal hearts are more aware of their VPCs, whereas those with sick hearts are less aware. Not uncommonly, individuals are more symptomatic when they are sitting around or watching TV or lying down and less so when they are active or exercising. This is because at rest the normal heart rate slows and the VPCs become manifest. While exercising, however, the heart rate is faster, and the VPCs are suppressed, a phenomenon called "overdrive suppression."

The Origins of VPCs

VPCs may arise anywhere from the right and left ventricle. The commonest sites include the right ventricular outflow tract (RVOT) followed by the aortic cusps, the papillary muscles, and the epicardial surface of the heart.

Martha: Anxiety Versus VPCs

Martha was a 35-year-old woman who came to see me because of a history of palpitations. When I asked her to describe her symptoms, they turned out to be due to extra beats. An ECG confirmed that she had VPCs arising in the right ventricle, near the pulmonary artery leading to the lungs. They tended to occur every other beat (Fig. 9.1 B), what is referred to as "bigeminy." Her portable monitor showed that 32% of the total beats were VPCs, but her symptoms did not always correlate with their presence. An echo showed mitral valve prolapse and normal heart function. Patients with "mitral valve prolapse" have a higher incidence of VPCs. These patients are also commonly very anxious. The next time I saw her, she was rather frantic with all sorts of nonspecific symptoms that sounded like panic attacks. She had read everything there was to read about VPCs, sudden cardiac death, and cardiomyopathy and was more informed than most doctors. She had just broken up with her boyfriend and worried about her child-bearing age, and these burdens compounded her anxiety. No reassurance was helpful. I told her that most of her symptoms were likely not related to the VPCs, but possibly to an underlying anxiety. I started her on an anti-anxiety drug and metoprolol, but she remained fixated on her VPCs.

The Rock and the Mountain

In patients like Martha, the doctor needs to correlate symptoms with the presence of VPCs. It is therefore important to track the heart for a day or two or, with an event monitor—which will turn on automatically and whenever they feel symptoms—over a 2–3-week period. The patient notes symptoms and their timing in a diary, and the doctor can then determine whether the symptoms are related to the arrhythmia.

But how can they do it? The solution came from, of all places, the small mining town of Helena, Montana. Norman J. "Jeff" Holter (1914–1983) was the scion of a Montana timber and mining dynasty, and he had trained in chemistry and physics, not medicine. He had a fierce independence and a voracious curiosity, and his passions included art, sculpture, and photography. He called himself an advocate of "non-goal-directed scientific research," meaning that he would work by intuition as much as logic and follow his hunches.

He clearly saw limitations in ECG recording. As he said, what if he owned all of Mt. Helena and he picked up a rock at the bottom and sent it to a lab for analysis? The lab might say it was 37% zinc and 11% lead. Should he conclude that the mountain itself was 37% zinc and 11% lead? "That's what's called poor sampling, in any kind of science," he said. "The idea that I should conclude that that mountain has those percentages of minerals is absurd. But that's exactly what you do when you take an ECG in the office. You take 12 to 14 heartbeats. But in the meantime, the heart beats 120,000 times a day. So, you look at 12 of them, and you say, 'Oh, you're very healthy.' Or 'You're a very unhealthy man. No smoking, please.'"

He knew that to assess the heart while people go about their daily activities, cardiac monitors had to be portable. Along with Dr. Bill Glasscock, he worked on the problem in a lab he had started in a former train station in Helena, far away from leading-edge places like New York. He developed his first heart monitor in 1947 and it was portable only in a technical sense. It was the size of a backpack and weighed 85 pounds. But eventually he made devices that fit in a coat pocket.

Holter released the invention for commercial production in 1962. Today, the Holter monitor is the size of an iPod and can record a heartbeat for days or even weeks. The monitors that our interns and Martha wore were Holters.

This device gave the VPC considerable importance and notoriety. For instance, though VPCs had been detected in 1–4% of people using one-time assessments, with 24- to 48-hour Holter monitoring, they were found in more than 40% of people (with a range of 40–70%). The rock is not the mountain after all.

VPC-Induced Cardiomyopathy

Sometimes, VPCs are only the tip of the iceberg. In 1998, Douglas F. Duffee of the Mayo Clinic and associates introduced the concept of VPC-induced cardiomyopathy, i.e., enlargement of the heart. As the name suggests, VPCs can impair the heart's function. Most patients with frequent VPCs will not develop this condition, but some will. Why does it strike some and not others? We're still debating the mechanisms and risk factors. In any case, if the echo reveals cardiomyopathy and a low ejection fraction, physicians must determine whether VPCs are the cause.

"VPC burden" provides one clue. It is the frequency at which you're having VPCs. More specifically, it's the number of VPCs divided by the number of heartbeats per hour. If you have 1200 VPCs and 4800 heartbeats in an hour, for instance, the VPC burden is 25%. And a VPC burden of 25% or higher suggests that VPCs may be causing the problem. Additionally, the absence of scar and heart wall thinning tends to rule out other causes. For instance, if a patient does have thin walls, the cause is likely not VPCs but rather the narrowing of coronary arteries, which thins the walls and makes the heart pump less effectively.

MRI findings can be diagnostic for other conditions that are causing the cardiomyopathy, such as scar due to a previous heart attack, inflammation of the heart (myocarditis), "infiltrative" diseases which deposit abnormal substances on the heart (like sarcoidosis), and a congenital condition in which fibrous tissue or fat replaces some of the heart muscle, called right ventricular dysplasia.

Fortunately, the treatment is obvious. Eliminating the VPCs helps the heart return to normal. Duffee and associates observed that the drug suppression of VPCs led to improvement in heart function. Radiofrequency ablation is also highly effective and preferred rather than lifelong drug treatment.

From Killer Treatments to No Treatment to Ablation

Dr. Bernard Lown was a Harvard cardiologist, known in the late Cold War for more than the study of arrhythmias. Together with his Russian counterpart, prominent cardiologist Dr. Yevgeny Chazov, he cofounded the organization *International Physicians for the Prevention of Nuclear War* in 1980, and in 1985, they received the Nobel Peace Prize. Dr. Lown worked in the Lown Cardiovascular Center in the Coolidge Corner area of Brookline, Massachusetts, where he saw patients and conducted his research. He was a believer in noninvasive testing for heart rhythm abnormalities using monitoring, stress tests, and antiarrhythmic drug treatment.

Along with Dr. Louis Wolff (1898–1972), he devised a grading system for VPCs in 1971 that depended on their frequency and severity on a 24-hour Holter monitor.

The higher the grade,[1] the more serious the condition. Grades I through III were considered benign and needed no treatment if the patient had no symptoms. In contrast, Grades IVA through V were considered potentially lethal and demanded attention.

Not surprisingly, physicians in practice readily embraced Dr. Lown's views on the subject. Hence, it was not uncommon in the early 1970s to see a person for some other problem and if it turned out that he or she had one of the upper-grade VPCs, to rush the person into the coronary care unit (CCU). Dr. Lown had hypothesized that abolition of VPCs with antiarrhythmic drugs would yield a better outcome, and the initially unsuspecting patient would now begin receiving intravenous medications. A sense of doom enveloped the individual who might have come in for a toothache or a headache and unexpectedly landed in the CCU.

As far back as 1973, when I was a medical resident rotating through the CCU of a New York City Hospital in Queens, I witnessed a transformational case that furthered my interest in the VPC. The case in point was Robert, a 70-year-old patient in whom a routine exam revealed VPCs and physicians ordered a 24-hour Holter monitor. The cardiologist reading the monitor found more than 30 VPCs per hour, and repetitive runs of non-sustained ventricular tachycardia: grade IVB. He sounded the alarm. The patient was immediately called and asked to report to the ER, from where he was admitted to the CCU.

Robert was a retired mechanic who was unaware of his VPCs and was entirely asymptomatic. He had no history of heart attack or heart failure. Doctors didn't know his ejection fraction (i.e., heart function), since in those days there was no ultrasound or echo technique available. In any event, the relation between heart function and VPCs remained obscure as well. The doctors administered all available drugs sequentially without benefit. Robert acquired pneumonia in the hospital and then succumbed to what we now refer to as a "pro-arrhythmic heart arrhythmia." That means that instead of suppressing the arrhythmia, the drugs worsened it. There is a lesson to be learned here: *every good drug has the potential of causing harm.* This case got me thinking. Did other factors, in addition to the VPCs, determine the fate of such patients?

In 1980, I embarked on a study and found that people with high-grade VPCs, but with otherwise normal heart function and no previous heart attack, had the same risk as those without VPCs. The patients with the highest risk of sudden cardiac death were those who had an old or a remote heart attack in association with depressed heart function (ejection fraction of 40% or less) and in whom a ventricular tachycardia was initiated in the electrophysiology lab. These observations were reported in the journal *Circulation*. At about the same time, Drs. Arthur Moss and

---

[1] Grade 0, no VPCs; grade I, less than 30 per hour; grade II, more than 30 per hour; grade III, multiform, that is, more than one ECG morphology. Three of our 20 interns had multiform VPCs; grade IVA, couplets or two VPCs in a row. Two of our interns had couplets. Grade IVB, three or more consecutive beats or non-sustained ventricular tachycardia ("non-sustained" because it terminates on its own); grade V, R on T VPCs (i.e., a VPC superimposed on the T wave of the preceding beat)

Thomas Bigger reported on the relationship between VPCs and poor heart function immediately after a heart attack. They observed that the association of more than ten VPCs per hour in subjects with heart attacks and poor heart function increased the risk of sudden death during follow-up. Our observations and those of Bigger and Moss were confirmed by a large multicenter study called the GISSI-2 trial in 1993.

The Lown-Wolff grading system had ignored the presence of heart disease, previous heart attack, or heart function. However, when the grading system was developed, echocardiography or ultrasound of the heart was not yet available to determine heart function.

That wasn't all. Between 1986 and 1989, a large landmark study took place that shocked the medical community. The Cardiac Arrhythmia Suppression Trial (CAST) revealed that antiarrhythmic drugs (flecainide, encainide, and moricizine) often did just the opposite of what they were supposed to do. They produced *lethal rhythms* in patients with heart attacks and depressed heart function. Although these drugs were potent "VPC killers," they risked killing the patient as well. The fact that abolition of VPCs with drugs did not prevent sudden cardiac death completely debunked Dr. Lown's hypothesis. As a matter of fact, the CAST study was prematurely stopped since more patients were dying on the drugs than on the placebo.

We learned several facts from CAST about the search for truth in medicine:

1. *Large, sound randomized studies are the foundation.* We should base conclusions about the effect of medical treatment on large, multicenter, randomized studies, using sound statistical analysis. We need small-scale studies too, but when they yield interesting findings, they should be catalysts for large, multicenter studies. A recent case in point is the use of the antimalarial drugs hydroxychloroquine and chloroquine for COVID-19, promoted on the basis of anecdotal evidence rather than a large-scale randomized study. The stockpiling of 66 million tablets of the drugs proved to be useless after randomized studies showed that the drug was ineffective for COVID-19.
2. *Anecdotes and hunches can do more harm than good.* We cannot base treatment of patients on anecdotal cases of success versus failure or on a hunch or hypothesis. This reasoning also applies to alternate forms of therapy. A technologist like Jeff Holter could rely on his hunches, but he was not treating patients.
3. *Best practices change.* A good and sound treatment at one moment in time may be considered harmful at a future date, and vice versa. Medical literature is full of such instances.

Today, VPCs as harbingers of sudden cardiac death are mostly viewed in the context of underlying heart disease and heart function and not as "separate independent entities."

In general, doctors will decide on treatment according to the following:

1. *If you have no heart disease or VPC-related symptoms*, medical treatment is not necessary. The treatment is reassurance.

2. *If you are symptomatic*, your doctors has to clearly establish a correlation between your symptoms and the VPCs. Often, there is no correlation at all, and the symptoms are anxiety-related. If this is established, then the treatment is usually reassurance.

Your heart rhythm expert will also check your VPC burden (number of VPCs divided by the number of heartbeats per hour). If it is 24% or above, the exact cutoff point has been controversial, or if the duration of the VPCs is greater than 150 milliseconds, they will check your heart for cardiomyopathy with an echo. If there is no cardiomyopathy, initially, physicians will give you a beta-blocker like metoprolol. If you do not respond or experience drug-related side effects, they will try calcium channel blockers such as verapamil or diltiazem or proceed to ablation.

In recent years, catheter ablation has evolved as a favorable treatment option for VPCs even as first-line treatment in young patients who prefer not to take drugs. Nonetheless, the ablative procedure should not be taken lightly. It is important to localize the VPCs using ECG algorithms prior to ablation, particularly since ablation at certain sites and a low VPC frequency can have a significant impact on the outcome as well as the complication from the procedure such as perforation and damage to coronary arteries. VPCs that originate from the right ventricular outflow tract have the highest success rates of around 90%, while those that originate from papillary muscles and left ventricular outflow tract or those arising near the coronary arteries in the coronary cusps and those arising in the epicardium and intramural VPCs can be challenging and have a lower success rate and higher complication rate. These VPCs are better tackled at major academic centers.

If ablation is not an option, the drug flecainide with a beta-blocker is my favorite combination. This combination has a high success rate of around 75%.

Coming back to Martha, I finally decided to proceed with ablation, but I told her I wasn't sure whether her symptoms would totally abate. The procedure was highly successful. Her Holter monitor showed no VPCs at all, but some of her symptoms did not entirely vanish. Finally, I convinced her to see a psychiatrist. A small dose of Zoloft seemed to have done the trick. But the abolition of the VPCs probably contributed to her well-being on the long run.

3. *If you have VPC-induced cardiomyopathy*, I favor amiodarone initially on a short-term basis. If the heart function improves along with a significant reduction in the VPC burden, then I favor proceeding to curative ablative therapy. However, some heart rhythm experts may opt for ablation at the outset.

4. *If you have significant heart failure, where it is felt that the VPCs are not the cause but perhaps a contributing factor*. Here the treatment is controversial and not adequately defined. Most heart failure specialists will tend to ignore the VPCs and treat the heart failure. If this approach does not yield benefit, I prefer the use of amiodarone on a short-term basis, and if there is significant clinical improvement in heart failure, I recommend ablation.

♥

Chapter 10
A Catastrophic Event: Sudden Cardiac Death

Sudden cardiac death has left no age untouched; sparing neither saint nor sinner, it has burdened man with a sense of insecurity and fragility.

—Bernard Lown

A death from a long illness is very different from a sudden death. It gives you time to say goodbye and time to adjust to the idea that the beloved will not be with you anymore.

—Meghan O'Rourke

Watkins was a perfectly healthy 59-year-old African American, a Con Edison employee in Flushing, New York. He collapsed while walking to his car accompanied by several of his coworkers after the evening shift.

At the hospital, a catheterization showed that he had extensive three-vessel coronary artery disease and a previous heart attack he was unaware of. He also had an aneurysm,[1] and it lay in the back wall of the heart (i.e., posteriorly). We subjected him to coronary bypass surgery and removal of the aneurysm.

Only about 10% of victims of sudden cardiac death (SCD) survive, and he did. Indeed, he had risen from the dead so to speak.

In fact, he'd been lucky to even reach the hospital.

When he collapsed, he recalled, "As I sank to the ground, a faceless hand waved good-bye."

His friends immediately began cardiopulmonary resuscitation (CPR) and called 911.

---

[1] An aneurysm is a bulge or ballooning of the wall of the heart, where a heart attack has thinned the tissue. The deformity is visible in the relaxed phase of the heart. In systole, when the heart muscle contracts, the thinned wall moves in the opposite direction. The presence of aneurysm can result in a marked decrease in ejection fraction and heart failure, as well as clot formation. Additionally, the border zone of an aneurysm can be the source of ventricular tachycardia.

© The Author(s), under exclusive license to Springer Nature Switzerland AG 2021
J. A. Gomes, *Rhythms of Broken Hearts*,
https://doi.org/10.1007/978-3-030-77382-3_10

"What happened next?" I asked.

"The paramedics arrived and apparently thought me dead and left—for somebody else close by was shot and stabbed."

"What?" I said, rather bewildered. Perhaps they felt no pulse, and seeing that he was not breathing, they believed he was already dead? But his friends did not give up.

"My friends continued the CPR. They were Con-Edison men: they climb poles, revive dead souls."

"Go on." I said.

"Pounding away on me chest, they radioed for another ambulance. The paramedics hooked me to an ECG machine. I was in ventricular fibrillation (VF). With bolts of electricity, they brought me back to life for a shot of Bourbon and a cigarette, Doc."

"You've got to stop smoking," I said.

"I know. I'll stop. It's my life, Doc. I was in the *twilight zone*…I had left my body and was traveling through a dark tunnel with intermittent flashes of light, when suddenly I was awakened by a jolt."

"You were on your way out, my friend," I said.

And indeed, he was. Death is so common from these events that the term "sudden cardiac death" is used universally in medicine *whether or not a person survives the episode.* It is the leading cause of death in the industrialized world accounting for approximately 350,000–400,000 deaths per year in the United States alone or about half of all cardiovascular-related deaths. Moreover, it is disconcerting that nearly 70–80% of individuals who die suddenly have no identifiable symptoms beforehand.

It is the Prince of Darkness in the realm of cardiovascular diseases.

Watkins's buddies had saved his life. Knowledge of CPR is highly important for family members when one or more of the family has a life-threatening cardiac condition. It needs to be encouraged in the community and taught in schools and colleges. It can be a *lifesaver.* More recently, automated external defibrillators (AEDs) that are portable, easy-to-use medical devices have been deployed in many public places. Many lives can be saved when bystanders use CPR and AEDs during a sudden cardiac death event. Recent data from the American Heart Association point to a 31.4% survival of 19,300 bystander witnessed cases in which individuals with ventricular tachycardia (VT) or ventricular fibrillation (VF) were treated effectively with a defibrillator.

Though Watkins did well after the operation, 10 years later he had an implantable defibrillator that saved his life twice. He survived for another 14 years and died of cancer at the age of 84.

Profile of the Dark Prince

SCD is defined when death occurs suddenly and unexpectedly within 1 hour of the onset of symptoms. It can occur in an individual with either known or previously undetected heart disease, in whom the mode and time of death are entirely unexpected like with Mr. Watkins. Although one of the key features is unexpectedness, in some patients, certain clinical markers such as a previous heart attack, heart failure, and transient ischemia due to coronary artery disease (CAD) have been identified. However, despite recognition of these predictors, a large proportion of SCDs occur as the first clinical manifestation of heart disease. It is usually due to a lethal heart arrhythmia: ventricular tachycardia (VT[2]) (Fig. 10.1) that degenerates into VF if not interrupted immediately.

It is the leading cause of death among men aged 20–64 years, with a threefold to fourfold greater incidence among men than women, and it accounts for the excess of female widows observed in retirement communities. It has been argued that in old age, the sudden and often unexpected mode of exit from life might be a blessing rather than a scourge, but today it occurs at a median age of only 66 years, exploding

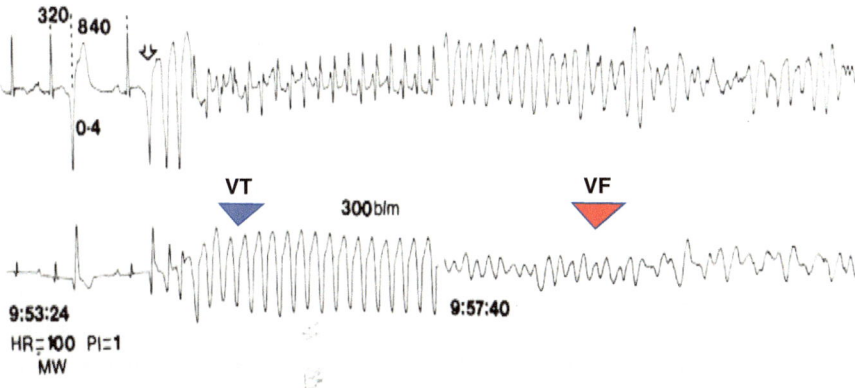

Fig. 10.1 Sudden cardiac death in a patient after a heart attack. Legend: Real-time ECG monitor strip, showing that at 9:53:24 AM the patient develops a close coupled VPC, followed by a pause and then a rapid VT at 300 beats per minute (blue arrow) that degenerates into VF (red arrow) approximately 4 minutes later, at 9:57:40. Note that the VPCs fall on the T wave (the vulnerable period) and the onset of VT is preceded by a short/long cycle that causes significant dispersion of refractoriness in ischemic Purkinje-muscle elements

---

[2] Ventricular tachycardia is a rapid heart rhythm of 110–300 beats per minute arising in the ventricles. It can stop on its own (non-sustained) or last for more than 30 seconds (sustained). Though it can occur in the absence of heart disease, in most cases, it occurs in patients with recent or previous heart attacks and cardiomyopathy, as well as a variety of other causes including genetic abnormalities in the cardiac electrical system. It usually causes palpitations, shortness of breath, and temporary loss of consciousness (syncope). It has the propensity of degenerating into ventricular fibrillation resulting in sudden death.

in the prime of life. Furthermore, SCD is becoming a global problem. Its incidence in developing countries is on a steep rise.

People have watched SCD with horror throughout history. A relief on the Tomb of Sesi (Sixth Dynasty, 2625–2475 BC) at Sakkara, entitled "Sudden Death" by Egyptologist F. W. von Bissing (1873–1956), shows a nobleman collapsing, like Watkins, in the presence of his shocked family and servants.

Who Is Most Susceptible?

The epidemiology and risk factors for SCD have been studied in recent years and reported by Dr. Robert Myerburg and his colleagues. They found three groups of patients: (A) SCD in the general population, (B) a high-risk subgroup with a prior low-risk coronary event, and (C) a high-risk group consisting of patients with previous heart attack or cardiomyopathy with low heart function. It is noteworthy that the general population group accounts for the majority of SCDs.

Age and male gender are also risk factors. In addition, individuals susceptible to a sudden life-threatening electrical instability include those with:

1. Asymptomatic CAD with a vulnerable soft atherosclerotic plaque that suddenly ruptures, resulting in acute thrombosis and ischemia[3] to the heart muscle with resultant VT and VF like my patient Pedro Sanchez. Approximately 75–80% of all SCDs in the United States and Western Europe are associated with CAD.
2. A previous heart attack with a significant drop in heart function to 35% or below.
3. Cardiac muscle weakness (cardiomyopathy) due to a viral infection of the heart.
4. Hypertrophy or overgrowth of the heart muscle.
5. Infiltrative diseases of the heart such as sarcoidosis.
6. Aortic and valvular heart diseases.
7. Genetic abnormalities in electrical impulse generation and conduction and in the muscle mechanics as in hypertrophic cardiomyopathy that often goes unrecognized.

In some individuals, the cause of ventricular fibrillation remains unknown ("idiopathic"), since all tests including autopsy findings are normal. It is felt that these patients have unrecognized genetic abnormalities in the electrical properties of the heart that we might decipher in the future.

Our studies and those of others have revealed an increase in heart rate suggesting a heightened adrenergic[4] activity, R on T VPCs,[5] and runs or short burst of VT

---

[3] Ischemia is an inadequate blood supply to an organ, in this case the heart due to blockage of blood vessel leading to part of it. If total, ischemia will result in death of muscle tissue.

[4] "Adrenergic" refers to nerve cells that transmit signals across the synapse with epinephrine, norepinephrine, or similar substances.

[5] R on T VPCs are extra beats that arise in the ventricles and fall on the T wave, the vulnerable phase of the heart's electrical system. The early VPC also results in a compensatory pause in sinus

1 hour before the fatal event (Fig. 10.1). These observations were made on Holter monitors during episodes of VT and VF. Similar observations have been confirmed in patients with implantable defibrillators.

Treatment of SCD

Acute Management

The acute management of a victim of cardiac arrest consists of chest compressions of 100/min referred to as cardiac cerebral resuscitation (CCR), instead of the past cardiopulmonary resuscitation (CPR) and defibrillation with an automatic external defibrillators (AED). On the other hand, for witnessed adult cardiac arrest, an AED should be used immediately if available.

For adults with unmonitored cardiac arrest or when an AED is not immediately available, CCR should be initiated while the AED is being retrieved and applied as soon as the device is ready for use. When two or more rescuers are present, one should begin chest compressions, while the other activates the emergency response system and gets the AED or a manual defibrillator. An increase in survival following SCD seems to be associated with an increase in bystander CPR. However, improvement in survival seems to be related mostly to shockable rhythm. These observations highlight the importance of a dense network of AEDs and community awareness of cardiac arrest and cardiopulmonary and cardiac cerebral resuscitation.

Management of Survivors of SCD

The treatment of patients lucky enough to survive SCD after successful defibrillation has been a difficult and complex undertaking, one that has evolved over time, and depicted in Fig. 10.2.

* In patients in whom the cause is ischemia due to CAD, revascularization consisting of coronary artery bypass surgery (CABG) or coronary stenting is recommended. For patients with severe LV dysfunction (EF $\leq$ 35%), a LifeVest Wearable Defibrillator is given for a 3-month period for protection. If a repeat echo done 3 months later does not show significant improvement in heart function (EF remains $\leq$35%) on optimal medical therapy, an ICD is recommended (see Chap. 14).

---

node discharge, which results in a short/long cycle sequence. That sequence causes dispersion of myocardial refractoriness, which predisposes to the development of fast polymorphic ventricular tachycardia that rapidly degenerates into ventricular fibrillation.

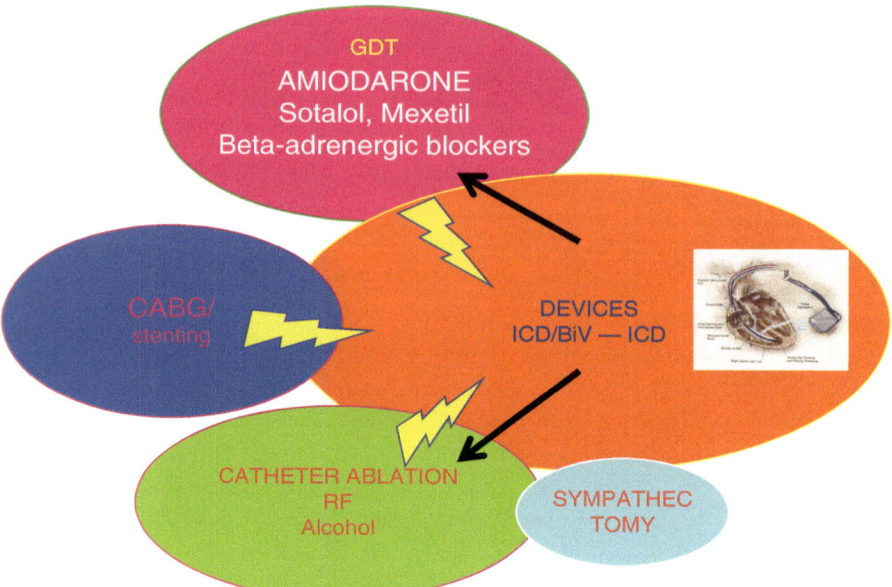

Fig. 10.2 Current modalities of treatment for survivors of SCD. Legend: Schema showing different treatment options. The orange oval represents the use of devices such as an ICD and biventricular ICD. Blue oval represents coronary bypass surgery (CABG)/stenting. Green represents catheter ablation; pink oval represents drugs. Light blue represents bilateral sympathectomy. (Reprinted from Fig. 17.10 by J. Anthony Gomes. *Heart Rhythm Disorders: History, Mechanisms and management Perspectives*. Springer 2020)

- In patients in whom SCD was due to a heart attack, following primary coronary intervention if this is feasible, the subsequent management follows the same principals as outlined above.
- In all other patients, an ICD is recommended as first-line treatment. Patients with an ICD have a better expected survival than patients who had arrhythmia surgery and drug therapy.
- In those who subsequently develop sustained VT requiring ICD shocks, amiodarone is administered initially; eventually they should be considered for catheter ablation of VT (see Chap. 13). Other antiarrhythmic drugs such as sotalol may be used particularly if LV function is relatively preserved. Amiodarone in combination with mexiletine or dofetilide is also another option in patients who have recurrent ICD shocks. Bilateral sympathectomy can be undertaken in those that are recalcitrant to antiarrhythmic drugs in combination with catheter ablation.
- In patients who have LV dysfunction (EF ≤ 35%) and left bundle branch block with a QRS duration of ≥150 milliseconds, a biventricular ICD is recommended.

♥

Chapter 11
Strange Occurrences in Life's Channels

Death is a distant rumor to the young.

—Andy A. Rooney

Your life was a hypothesis. Those who die old are made of the past. Thinking of them, one thinks of what they have done. Thinking of you, one thinks of what you could have become. You were, and you will remain, made up of possibilities.

—Édouard Levé

It is sad, mystifying, and astounding that some young children, otherwise entirely healthy, are born with genetic abnormalities in the heart's electrical system commonly known as *channelopathies* that determine their fate at an early age. Only a few decades ago, the sudden unexpected death of otherwise healthy young individuals remained a mystery often attributed to divine intervention, either a curse on the family, an evil eye, or the will of God. I can only imagine the pain and suffering of the parents of these children: *Why did it happen? What did I do wrong? She was such a healthy and happy child—why, why, why?*—a lifetime question.

These inherited maladies are among the most baffling, with tragic occurrences, and yet, from a medical perspective, they are fascinating diseases, which a heart rhythm expert sometimes encounters.

The Magic of DNA

Every living cell has a recipe for life: the *chromosomes* made of strands of deoxyribonucleic acid (DNA). Segments of DNA are called genes, and each gene directs production of a specific protein. Most human cells contain 46 chromosomes, in 23 pairs of threadlike segments, and each chromosome has thousands of genes. Genes are the hallmark of inheritance from our parents and our species. It was the Austrian

© The Author(s), under exclusive license to Springer Nature Switzerland AG 2021
J. A. Gomes, *Rhythms of Broken Hearts*,
https://doi.org/10.1007/978-3-030-77382-3_11

monk Gregor Mendel (1822–1884) who first described traits and inheritance from one generation to another.

A gene can exist in different forms called alleles (from the Greek word *allos* or "other"). One inherits one allele from one's mother and one from one's father. An allele may be *strong* referred to as *dominant* or *weak* termed *recessive*. While one dominant allele alone will express a trait, two recessive alleles are necessary to express a recessive trait.

Every living cell contains a full copy of DNA in its nucleus (Fig. 10.1). It is a tiny, balled up molecule, and it would extend 6.5 feet if you unwound it. It has 23 pairs of threadlike segments called chromosomes. If we think of DNA as a city, each chromosome is like a neighborhood. Twenty-two of them are strands lying parallel, with their genes matched up, and each matched pair of genes can have the dominant and/or recessive gene. The remaining two, the X and Y sex chromosomes, look quite different, and the X is much longer than the male Y chromosome.

The genes in DNA are our most essential gift from our parents and our species. These instructions that evolved over billions of years create us physically—our hands, hair, stomach, heart, and everything else. They are a code, comprising four chemical bases: cytosine (C), guanine (G), adenine (A), and thymine (T) (Fig. 11.1). Each DNA molecule has about three billion of these bases total. String each letter together in normal size font and they'd fill 1.5 million book pages. Since genes contain instructions to build specific proteins, they make our substance. But most of the DNA molecules aren't technically genes at all. Instead, they regulate genes, turning them on and off as needed, in ways we don't yet fully understand. As the author and physician, Siddhartha Mukherjee said, it's "not a matter of gene numbers, but of the sophistication of gene networks. It's not what we have; it's how we use it… it is the *ingenuity* of our genome that is the secret to our complexity."

It is all vastly intricate, and usually it works. Usually.

Since genes make us, they can unmake us too. The genetic code that determines who we are and what diseases we might inherit depends on the genetic information provided by our parents and on genetic mutations. Hereditary mutations are inherited from a parent and are related to errors during DNA replication and exposure to by-products of cellular metabolism. The inherited mutations are present throughout one's life in virtually every cell. On the other hand, mutations can occur due to exogenous or environmental factors such as exposure to radiation, ultraviolet light, tobacco smoke, other chemicals, and during DNA replication. These mutations are present in certain body cells and cannot be passed on to the next generation if they do not involve sperm and egg cells.

Thus, the alteration of the genetic code occurs when genes are deleted or they wind up in the wrong place on a chromosome or when they get swapped between chromosomes. Under these circumstances, a protein may be substituted with another or be deleted altogether, and the gene may not work or may turn on elsewhere. Gene mapping has been used to determine the *locus* or the specific location or position of a gene to isolate a particular biological trait.

Fig. 11.1 DNA double helix. Legend: Double helix is the description of the structure of a DNA molecule. A DNA molecule consists of two strands that wind around each other like a twisted ladder. Each strand has a backbone made of alternating groups of sugar (deoxyribose) and phosphate groups. Attached to each sugar is one of the four bases: adenine (A), cytosine (C), guanine (G), or thymine (T). The two strands are held together by bonds between the bases, adenine forming a base pair with thymine and cytosine forming a base pair with guanine. (Source: https://www.genome.gov/genetics-glossary/Double-Helix)

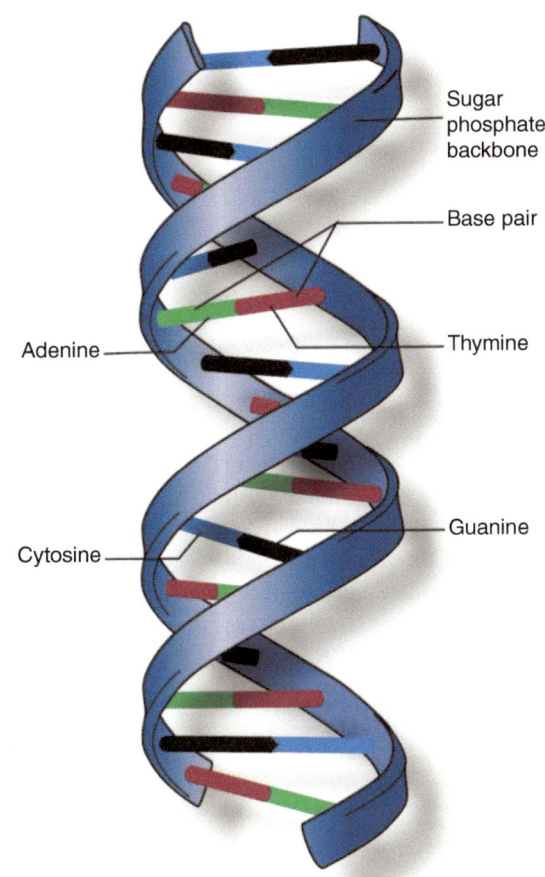

Lights, Cameras, and Sudden Death

In December 1970, in the days of black-and-white TV in Italy, during a live show, the anchorman pointed to an 18-year-old girl and asked her a question: "What is your name and what do you do?" All cameras turned toward the girl.

She jumped up all excited and then collapsed and died instantaneously. This event was watched on TV in sheer horror by millions of Italians.

She had lost consciousness several times before whenever she became emotional, but no definitive diagnosis was entertained. Her local practitioner probably attributed her fainting spells to psychogenic anxiety or felt they were just run of the mill fainting spells. Her story was told to me by Professor Dr. Peter Schwartz of the University of Milan, one of the pioneers of the long QT syndrome. He had later found an ECG of the girl, taken after a fainting episode. It showed prolongation of the "QT interval" of the electrocardiogram (ECG) (Fig. 11.2a and b) that had gone

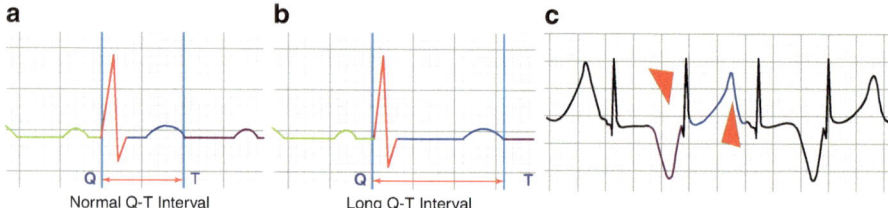

Fig. 11.2 The QT interval and T-wave alternans. Legend: The QT interval is measured from the onset of the Q-wave to the end of the T wave. Panel "**a**" shows a normal QT interval, panel "**b**" shows a markedly prolonged QT interval, and panel "**c**" shows macrolevel T-wave alternans. Note that one T wave is going downward, and the next T wave is going upward (shown by red arrows). Alternans produces spatial gradients of repolarization of sufficient magnitude to cause unidirectional block and reentrant ventricular fibrillation and sudden cardiac death

completely unnoticed. The QT interval is the period between when the heart begins to contract and when it refills with blood again. Since the QT interval varies with heart rate, it has to be corrected for this factor and expressed as "QTc," meaning QT corrected (c) for rate. The QTc is prolonged if it is >0.44 seconds in men and >0.46 seconds in women. The association of QT prolongation and sudden cardiac death (SCD) had remained an enigma for decades. Although British physician Henry Cuthbert Bazett developed and published the "Bazett formula" for QT measurement at Oxford in 1920, the very significance of the long QT interval remained a mystery.

The dead girl's younger sister, Agostina, began having the same symptoms: sudden loss of consciousness, especially during emotional stress. Her mother, fearful of a similar fate, insisted on having the 9-year-old Agostina admitted to a leading Italian hospital. She was finally admitted to the Department of Medicine of the University Hospital in Milan for evaluation. She occupied one of the four beds in the ward for which Dr. Schwartz then a rookie barely out of medical school was responsible for delivering care in the process of learning practical medicine and cardiology. The only obvious finding on the girl was a very long QT interval and the history of frequent blackout spells always associated with physical or emotional stress. At the time, no one had any idea of what disease little Agostina had. While Agostina was in the hospital, she was brought to the exercise stress test laboratory but frightened by the instrumentation, she almost fainted: the ECG showed bizarre T-wave changes, which prompted one of the senior cardiologists in the lab, to utter—"She has ugly T waves." Young Dr. Schwartz had no idea what was going on but was quick enough to make a long recording of the episode of a rapid rhythm. After looking at these strange T waves, which none of his seniors had been able to explain, he returned to the library. It did not take long for the inquisitive Dr. Schwartz to learn that the phenomenon was called "T-wave alternans" (Fig. 11.2c) and was both rare and of uncertain significance. It took him little time to review all of the few publications dealing with the long QT syndrome and to discover with great excitement that in half of them episodes of T-wave alternans had been noted. A rare phenomenon in an extremely rare disease? Very unlikely. Since her syncopal episodes were clearly triggered by sympathetic activation during emotional stress, the doctors decided to initiate treatment with a drug known as propranolol, a beta-adrenergic blocker, a commonly used drug that blocks sympathetic traffic to the heart. Beta-blocker therapy markedly reduced Agostina's syncopal episodes, but in the summer of 1972, she had a frank cardiac arrest and was resuscitated by her mother, who performed thump version following the doctors' previous instructions. After having decided that neural activity through the left stellate ganglion was playing an important detrimental role, after convincing her parents, on March 25, 1973, Agostina underwent left cardiac sympathetic denervation.[1] The method was pioneered by Drs. Moss and McDonald in 1971 at the University of Rochester, New York. They performed left sympathectomy in a woman with severe long QT syndrome and demonstrated dramatic shortening of her QT interval and arrhythmia suppression.

It was gratifying that for almost 40 subsequent years, Agostina had no more cardiac events, and Dr. Schwartz served as best man at her wedding. Professor Dr. Peter Schwartz of Milan, who would ultimately become one of the world's authorities on the "congenital long QT-syndrome" told me that by chance, Agostina's and his life crossed at the right time and that it affected each other's future in a unique way. He had saved her life, and she, by stimulating him to study the intriguing disease that was affecting her, shifted his professional life and career in an unforeseen direction with long-lasting consequences that he does not regret. The creation of the International Long QT Syndrome Registry in 1979 by Drs. Peter J. Schwartz and the late Arthur J. Moss of New York played a pivotal role in understanding the phenotype-genotype relationship, treatment, and outcome of this lethal congenital disorder. In 2019, Dr. Peter Schwartz was awarded the prestigious Lefoulon-Delalande Foundation Scientific Prize in France for his significant contributions on the congenital long QT syndrome.

Killer Alarm Clocks

In 1972, Dr. Hein J.J. Wellens of Amsterdam, Holland, reported the case of a 14-year-old Dutch girl who first lost consciousness when she was awakened by a thunderclap, and subsequently she would faint when awakened in the morning with the clang of her bedside alarm. Dr. Wellens had the presence of mind to attach an ECG monitor to the young patient (Fig. 11.3). He found that when the alarm went off in the early morning hours, she developed the dreaded rhythm called *torsade des pointes* (from the French "twisting of the points," used in ballet when the dancer twists around the tips of her shoes), during which, she fainted. This abnormality seen on the ECG, first colorfully described by French physician François Dessertenne, can degenerate into ventricular fibrillation and result in sudden death.

---

[1] Surgical removal of the lower half of the left stellate ganglion and the first four thoracic ganglia currently performed by video-assisted thoracoscopy

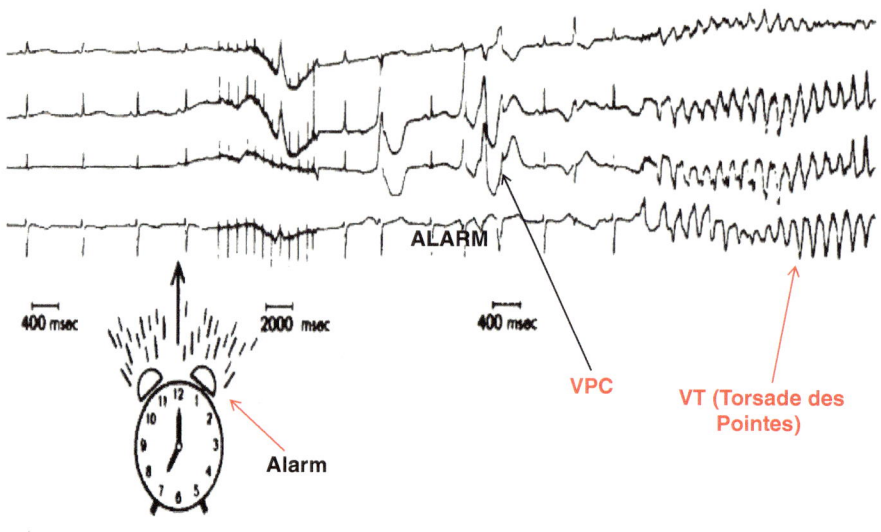

Fig. 11.3 Bedside alarm inducing VT and syncope in a patient with the long QT syndrome. Legend: From ringing alarm to ventricular tachycardia—an ECG monitor recording showing the VPCs and VT (extreme right: torsade des pointes) after the alarm clock goes off

Dr. Wellens placed the girl on a beta-blocker and initially she did well. But later, she had another syncopal attack, and he bolstered the regimen with Dilantin, an anti-seizure drug that also has effects on the electrical system of the heart. He stressed that she should be on the medications for the rest of her life. Three years later, when she was 17, at the suggestion of her boyfriend, she stopped the medications and died suddenly in bed 2 weeks later. Dr. Wellens, a good friend and an esteemed colleague, wrote to me: "What I learned from that case, and since then always tell my students, is that children and adolescents suffering from a life-threatening arrhythmia should be told to come back to the out-patient clinic often, again and again, telling them, but also the parents and eventual partners, that taking their medication is crucial." Dr. Hein J.J. Wellens, a legend in Dutch and European cardiology who wrote the foreword for my book, *Heart Rhythm Disorders*, passed away in the month of June 2020.

Today, however, besides a beta-blocker, an implantable cardioverter-defibrillator (ICD) can be lifesaving in such patients.

Startling sounds are often triggers in this ailment. I know the tragic story of a 10-year-old girl who dropped dead at home when she heard a loud honk of the car of a friend who had come to pick her up. It turned out that her father and two of her siblings had the genetic abnormality too, and all three subsequently received an ICD. I was honored to deliver the "Memorial Lecture on Sudden Cardiac Death" in her name in a New Jersey institution that was funded and attended by her parents and her siblings.

LQTS appears in both children and adults, and it causes *torsade de pointes* and fainting spells. It can be associated with congenital deafness (Jervell and Lange-Nielsen syndrome)[2] or can exist without it (Romano-Ward syndrome).[3] In LQTS, triggers, such as swimming and sudden loud noises from a car horn, an alarm clock, or thunderclap, can precipitate an arrhythmia and even death. Tragically, SCD can be its first manifestation.

In the past, these young sufferers were often treated for seizure disorders. Indeed, in my own practice, I encountered a 25-year-old man in 1984 with long QT who had come to the emergency room of the Mount Sinai Hospital for a fainting spell with a diagnosis of a seizure disorder. When I told him the correct diagnosis, he was surprised. Since the ICD was not yet invented at the time, I placed him on a beta-blocker in addition to the Dilantin he was taking and asked him to see me in the clinic. I never heard from him again.

What is actually going on in these baffling cases?

In 1985, Dr. Mark Keating was an ambitious research associate at the University of California in San Francisco. After much debate, he felt that unfortunately for him, the revolutions in basic medical science weren't happening in San Francisco. They were happening in Utah. He relocated to the University of Utah, a career move some deemed hazardous both because the institution was less prestigious and because he was switching his focus from cell biology to molecular genetics. "I was viewed as going a little bit off the deep end academically," he said. "I wasn't so anxious about it because it was what I really wanted to do. But all this angst that everybody else had was making me a bit nervous." Yet Utah had key advantages. The university possessed one of the world's few genetic probes—short stretches of single-stranded DNA used to search for a particular gene. Moreover, the largely Mormon population kept careful genealogies, important to track the genetic heritage of ailments. In 1989, Keating began his first genetic linkage analysis, focusing on the dreaded entity—the long QT syndrome (LQTS) that the Dutch and Italian girl had.

When Dr. Keating began researching LQTS, we knew of the ECG pattern but had little understanding of its cause. And gene mapping technology was in its primitive stages. He later said that this study was the most exciting of his career, and well he might. He had a total of 250 gene probes, and as he tested them, one by one they yielded no result. "I was doing it all with my own hands. At the time, it wasn't clear

---

[2] *Jervell and Lange-Nielsen syndrome is a condition that causes profound hearing loss from birth and a disruption of the heart's normal rhythm. This disorder is a form of long QT syndrome, which causes the heart muscle to take longer than usual to recharge between beats. Right from early childhood, there is an increase in risk of fainting (syncope) and sudden death. It affects an estimated 1.6 to 6 per million people worldwide and has a higher prevalence in Denmark where it affects at least 1 in 200,000 people. Mutations in the KCNE1 and KCNQ1 are responsible for the syndrome.*

[3] *The Romano-Ward syndrome is the most common form of inherited long QT syndrome, affecting an estimated 1 in 7000 people worldwide. It can cause fainting episodes, cardiac arrest, and sudden death. Mutations in the KCNE1, KCNE2, KCNH2, KCNQ1, and SCN5A genes are the culprits in the Romano-Ward syndrome.*

we would ever succeed. I was getting anxious about the whole process." Finally, with the 242nd probe, he discovered the general location, the "locus," in 1991 on chromosome 11, ultimately pointing to the Harvey-ras-1 gene in three large families with LQTS residing in Utah. However, this proved to be the wrong gene as Harvey-ras1 happened to be near the true culprit gene, KCNQ1, which encodes the main component of the potassium channel (IKs) in the heart. Keating's monumental work shifted the attention to genes encoding the ion channels and the birth of "channelopathies."

He had sourced the first channelopathy (i.e., genes damaging ion channels) of the heart. The commonest of these include long QT syndrome, catecholaminergic polymorphic ventricular tachycardia (CVPT), and Brugada syndrome. There is also a short QT syndrome, but it is extremely rare; I have yet to encounter a case. In many of these maladies, family members have a history of fainting spells or sudden death due to an inherited channelopathy. But at other times, the mutation arises spontaneously in the individual, with tragic consequences.

Long QT comes in at least ten forms, but three accounts for over 90% of cases. They have alphanumerical names: LQT1, LQT2, and LQT3. Each has special hazards. Italian Drs. Peter Schwartz, Silvia Priori, and their associates, pioneers in the field, correlated genetic expression with clinical presentation in 670 LQTS patients with major cardiac events. These researchers found that exercise was the trigger in 62% of LQT1 patients, and in only 3% did a cardiac event occur during rest or sleep. Of the lethal events in patients with LQT1, about two-thirds (68%) occurred during exercise. Patients with LQT2 are like Wellens' Dutch girl, Agostina, and the 10 years old I mentioned. They're the ones most likely to die after startling sounds like thunderclaps and loud honks or alarms going off. Dr. Keating even knew of a student who had a cardiac event after a teacher scolded her in class. Forty-three percent of these episodes occurred during emotional stress and 13% during exercise. Exercise, however, played no role at all in LQT2 deaths. And for people with LQT3, intriguingly, sleep is a hazard. Thirty-nine percent of events occurred during sleep or rest, when the heart beats more slowly, and only 13% during exercise. The likelihood of dying from a cardiac event is significantly higher (20%) with LQT3 as compared to 4% for both LQT1 and LQT2.

Long QT syndrome can result from any of an array of mutations, over 130 identified so far. And they can occur in a variety of genes, 17 at last count. But the primary ones are KVLQT1, hERG, and SCN5A—the former two impact the potassium channel and the latter the sodium channel in the heart. If these names seem to lack resonance, it's because there are so many genes in DNA that, like the less visible stars in the sky, they challenge imagination and we fall back on clusters of letters or numbers.

The sodium-related LQTS is less frequent than potassium-related LQTS in adulthood; however, they are associated with LQTS-related perinatal mortality, including life-threatening arrhythmias in the first year of life, sudden infant death syndrome (SIDS), and sudden unexplained intrauterine fetal demise (IUFD).

The value of genetic testing and lifestyle modification in these patients is of paramount importance. Genetic testing should be performed when the diagnosis of

LQTS is suspected and in siblings of an affected member. This allows for the confirmation of the genetic abnormality and the institution of preventive measures including recommendation to avoid QT-prolonging drugs as well as avoiding low levels of potassium and magnesium and other precipitating factors. For instance, LQT1 patients should not engage in competitive sports, and should avoid swimming and all physical stress. Since auditory stimuli are strong triggers in LQT2 patients, the removal of alarm clocks and loud telephone rings is paramount.

Today, the lethal consequences of the LQTS are treatable with an ICD, drugs, and sympathectomy if necessary.

In June of 1993, a 33-year-old Russian émigré, Alexei, a construction worker, presented to a hospital with severe abdominal pain. He was diagnosed with acute inflammation of the gallbladder, called cholecystitis, and had the organ removed. While in the surgical intensive care unit, he developed recurrent cardiac arrest requiring cardiopulmonary resuscitation, electrical shocks, and intubation. His ECG showed a very long QTc interval of 0.6 seconds (Fig. 11.4).

He was transferred to Mount Sinai Medical Center under my care. I placed him on a beta-adrenergic blocker and implanted an ICD. I instructed Alexei to call his only brother in Russia and ask him to see a cardiologist and have his ECG analyzed for the long QT syndrome. Alexei did, but the brother was unconcerned and did not seek the advice. A few years later, I received a call from an outside hospital requesting the transfer of the brother who after arrival in the United States developed a cardiac arrest. He was resuscitated but remained brain dead and subsequently passed away.

Alexei did very well until 14 years later in 2007, when he had dizzy spells and multiple shocks from the ICD, resulting in transient unconsciousness. If not for the ICD, he would have died. In view of the recurrent episodes of the lethal arrhythmia, due to a sympathetic imbalance seen in this syndrome, I subjected him to left cardiac sympathetic denervation, which consisted of cutting the left cervicothoracic

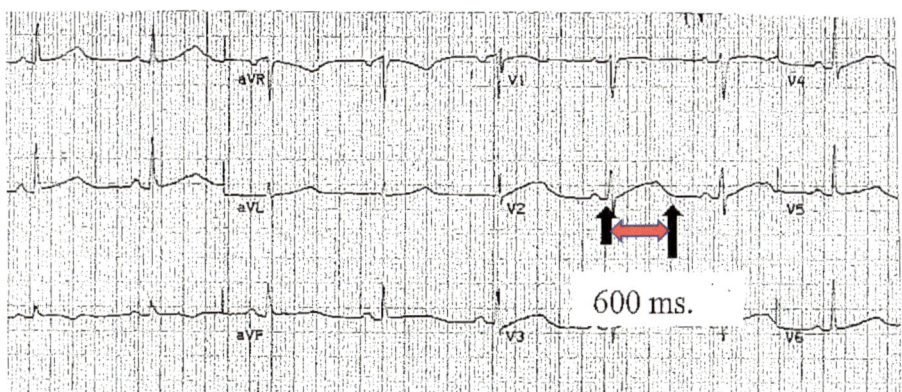

Fig. 11.4 Alexei's 12-lead ECG showing the long QTC. Legend: Alexei's ECG. His markedly prolonged QTc of 0.6 seconds is shown by arrows. He developed ventricular fibrillation and recurrent cardiac arrests

sympathetic nerve. His QTc shortened and he has remained free of arrhythmia to this day. Similar observations were reported by Dr. Peter J. Schwartz and his associates from a worldwide registry report in 1991.

A Lethal Request: CVPT

A 14-year-old boy once tried to ask a girl to a school dance. He was in a highly emotional state and his heart rate went up. And suddenly, he went into cardiac arrest. His symptoms resembled those in LQT2, but his ECG was entirely normal. There was no QT prolongation.

In 1978, the late Dr. Philippe Coumel (1935–2004) of Paris, France, another giant in cardiology and heart rhythm disorders, and his coworkers reported on this condition. It is much rarer than long QT, usually has no warning signs, and tends to strike during exercise or emotional stress. It generally appears as a blackout spell in young children, and if untreated, sudden death ensues. Coumel named it *catecholaminergic polymorphic ventricular tachycardia*. That's a good description, but its 20 syllables are unfriendly to the tongue, and we abbreviate it CPVT.

This syndrome is highly lethal and sudden death may be its first manifestation. The mean age of onset of symptoms is between 7 and 12 years. However, onset as late as the fourth decade of life has been reported.

About half of the cases stem from mutations in the cardiac ryanodine receptor (RYR2) gene and another 1–2% from damage to the cardiac calsequestrin (CASQ2) gene. We don't know the genetic causes in the rest. Both of these two genes handle calcium in the heart muscle cells.

Beta-blockers are the firs-line therapy and are effective in about 60% of individuals with CPVT. Flecainide in combination with a beta-blocker is recommended in those with recurrence of syncope or complex arrhythmias during exercise. An ICD is recommended in individuals with cardiac arrest and recurrent syncope despite optimal therapy. Lifestyle changes that include avoiding sports activity, strenuous exercise, and emotionally stressful situations are recommended.

Death Preceded by a Scream in Sleep: The Brugada Syndrome

When Dr. Pedro Brugada graduated from medical school in Barcelona in 1975, he decided to study electrophysiology in the Netherlands with Dr. Hein J.J. Wellens. A friend shook his head. "There is nothing new," he said. "Everything has already been done." The defibrillator was not yet invented, and decoding the human genome was a dream. "Just imagine what a bad prediction that was," said Dr. Brugada much later.

In 1987, he saw a new patient, a 3-year-old son of Polish parents. The boy had had repeated fainting spells and cardiac arrest, and his sister had died at the age of 3 with similar symptoms. When Dr. Brugada took the child's ECG, he was surprised. In fact, he had never seen anything like it before, and could not find the pattern in any publication. He wondered if he could also get the sister's ECG. The father traveled back to Poland and returned with it. "It was 1987," Dr. Brugada recalled. "The Berlin Wall was still there, so everything this guy was doing was illegal." The sister's ECG completely matched the boy's. After scanning records for the next 4 years, he and his brother Josep, also a physician, found only two more cases like it. They presented them at a conference of the American Heart Association in 1991, and doctors came forth with four more cases. In 1992, the Brugada brothers reported on a series of eight patients (six male and two female), from Aalst, Belgium, and Barcelona, Spain, who had ECG abnormalities consisting of a right bundle branch block pattern and persistent ST segment elevations in leads V1–V3 of the ECG (see Fig. 11.5). They suffered from repeated episodes of syncope or aborted sudden death.

"Since then, it has become an explosion," Pedro Brugada said. "We thought it was a curiosity, but it has become very important in epidemiology because the major contribution of that boy was to put the whole genetics of cardiac arrhythmias (into) another context." Six years later, with a third physician brother, Dr. Ramón Brugada, they published its genetic base. In 2019, Dr. Pedro Brugada shared with Dr. Peter J. Schwartz the prestigious Lefoulon-Delalande Foundation Scientific Prize for his significant contributions on the Brugada syndrome.

In the 1980s, the Center for Disease Control in Atlanta observed a high incidence of sudden death in Asian refugees from the northeast of Thailand. Indeed, the clinical phenomenon of Brugada syndrome had actually been known in Southeast Asia for decades, where people knew it under various names: *bangungut* in the Philippines meaning "scream followed by sudden death in sleep," *lai tai* in Thailand meaning "death during sleep" or SUDS, and *pokkuri* in Japan meaning "unexpected sudden death at night." In northeast Thailand, the incidence is 26–38 cases per 100,000 inhabitants per year, while in Laos it causes 100 sudden deaths per 100,000 inhabitants per year.

In the late 1990s, I encountered a young Jamaican man in my practice. He had suffered a blackout spell and told me that his father had died suddenly at the young age of 33, an event people attributed to a voodoo curse. He had a classic Brugada ECG (Fig. 11.5, coved pattern). An electrophysiological study revealed an inducible rapid ventricular tachycardia, with lethal consequences if it occurred spontaneously. I implanted an ICD to keep him from dying suddenly. His father had almost certainly died of SCD rather than the voodoo curse, and he passed the faulty gene on to Brandon.

That gene is the same one that causes LQT3: SCN5A. Physicians have identified a host of mutations in it since the genetic studies of Quiyun Chen and coworkers in

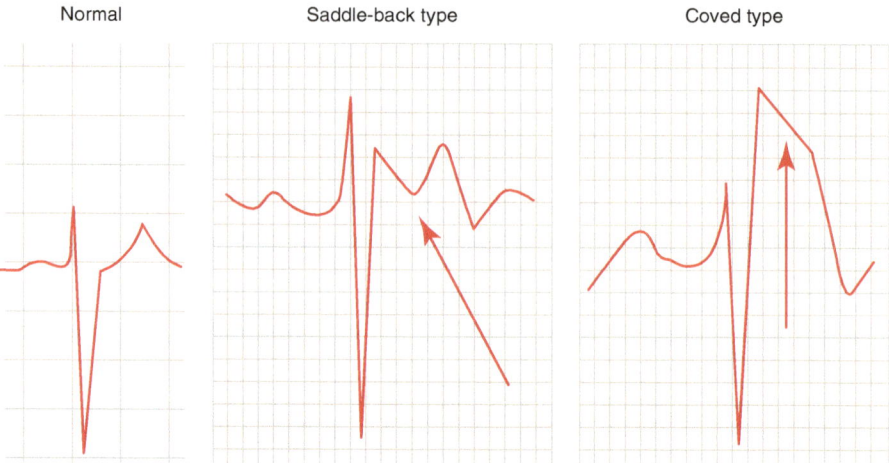

Fig. 11.5 The Brugada ECG pattern. Legend. The left vertical panel shows a normal ECG lead V2 tracing. The middle panel shows the saddleback type of ECG in lead V2, also referred to as type II. The right vertical one shows a coved-type pattern (arrow) best seen in lead V2, also referred to as type I. The coved pattern has an ominous prognosis in Brugada syndrome, yet the two patterns may be present interchangeably at various times

1998. Some alter the structure of sodium ion channels that the SCN5A protein normally makes and thus disrupt the flow of ions into cardiac cells. Other mutations prevent the SCN5A gene from producing any functional ion channels, which also reduces the inward flow of sodium ions. Such disruptions can lead to ventricular fibrillation and sudden death. Notably, a high fever and certain drugs such as procainamide can unmask the Brugada ECG pattern from the "saddleback" to "coved-type" (Fig. 11.5) in patients with this syndrome. Procainamide is often used as a provocative agent in patients suspected of the Brugada syndrome. In patients who survived a cardiac arrest or a syncopal episode, an ICD is recommended.

The genetic revolution in ion channelopathies is attributable to the knowledge of the human genome and has the potential of advancement with the development of new genomic technologies. Ultimately, correction of the genetic abnormality will be the tour de force in channelopathies described above. However, this ambitious undertaking of altering or fixing one's genes is probably decades away.

♥

Chapter 12
A Heartbreaking Calamity: Sudden Death in the Athlete

> *Today, the road all runners come,*
> *Shoulder-high we bring you home,*
> *And set you at your threshold down,*
> *Townsman of a stiller town.*

—A.E. Housman

> *Sudden death in young competitive athletes usually is*
> *precipitated by physical activity and may be due to a*
> *heterogeneous spectrum of cardiovascular disease, most*
> *commonly hypertrophic cardiomyopathy.*

—Dr. Barry J. Maron

In 490 BC, Pheidippides, a long-distance runner-messenger, arrived in Athens on the run to report the defeat of the Persian army by the Athenians in a battle in the plain of Marathon located roughly 26 miles from Athens and dropped dead. The marathon was created in 1896 to honor his legendary run. He is presumably the first documented case of an athlete dying suddenly.

On March 4, 1990, the Loyola Marymount University basketball team was playing the University of Portland in the second round of the West Coast Conference tournament. Loyola had the advantage with its 6-foot-7 star Hank Gathers—the nation's most dominant player in college basketball. During the match, as he began running back down the court, suddenly he collapsed and lay inert on the hardwood floor. A ghastly silence filled the arena. However, some thought that it was possibly a prank. Gathers was rushed to the hospital where he died soon after. He was only 23 years old.

His death shocked the nation.

Besides Hank Gathers, the sudden deaths of other prominent athletes in recent years have drawn intense attention to sudden cardiac death (SCD) in sports. We rarely imagine young athletes dying suddenly while partaking in sports activity. Most recently on June 12th 2021, Christian Ericksen suffered a cardiac arrest during

J. A. Gomes, *Rhythms of Broken Hearts*, https://doi.org/10.1007/978-3-030-77382-3_12

the EURO 2020 soccer tournament between Denmark and Finland. He was resuscitated on the field and survived while millions watched on TV. Sudden cardiac death (SCD) is usually the way of exit of older individuals, and it can even be a blessing in disguise to those suffering from terminal heart failure or cancer. But SCD can strike young athletes in the springtime of life; when the future smiles and beckons, love is just around the corner, and good health seems a given, until it all comes crashing down leaving families and friends bereft and devastated.

The Effect of Athletics on the Heart

Before we discuss SCD in athletes, it is important to understand how athletics affects the heart. There are two main kinds of fitness: endurance and strength. People train for endurance in long-distance running and swimming and for strength in wrestling, weightlifting, and shot put. Sports such as cycling and rowing involve both types. Endurance training substantially increases cardiac output, systolic blood pressure, and oxygen consumption. On the other hand, strength training mildly increases cardiac output and oxygen consumption but significantly increases blood pressure, heart rate, and resistance of the peripheral arteries and veins. All of these changes can have an acute as well as long-lasting impact on the heart. Thus, we see ECG abnormalities and enlargement of the heart chambers by echocardiography in over 40% of endurance athletes—the phenomenon called *athlete's heart*. It is essentially benign and does not lead to lethal heart rhythms.

However, athletes who die suddenly, suffer from genetic abnormalities they are born with, are usually unaware of, resulting in tragic consequences.

Causes of SCD in Athletes

In the United States, most athletes who die suddenly suffer from hypertrophic cardiomyopathy (HCM), a genetic abnormality that causes marked thickening of the heart muscle (Fig. 12.1) and is usually diagnosed by ultrasound examination of the heart commonly referred to as echocardiography. HCM can be inherited from just one parent, and a host of genes and numerous mutations can be responsible. Two genes in particular[1] account for approximately 82% of families with such mutations. The condition often goes unrecognized until death comes abruptly while competing in sports such as basketball or soccer. HCM accounts for at least one-third of the mortality in autopsy-based athlete study populations in the United States. Hank Gathers and Reggie Lewis had it.

---

[1] The cardiac myosin-binding protein C (MYBPC3) and beta-myosin heavy-chain (MYH7) genes

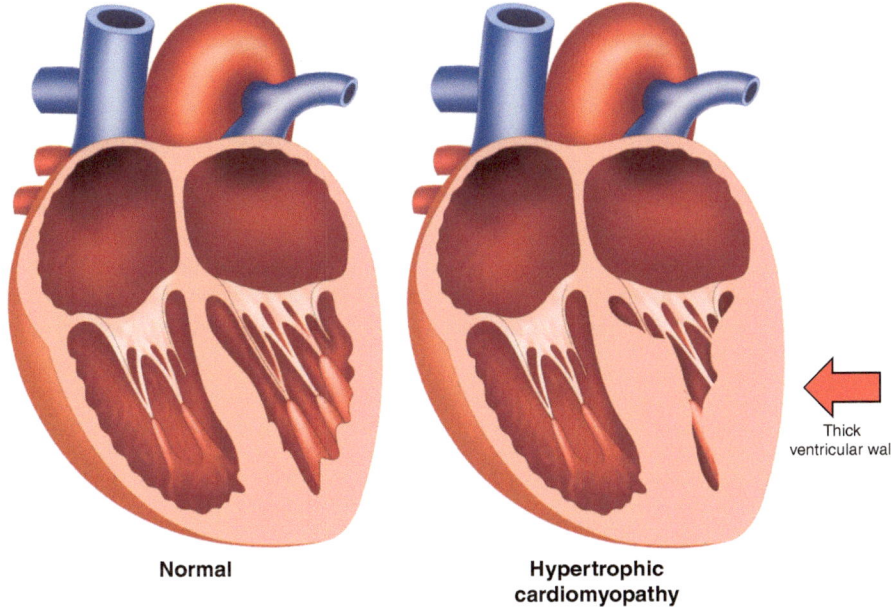

Normal   **Hypertrophic**
                                        cardiomyopathy

Fig. 12.1 The heart muscle in normal versus hypertrophic cardiomyopathy. Legend: Note the marked thickening of the left ventricular walls and cavity obliteration in hypertrophic cardiomyopathy

The case of Reggie Lewis is worth remembering. He was an NBA All-Star and a Boston Celtics player from 1987 to 1993, an outstanding athlete who once blocked all-time great Michael Jordan four times in one game. Notwithstanding, he suddenly blacked out during the Celtics' first-round playoff series with Charlotte Hornets.

After this episode, a "dream team" of 12 top Boston heart specialists consulted on him at the New England Baptist Hospital. Heart rhythm experts Dr. Mark Estes and the late Dr. Mark Josephson felt that he had a cardiomyopathy. Dr. Josephson said, "I still think ventricular arrhythmia is a more likely cause of his collapse than neurocardiogenic syncope," that is, a common, typically harmless faint. On this reasoning, he should have had a defibrillator and given up competitive sports.

But Lewis found this opinion hard to accept. Even noncompetitive athletes find it disheartening and heartbreaking to abandon sports, and for professional athletes, it can mean the end of a career after a near lifetime of hard training. Basketball was Lewis's world and livelihood. It had made him famous. It was his identity.

Lewis turned to Dr. Gilbert Mudge, director of Clinical Cardiology at Brigham and Woman's Hospital in Boston. In a TV news conference, Dr. Mudge announced that his collapse was probably from "neurocardiogenic syncope" —a common faint. "I am confident," Dr. Mudge said, "he can return to professional basketball without limitations." Dr. Mudge's opinion carried the day and Lewis returned to play.

Two months later, on the afternoon of July 27, 1993, he was shooting jumpers with friends at Brandeis University when he passed out again. He died 2 hours later. It was alleged that he used cocaine, but the doctor who performed the autopsy observed that the scarring of his heart was consistent with HCM, and not cocaine. *Needless to say, athletes with HCM should not participate in competitive sports, with the exception of low-intensity sports.*

The second most common cause of SCD in US athletes is congenital anomalies in the coronary arteries, seen in 15–20% of cases. Other diseases account for at most 5% of sudden deaths each. They include arrhythmogenic right ventricular dysplasia (ARVD), ion channelopathies,[2] myocarditis,[3] aortic valve stenosis, aortic dissection/rupture (including cases of Marfan's syndrome[4]), and atherosclerotic coronary artery disease.

The Ungluing Disease: ARVD

On August 25, 2007, around the 35th minute of a soccer game between Sevilla and Getafe at the Sánchez Pizjuán Stadium, the ball got kicked off the field near the penalty box. As a Getafe player brought it back to play, 22-year-old Sevilla defender, Antonio Puerta, crouched and then lay flat on his back. He was in cardiac arrest and was resuscitated on the field. Back in the locker room, he collapsed again. He was pronounced dead at the Virgen del Rocío University Hospital. An autopsy revealed ARVD.

Diamond, a patient of mine, was 59 years old when he blacked out for the first time while vacationing in Bali. When I saw him in 1992, I initially did not suspect ARVD because his syncope had manifested at such a late age. However, after a host

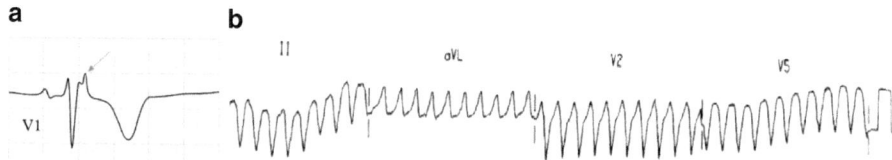

Fig. 12.2 The epsilon wave and a rapid VT in ARVD. Legend: **Panel A** shows a deflection in the terminal part of the QRS complex called the "epsilon wave" seen in patients with advanced ARVD. **Panel B** shows a rapid VT of 260 beats per minutes in a patient with syncope and ARVD

---

[2] Diseases caused by disturbed function of ion channels or the proteins that regulate them

[3] Inflammation of the heart muscle, usually due to a virus

[4] A genetic disorder of connective tissue. People with the condition tend to be tall and thin, with long arms and flexible joints. The most serious complication includes the involvement of the heart and aorta with increased risk of valve prolapse (a flop back into the left atrial chamber) and an aortic aneurysm that is prone to rupture.

of tests, it was clear that he had it (Fig. 12.2). Today, the MRI of the heart is useful in making a definitive diagnosis.

I implanted a defibrillator on Diamond and placed him on the drug amiodarone for recurrent bouts of VT (Fig. 12.2b). He did very well on this regimen and maintained an active and productive professional life, well into his retirement. He ultimately developed left heart involvement besides the right heart disease, went into heart failure to which he succumbed at the age of 82.

ARVD was first described by the talented French electrophysiologist Dr. Guy Fontaine, who was born in Corbeil-Essonnes, a suburb of Paris, the son of a banker. His training in electrical engineering and medicine enabled a thorough understanding of cardiac electrophysiology when he started his career in the 1960s. Using handheld probes, together with his brainy surgeon Guiraudon, he began mapping the reentrant circuits in patients with VT during open heart surgery with the aim of interrupting the arrhythmia by cutting the muscle involved in the circuit. It was during these endeavors in 1977 at the Pitié Salpêtrière Hospital that he recognized that some patients with sustained VT had a peculiar condition characterized by fatty replacement of the free wall of the right ventricle, which was the site of origin of the tachycardia, whereas the left ventricle appeared normal. This led to the discovery of a new disease entity called, "arrhythmogenic right ventricular dysplasia," which resulted in the publication of some of the first clinical descriptions of this condition.

ARVD is a genetic abnormality commonly seen in the Veneto region of Italy, around Venice, Verona, and Padua, where it is the most frequent cause of SCD. It is also the predominant cause of death in Spanish athletes under 30 years of age, like Antonio Puerta.

The first causative gene for ARVD was identified in people on the Greek island of Naxos. These individuals also had woolly hair and unusual thickening of the palms and soles,[5] and the condition gained the name Naxos disease. Intriguingly, Venetian Marco Sanudo (c. 1153–c. 1227) and his men had landed on Naxos in 1207, conquered both it and the island of Andros, and founded the Duchy of the Aegean Sea with Naxos as its capital. They occupied Naxos for over three centuries, from 1207 to 1537. The mixture of Venetian genes into the local population explains the high incidence of the disease on the island.

In all cases, ARVD affects the desmosomes, which are proteins that act as a kind of glue to keep the heart muscles attached to each other. They're essential, given the stress these muscle fibers endure. In ARVD, the muscle cells pull apart and die. Fatty or fibrous cells replace them, and the walls become weaker and extremely thin.

Whereas in some patients like Antonio Puerta SCD is the first unfortunate manifestation, in others like Diamond, it presents with syncope, and still others might present with VPCs and VT. For instance, another young patient of mine blacked out while running in Central Park but did not suffer from a cardiac arrest. He was in VT in the ER, which was terminated with a shock. Ultimately, he received a heart transplant.

---

[5] Technically, non-epidermolytic palmoplantar keratoderma

An ICD is a class I recommendation in patients presenting with syncope, sustained VT, or SCD. In patients with recurrent VT unresponsive to drug therapy, ablation on the outer surface of the heart (epicardium), as well as the endocardium (inner surface), is successful when performed at major institutions with a high volume of ablations. We now know that competitive sports and intense exercise are not good for those suffering from this disease, and should be avoided to prevent progression of the disease. Thus, athletes with a diagnosis of ARVD should not participate in competitive sports. If they have a defibrillator, they may partake in low-intensity sports.

Commotio Cordis

Commotio cordis (Latin for "agitation of the heart") is a condition so strange that some once doubted its existence. It occurs when a seemingly innocent item like a football strikes the chest, leading to ventricular fibrillation and sudden death. It has been reported in the United States after being hit with a baseball and softball and in the rest of the world with a soccer, cricket, and hockey ball. The blow from the ball falls on the upstroke of the T wave of the ECG, the vulnerable period of the heart, and triggers an extra beat (VPC), which causes ventricular fibrillation. It is, thankfully, very rare.

Which Athletes Are at Risk?

SCD in young otherwise healthy athletes is a tragic event, often one with high public visibility, intense media scrutiny, and potential legal liability. Therefore, strong reasons exist to identify high-risk athletes. Indeed, there is an ever-expanding population of competitive athletes, as well as people with implanted defibrillators, who wish to take part in competitive sports and long-distance running.

The intensity of the sport and the type of sport matter much more than the region. In the United States, SCD mainly occurs in the demanding sports of basketball and American football, while in the rest of the world, it is soccer. A UK study, for instance, reported that soccer was the most common sport associated with SCD in athletes aged 11–35 years. These differences seem less related to hazards in the sports themselves than to their popularity. The same person who died playing soccer in Europe might have died playing basketball in the United States.

Some athletes are more at risk than others. A large American registry was developed over 27 years from 1980 to 2006, spearheaded by Dr. Barry J. Maron from the Hypertrophic Cardiomyopathy Center, Minneapolis Heart Institute Foundation. It contained data on 1866 athletes who died suddenly (or survived cardiac arrest) in 38

US sports. The number of events per year was small, ranging from 50 to 76 between 2001 and 2006, with an average of 66 deaths per year. Males and African Americans were especially predisposed; 89% of deaths occurred in males and 29% in African Americans. High school students were also prone, with 54% of fatalities occurring among them. And 82% succumbed during competition or training, presumably because of the extra demands made on the heart.

SCD accounted for 31% from 1980 to 1993 but 69% from 1994 to 2006, increasing at a rate of 6% per year. The deaths mainly stemmed from cardiovascular disease (56%), but other conditions afflicted athletes too, such as blunt trauma usually to the head and neck (22%), heatstroke (2%), and commotio cordis (3%). Among the cardiovascular causes of SCD alone, the most common were HCM (36%) and congenital coronary artery anomalies (17%).

These observations are in sharp contrast to those found in a large and important 2016 report from a United Kingdom Regional Registry. Between 1994 and 2014, the team studied 357 hearts of athletes whose age at sudden death ranged from 7 to 67, with a median of 27 years. About two-thirds (69%) were competitive athletes, while the rest were recreational. *The study found that 81% of the athletes had no symptoms before the tragic event.* Heart disease was present in 40% of cases, while structurally normal hearts were found in 56% of children and adolescents under 18 years, 44% of young adults under 35, and 26% of individuals older than 35. It is noteworthy that in channelopathies, anatomically, the hearts are usually structurally normal.

Intriguingly, the study found that 40% of athletes died while at rest. Those who died during exertion were much more likely to have ARVD. On the other hand, and surprisingly, HCM was present in a mere 6% of deaths, compared to 36% in the American registry. Since this finding runs counter to many others, the authors urged caution in its interpretation. They noted that it might have resulted from their own stricter definition of HCM as well as selection bias.

The authors reiterated the need for early detection and further research.

The Pre-screening Battle

Since SCD can strike unexpectedly with no obvious symptoms, athletes in competitive sports—including soccer, track and field, American football, and basketball—should undergo pre-screening. But the best method has been the subject of much controversy.

In 2005, the European Society of Cardiology and International Olympic Committee published the Lausanne Recommendations, which consisted of two steps:

1. A questionnaire about personal and family history of inheritable cardiac disease, a physical examination, and a 12-lead ECG.

2. If a person shows a risk in any of these areas, he or she must see an age-appropriate cardiac specialist for an evaluation. It may include echocardiography, maximal exercise testing, and 24-hour ECG monitoring. In addition, family members may have noninvasive screening to provide information about inherited cardiovascular diseases.

However, the most effective strategy for screening, and nationally sponsored and mandated cardiovascular screening, varies from country to country. For instance, Italian law mandates screening with a routine 12-lead ECG as well as history and physical examination, based on a unique program now over 30 years old and supported by sports medicine physicians. Israel has had a similar, obligatory ECG-based initiative and national sports law since 1997. Japan employs a broad-based cardiovascular screening in the healthy population not limited to athletes. *However, the American guidelines established by the American Heart Association (AHA) in 1996, 2007, and 2014 do not include a 12-lead ECG. They only require history and physical examination of high school and college-aged athletes.* The argument against the 12-lead ECG is that it is an unproven diagnostic tool with a low specificity. Furthermore, nearly 40% of US-trained athletes may have ECG abnormalities, which can result in more tests.

It is noteworthy that the incidence of SCD in competitive athletes is low, though they are calamitous in each case. Its incidence ranges from 1 in 80,000 to 1 in 200,000 participants per year, about the same as fatal lightning strikes and much lower than motor vehicle accidents and other tragic events. In the United States, the 33-year Sudden Death in Athletes Registry reported a maximum of 75 such fatalities nationwide in any given year, far lower than from the use of recreational drugs now on an epidemic rise in the country, suicides, homicides, or cancers in the same age group. The Veneto database has reported even fewer, 55 sudden deaths in 26 years or only 2 per year; the low incidence may stem from strict screening.

The feeling against ECG testing runs deep in the United States. After it was observed that SCD was much more common than previously believed in Division I basketball players, striking about 1 in 5200 per year and killing some 4–9 athletes annually, Brian Hainline, the chief medical officer of the National Collegiate Athletic Association (NCAA), announced in March 2016 that he was going to recommend ECG screening for all college basketball players in the 1100 NCAA schools. He backed off after an outcry by nearly 100 college team physicians.

Looking Forward

On March 17, 2012, 23-year-old Fabrice Muamba collapsed on the field during a soccer game between Bolton and Tottenham of the English Premier League. According to a reporter, he "fell like a tree trunk. He didn't put his arms out to break his fall, or anything, he just dropped." Millions saw it on TV and the 35,000 spectators in the stadium fell hushed. Resuscitation began right away on the field. Muamba was in cardiac arrest for 78 minutes and received a total of 15 defibrillator shocks. He was later found to have ARVD like Antonio Puerta, but remarkably, he made a full recovery with no neurological deficits. Similarly, as mentioned previously, resuscitation on Christian Ericksen began instantaneously on the field by medical personel. He survived the cardiac arrest to be dischrged from the hospital.

Undoubtedly, these miracles occurred because automated external defibrillators (AEDs) and well-trained personnel were available. Indeed, after the death of Marc-Vivien Foé in 2003, the Fédération Internationale de Football Association (FIFA) mandated that all stadiums be equipped with AEDs and have trained medical professionals available for emergencies such as cardiac arrest. It also developed and implemented a comprehensive precompetition assessment plan that resembled the Lausanne Recommendations but added both an exercise ECG and an echocardiogram.

Finally, it is important to keep in mind that for any athlete, it is demoralizing to abstain from sports activities. For professional athletes, it is the death knell of their professional carrier notwithstanding the amount of hard work they have put in and the financial loss. Thus, the doctor can be subjected to intense pressure from the individual and the team. Not uncommonly individuals may seek other favorable opinions to go ahead and partake in competitive sports.

♥

Chapter 13
Conquering the Arrhythmic Substrate: The Scalpel and the Source

> *In order to conquer, what we need is to dare, still to dare, and always to dare.*
>
> —Georges Jacques Danton.

Defibrillation of the heart with an electrical shock was capable of summarily stopping ventricular fibrillation (VF), while a shock synchronized to the QRS complex was able to instantaneously terminate ventricular tachycardia (VT). However, these creative interventions developed in the twentieth century could not prevent the recurrence of VT, which in some patients was recurrent and refractory to available drug therapy.

Deciphering Mechanisms: The Search for the Substrate

Dr. Hein J.J. Wellens: Starting and Stopping VT

In 1972, the late Dr. Hein J. J. Wellens (Fig. 13.1), then a dashing young man working with renowned Dutch electrophysiologist Dr. Durk Durrer at the University of Amsterdam, reported important new findings in the prestigious journal *Circulation*. He was able to initiate and terminate VT with programmed extra beats in five patients who suffered periodic attacks of it, four of whom had previous heart attacks. He induced the VTs by using a single ventricular extra beat, delivered into the right ventricle through a catheter connected to an external stimulator. He could terminate the VT since it arose from circular pathways, and thus a well-timed premature beat would make a pathway unresponsive and halt the rhythm. This finding pointed to the presence of a substrate (scarred muscle from a previous heart attack).

The experimentation was a rather courageous undertaking, which was much criticized at the time. Many academic cardiologists in the United States and abroad

J. A. Gomes, *Rhythms of Broken Hearts*,
https://doi.org/10.1007/978-3-030-77382-3_13

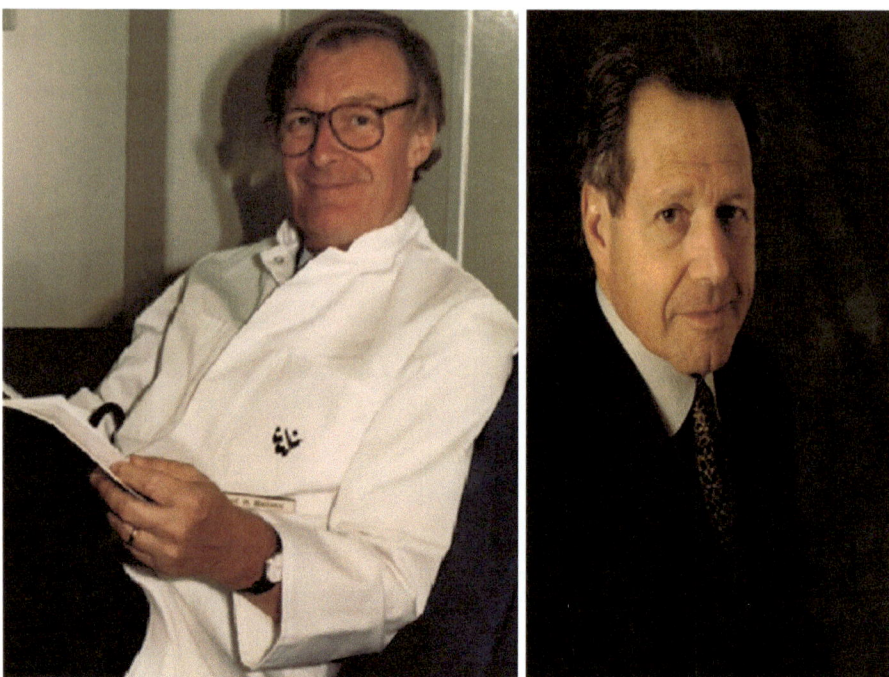

Fig. 13.1 The late Drs. Hein J.J. Wellens and Mark Josephson. Legend: Left-hand panel, Dr. Hein J.J. Wellens. Right-hand panel, Dr. Mark Josephson. (Courtesy of Drs. Wellens and Josephson)

questioned its purpose. Indeed, some even felt it unethical to perform such experiments in patients with previous heart attacks. It is noteworthy that in those times, the treatment of victims of heart attacks and VT was rudimentary at best. Most patients with recurrent VT after a heart attack were doomed to die.

I asked Hein what prompted him to study patients with VT and how those studies were received.

"These patients had a well-tolerated VT, due to a previous heart attack or unknown causes," he said. "None of them developed VF during stimulation in the laboratory. And VT could reproducibly be initiated in them. It was very difficult to get the first manuscript published. Several reviewers considered stimulation in VT dangerous and unethical. But one-and-a-half years after submission, Howard Burchell, the new editor of *Circulation*, decided that the manuscript was of value and publication followed."

Wellens made an important contribution, unrecognized at the time. He passed away on June 9, 2020, at the age of 85. Undoubtedly, his observations stimulated other investigators to determine the mechanism of this lethal arrhythmia, its response to drug treatment, and the best treatment options.

Mark Josephson: The Scalpel and the Source

Mark Josephson (Fig. 13.1), a brilliant, cerebral, and rather brash young physician, had finished his internship and residencies at the Mount Sinai Hospital in New York, where I first came to know him. He subsequently joined the USPHS Hospital in Staten Island. There, he studied electrophysiology under the direction of Dr. Anthony N. Damato and Sun H. Lau. Like me, Josephson was recommended to Anthony N. Damato by Dr. Jacob Haft, another disciple of Dr. Damato.

Mark was captivated with the work of Dr. Wellens and was anxious to proceed with his own studies in VT. After finishing his commission at the USPHS, Mark joined the University of Pennsylvania and ultimately took over the leadership and directorship of the electrophysiology lab, where he performed research deciphering the mechanism of VT in humans.

He took the bold step of introducing electrode catheters into the left ventricle of patients to map the origin of the tachycardia, an undertaking no one had attempted before. As with the reception that Wellens at first received for initiating VT, Mark's dabbling in VT in patients with previous heart attacks was controversial. In an interview he gave to Dr. Douglas Zipes on the history of electrophysiology for the Heart Rhythm Society, Mark said that one doctor told him that his experimentation was similar to those at Auschwitz. Mark being Jewish, the comment was highly insulting and traumatic, but he persevered.

Mark found that in patients with old heart attacks, the VT arose in the endocardial surface (the inside wall of the left ventricle that is in contact with blood), near the border zone of the aneurysm. He surmised that the electrical wave fronts during VT that defined its mechanism consisted of a circulating wave front (reentry) in the heart muscle damaged from a heart attack.

Historical Evolution of Surgery: The Philadelphia Peel

In the past, in patients with VT, surgeons often cut out the damaged bulging heart muscle after a heart attack, only to see a confounding recurrence of VT in over 50% of patients. In 1978, creative French surgeon Gerard Guiraudon and his coworkers had devised an operation called "encircling endocardial ventriculotomy" (Fig. 13.2a) where an incision was carried out through the whole length of the deceased heart muscle, thus isolating it.

Having deciphered the site of origin and mechanism of VT in patients with previous heart attacks, in 1979, Mark and his associate, Dr. Leonard Horowitz, together with surgeon Dr. Alden Harken, devised an operation to excise the area where the tachycardia arose. This operation—often accompanied by aneurysmectomy[1] and

---

[1] A surgical procedure to cut out the weak bulging heart muscle that has arisen from a heart attack. It requires open heart surgery and cardiopulmonary bypass.

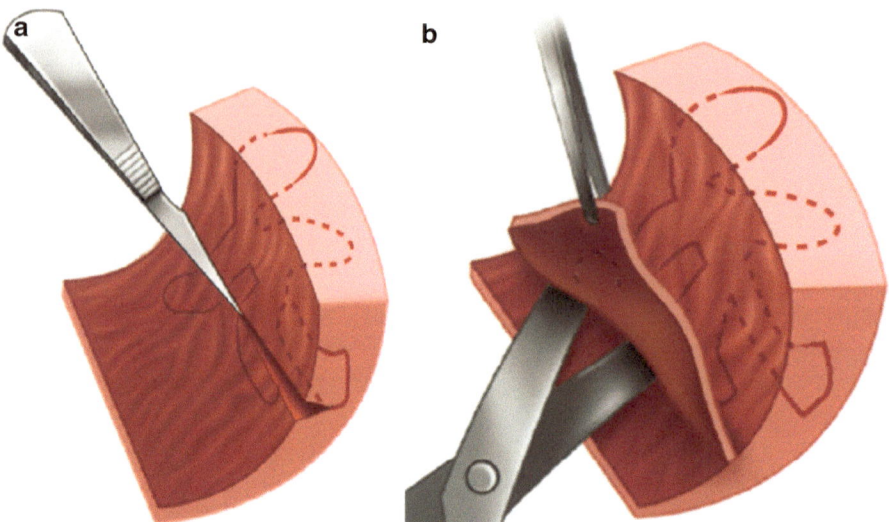

Fig. 13.2 Cartoon of surgical ablation of the VT substrate. Legend: **Panel A** shows the encircling endocardial ventriculotomy. The stippled line shows the reentrant circuit. **Panel B** shows subendocardial resection. The stippled line shows the reentrant circuit (for further explanation, see text)

coronary bypass surgery when necessary—came to be known as "endocardial resection" or, more colorfully, "the Philadelphia peel" (Fig. 13.2b). However, these open heart surgical techniques invented by Dr. Guiraudon in Paris and Drs. Josephson, Horowitz, and Harken in Philadelphia required a dedicated heart surgeon, and it was consequently performed in just a few academic centers in the United States and in Europe. Nonetheless, it was a significant advance in the treatment of this malignant rhythm abnormality.

The Josephson School of electrophysiology, as it is referred to, has left an important legacy in heart rhythm disorders in the United States and abroad. Of interest, and perhaps not surprisingly, the two giants in heart rhythm disorders, Drs. Josephson and Wellens, would ultimately establish a course for young trainees in Europe and the United States that started about 30 years ago and continued until recently. Dr. Mark Josephson passed away on January 11, 2017, at the age of 74 after a long battle with cancer. I met him at a symposium held in New York a couple of months before he passed away, where he was honored by Dr. Vivek Y. Reddy and Mark's past fellows, now cutting-edge experts in the field. He was well aware that the end was near, and we said our goodbyes. His wife had passed away a year or so before, and he was still mourning her. He remembered my wife's passing away more than 20 years ago and commented on our mutual loss.

Evelyn and the Countless Shocks

One of the most challenging patients I encountered in my practice in the mid-1980s was a middle-aged woman, Evelyn, who had a heart attack that destroyed the anterior (front) wall of her heart. She was recuperating rather well, when on the eighth day of her heart attack she unexpectedly collapsed from a rapid VT.

She was promptly transferred to our institution under my care. In our CCU, she again went into the lethal rhythm. We applied an electrical shock to her chest, put a breathing tube down her lungs, placed her on a respirator, and sedated her. We also gave her a host of drugs to prevent the episodes.

Sometimes, she went for a few days without VT, but when I thought she was on the home stretch and was about to pat myself on the back, it recurred. She repeatedly went into this death twister and was shocked with electrical current over 50 times in a 6-week period. We tried all possible medications—to no avail. She was in the CCU for almost 6 weeks. I was desperate. A scan of her heart had shown an aneurysm of the dead tissue of the heart. A coronary angiogram showed blockage of one of the main arteries to the heart; the other arteries were normal.

Finally, I got together with my associate, Dr. Stephen Winters, a most dedicated, highly motivated, and intelligent doctor, a man I was lucky to have as my associate at a critical juncture in my career. We approached our heart surgeon, Dr. Arisan Ergin, and told him that we had to operate.

"She's high-risk," he said. "Her ejection fraction is only 18%. Besides, she is only 6 weeks post a massive heart attack."

"I agree, but do we have a choice?" I said. Finally, Dr. Ergin was convinced, and we scheduled her for the surgery.

It was complex surgery since her infarct was rather recent, and we had to map the activation of the rapid tachycardia in the operating room on her beating heart. To do this, the surgeon had to enter her heart through an incision in the dead muscle and map the activation sequence of the tachycardia before cooling the heart, thus showing us where the tachycardia was coming from. Then we could cut out the culprit area as well as the aneurysm.

I had explained to Evelyn and her family that the mortality was over 10%, but that we had no choice; we had exhausted all possible medications. If the procedure was successful, it could be lifesaving. *Previous studies had shown that such patients have a dismal survival record, with high in-hospital and 1-year mortality rates of 50–80%.*

The next morning, we expectantly waited all gowned as the anesthesiologist, and the cardiothoracic resident went about preparing for surgery.

As soon as we placed Evelyn on the bypass machine and before cooling her heart, we induced VT by stimulating the heart via electrodes on its surface. The surgeon made an incision in the wall of the heart that was thinned from the heart attack and rapidly mapped the activation sequence of the tachycardia with an electrical probe attached to his three fingers held together with a rubber band. We only had a few minutes to accomplish this.

Dr. Winters and I rapidly analyzed the electrical tracings from inside the heart. We concluded that the tachycardia arose in the septal wall between the right and left ventricles. We lowered her body temperature to 25 °C (77 °F.). The heart quivered like a dying jellyfish and then stopped and collapsed like an empty sac.

Ready to cut out the aneurysm and shave the septum, the surgeon asked for the knife. He did it with care so that he wouldn't create a hole in the septum. Then he reinforced the septum with a Dacron patch.

It was now the moment of truth. Dr. Winters and I stared at each other.

The heart looked broken, amputated, the stump sutured together with a Dacron patch.

The surgeon asked the heart-lung machine technologist to warm her up. We waited anxiously for her heart to beat. The heart engorged with blood. A bluish hue appeared on it. The surgeon squeezed the heart several times. "Give her some calcium," he ordered. I requested he inject some epinephrine.

The heart began quivering. The monitor showed ventricular fibrillation. The surgeon took two metal pedals and shocked the heart with electricity.

We all waited in anticipation. Would her heart resume its rhythm? Would it generate a blood pressure? Would she come off the pump? Would she need the support of intra-aortic balloon counter pulsation?[2] These were anxious moments, and we all looked at the monitors and at each other.

"She's in sinus rhythm," I said.

"Let's pace her heart at 110 beats per minute," ordered the surgeon.

"The blood pressure is 110/70," said the anesthesiologist.

"Let's take her off bypass," ordered the surgeon.

"Great, we got this one going," said the surgeon.

"I'm dying for a drink," I said. It was 10 o'clock at night.

We all smiled, relieved! It was our first case of endocardial resection and removal of an aneurysm in a patient after a recent heart attack.

We soon became the prime center in New York for this complex lifesaving procedure in patients with recent heart attacks, 8–60 days prior, and with recurrent, drug-resistant VT. We did a whole lot of these procedures, with a success rate of over 75% and no surgical mortality. A couple of years later, we published our findings in the *Journal of the American College of Cardiology* on a large series of patients.

Evelyn came off the pump without the need of any support, and best of all she was awake in the cardiothoracic ICU the following morning and taken off the respirator. There was no sign of the tachycardia. Not even an extra beat. I was euphoric, but cautious. Eight days later, I took her to the laboratory and tried to induce the tachycardia. To no avail! The procedure was a remarkable success. Her heart function improved to 29% after cutting out the aneurysm. Within a week or so, she was discharged from the hospital.

---

[2] In intra-aortic balloon counter pulsation (IABP), physicians insert a catheter with a balloon mounted on it into the aorta via the femoral artery in the groin. It helps maintain blood pressure and coronary flow.

Fig. 13.3 Cartoon of catheter ablation. Legend: A schematic representation of a slice of the left ventricular muscle showing the catheter for ablation of the substrate of ventricular tachycardia. The solid circles represent the radiofrequency lesions

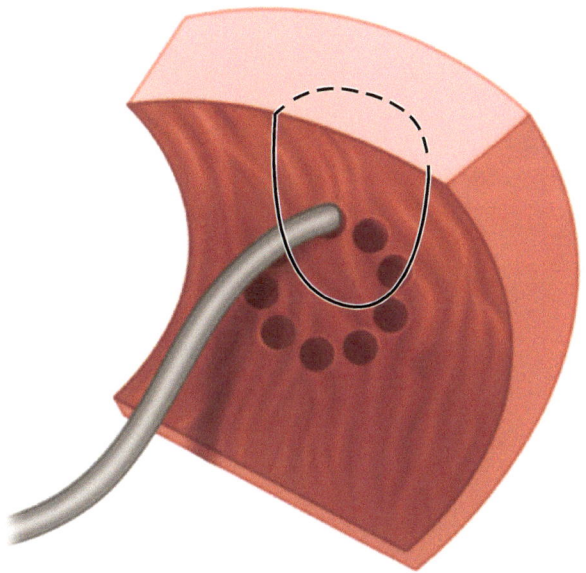

This was a huge accomplishment considering that without surgery she had a high in-hospital and long-term mortality of over 50%. I have never encountered a patient who was shocked externally over 50 times and survived to walk out of the hospital.

In today's day and age with the advent of novel therapies directed at decreasing the size of the heart attack and even preventing the heart muscle from dying with immediate restoration of blood flow ("reperfusion") and stenting, it is uncommon to see patients like Evelyn with recurrent VT either immediately or a couple of weeks after a heart attack. However, patients with remote heart attacks and those with implantable defibrillators will often develop recurrent VT. These patients when recalcitrant to drug treatment are subjected to catheter ablation (Fig. 13.3) which consists of delivering a localized burst of radiofrequency energy that produces a tiny burn about 4–5 mm in diameter. Most patients with scars will need multiple burns. The scars can be extensive and or patchy, and more recently we identify the entire scar by its electrical characteristics and ablate it sequentially. The success rate of VT ablation in patients after remote heart attack is around 70%.

♥

Chapter 14
A Revolutionary Idea: The Implantable Defibrillator: A Lifesaver

> *Political revolutions, the writer Amitav Ghosh writes, often occur in the courtyards of palaces, in spaces on the cusp of power, located neither outside nor inside. Scientific revolutions, in contrast, typically occur in basements, in buried-away places removed from mainstream corridors of thought.*
>
> —Siddhartha Mukherjee, The Emperor of All Maladies

Sometime in 1985, when cardiac electrophysiological studies (EPS) were still in its infancy, I saw Ann, a young woman aged 35 years, who suffered from angina pectoris during delivery of her first baby, caused by an abnormality in one of the main coronary arteries. She underwent bypass surgery but had a massive heart attack during the operation and ended up with a weakened heart muscle and an ejection fraction of 20%. This unfortunate woman was referred to me because her doctors noticed that she'd had runs of non-sustained VT, and a sustained one could result in sudden death. That same year, I had published an original research article in *Circulation*, the official journal of the American Heart Association, showing that induction of a sustained VT in the electrophysiology laboratory in such patients could predict dire future outcome, while non-inducibility would portend a favorable outcome.

I performed an electrophysiological study on her, and by artificially pacing her heart and introducing up to two extra beats, she developed a sustained VT—a rather bad omen. I placed her on the antiarrhythmic drug amiodarone, which had shown to be effective at preventing sustained VT and SCD in an Argentinian study. About 3 months later, she developed a rash, and her primary doctor decided to stop the medication. A month later, after having breakfast, she collapsed suddenly and died.

Around the same time, Jeff, a young lawyer in his early 40s, had fainted while playing tennis on a hot day in Connecticut. There was a doctor on the court who had witnessed the episode and found Jeff pulseless for a couple of minutes. He was

J. A. Gomes, *Rhythms of Broken Hearts*,
https://doi.org/10.1007/978-3-030-77382-3_14

admitted to a local hospital and worked up rather extensively, but the tests all came back normal. Because it was a hot humid day, his doctor dismissed the episode, thinking it was related to dehydration.

At the coaxing of his wife, Jeff sought a second opinion from a Mount Sinai cardiologist, who performed a catheterization to check his coronary arteries. The arteries were normal, but there was some sluggish movement of one of the walls of the heart, what we call in medical jargon *hypokinesis* ("hypo" = less than normal; "kinesis" = movement). Otherwise, his heart function was normal. His cardiologist requested my opinion.

I saw Jeff and requested a signal-averaged ECG, a more detailed high-resolution and revealing kind. I was looking for "late potentials" (micro signals from damaged heart muscle), on which I was researching at the time. I was totally surprised when the test came back positive, implying that he might have had VT secondary to a scar in his heart. I suggested that he undergo an electrophysiologic study. After introducing a couple of extra beats in his heart (as I had done with Ann), to my great surprise and astonishment, and Jeff's as well, he went into a rapid VT. He passed out and I swiftly used electrical shock to get him back. I placed him on the drug procainamide, which was successful in preventing reinduction of the tachycardia.

Jeff had difficulty accepting the diagnosis—that he may have fainted because of a dangerous heart rhythm that could kill. For a young active person like Jeff, it was obviously difficult to accept such a diagnosis. He wanted to run and ski on high slopes, and when I told him to avoid these activities, he became upset and sought other opinions. Almost a year went by and he did not faint again. He asked me whether he could stop the medications, and I gave him an emphatic no.

Apparently, some months later, he enrolled in a gym close to his office in Midtown Manhattan that had no monitoring system and no defibrillator. He had changed his care to another cardiologist, perhaps someone who agreed with him about physical activity, and had stopped seeing me or my associate altogether. A year or so later, I received a call from his wife that he collapsed in the gym while exercising. He was taken by an ambulance to a hospital across town on the West Side but was pronounced dead on arrival.

In the 1980s, we fought VT and cardiac arrest with drugs and other heroic procedures such as coronary artery bypass surgery and resection of the heart muscle known as endocardial resection—the source of the VT. However, we could perform these daring interventions in only a few patients with recent and previous heart attacks, or with aneurysms, and in a limited number of tertiary health centers. This left most patients vulnerable.

I have never forgotten the tragic fate of Ann, a wonderful young woman with a newborn baby and a devoted husband and family. Nor have I forgotten Jeff, who I suspect had myocarditis or heart inflammation due to a viral infection. They were the unlucky ones among many more. If they had presented several years later, they might still be alive, because of an extraordinary man.

From Mordechai Friedman to Michel Mirowski

The war against SCD raged sporadically, but the opposing generals—the heart rhythm experts with their respective armies of drugs—often turned their big "drug guns" on the patient's heart itself and made matters worse in the sense that the drugs themselves had the potential of initiating VT and SCD in the damaged post-infarct heart, what we later came to call: "proarrhythmia." Then a new soldier, Dr. Michel (Mieczyslaw) Mirowski, entered the battlefield. He was no Sir Lancelot, nor a prince in search of the dragon, but a plebeian with a dream.

He was born Mordechai Friedman on October 14, 1924, in Warsaw, Poland, growing up in a middle-class family among the city's Jewish population. The outbreak of World War II changed his life dramatically. When the Nazis invaded Poland in 1939, 15-year-old Mordechai and a friend escaped first to Lvov in the Ukraine and then to Rostov in the Soviet Union, where they intended to join the army and fight the Germans. He had changed his name to Mieczysław Mirowski to obtain a Russian passport, but he was too young to become a soldier in the Soviet army. He fled further by ship and train to Krasnodar and then to Andijan, an agricultural town in Uzbekistan brimming with factories built beyond German reach. There he worked 11 hours a day in an airplane factory, making his first contribution to the war. It was here, 2500 miles from Warsaw, that he successfully volunteered for the army as a Pole and became a junior officer in the support forces.

By the fall of 1945, Mirowski returned to Poland, the only member of his family to survive the war. He began medical school in Gdansk, and after a year, he left to pursue his medical education in Lyon, France, though he knew almost no French or English. It was in Lyon where Dr. Mirowski was first attracted to cardiology, and it was here where he met his wife Anna, who called him Michel, by which he became generally known.

The Inspiration

Upon graduation in 1954, he worked initially in Tel Aviv, Israel, at the Tel HaShomer Hospital under Dr. Henry Heller, professor and chief of Medicine. He admired Professor Heller for his medical acumen but had a rather poor opinion of him as a person. "Heller was smart but very Nietzschean and not personally helpful," he said. "I think he didn't care much about people. He'd fire someone by putting a letter on his desk. I saw him as a stereotype of the German culture of his time." But Heller would turn out to be the inspiration for Mirowski's life's work.

Subsequently, Mirowski pursued further training in Mexico City at the National Institute of Cardiology, spent a couple of years doing a fellowship in Baltimore, and he also worked at the US Cardiopulmonary Laboratory on Staten Island, NY, with Dr. Anthony N. Damato.

In 1963, Mirowski went back to Israel to work as chief of Cardiology in a small community hospital in Assaf Harofeh. And there in Israel, in 1966, Professor Harry Heller began having episodes of VT and died suddenly a few weeks later. It was with Heller's death that the idea of an implantable cardioverter-defibrillator (ICD) was born. He surmised that a small defibrillator embedded in the body, with electrodes connected to the patient's heart, could quickly detect and interrupt ventricular fibrillation before it resulted in death. It would thus save many lives, though it wouldn't prevent ventricular fibrillation from occurring in the first place.

This was a revolutionary idea and a tall task. He soon decided that the best place to develop such a device was the United States. However, the idea of an ICD was vehemently rejected and even ridiculed by the influential pundits and gurus in the halls of academic cardiovascular medicine in the United States and abroad. This attitude is not uncommon in science as well as in the arts—novel and unconventional ideas are often rejected by those dominant in the field.

Development of the Implantable Cardioverter-Defibrillator (ICD)

Dr. Mirowski returned to the United States in 1968 to direct the newly formed coronary care unit at the Sinai Hospital in Baltimore, an affiliate of Johns Hopkins University Hospital. He was given protected time for research, and fortunately for him, the hospital had a division of biomedical engineering and an animal laboratory. There, together with Dr. Morton Mower (Fig. 14.1), a junior cardiologist on staff with extensive animal research experience, he began work on the defibrillator in the basement of the hospital. It is noteworthy that Mower himself had envisioned the possibility of an internal defibrillator but considered it unfeasible. Undoubtedly, Mower was thrilled to find out that two people of entirely different backgrounds would think alike.

Fig. 14.1 Dr. Michel Mirowski (R) with Dr. Morton Mover (L). (Reprinted with permission from John A. Kastor: Michel Mirowski and the automatic implantable defibrillator. *The American Journal of Cardiology*, 1989; 63 (15): 1121–1126)

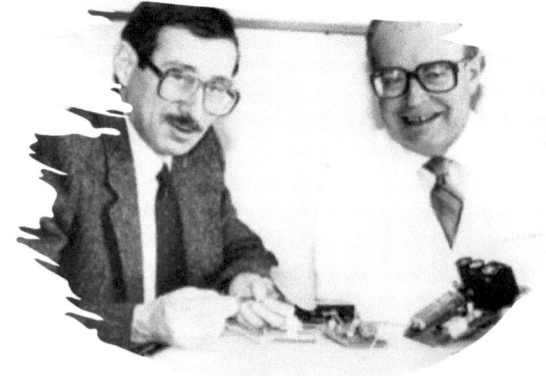

After many rejections, in 1970, they published the scientific manuscript in a medical journal describing their initial work. But considerable antagonism remained in the cardiology community toward the concept, and it made securing funds hard. Furthermore, a scathing editorial appeared in 1972 in *Circulation*, written by the co-inventor of the external DC defibrillator, Dr. Bernard Lown, then considered the ultimate guru of SCD. Mirowski was unbowed, perhaps because he had overcome worse opposition. "I was always slightly outside the mainstream of academic medicine," he once said. "There are those who are accepted, whose futures are planned, whose promise is appreciated. But that's not me. Nobody nursed me along."

The skepticism of the concept kept other doctors in academia and the device industry uninterested. There was hardly any competition in the United States or abroad, except for John Schuder, an electrical engineer at the University of Missouri in Columbia. He also began work on an implantable defibrillator and was the first to implant a cardiac defibrillator in a dog in January 1970. For unknown reasons, he subsequently abandoned the project concentrating on optimization of shocking waveforms.

In 1972, at a conference in Singapore, a mutual friend introduced Mirowski to Dr. Stephen Heilman. He was a physician and engineer who had formed a small medical equipment company called Medrad Inc. Heilman met Mirowski for dinner and immediately grasped the possibilities of the ICD. He then placed the company's engineers at Mirowski and Mower's disposal.

As a spin-off from Medrad, in 1975, Intec Systems developed the world's first ICD prototype, small enough to be completely implanted in a dog. A series of 25 long-term dog experiments proved the viability of the device. A film of the first successful defibrillation of a dog implanted with the device was shown; however, many in scientific community remained skeptical. As sociologist Robert Nisbet once said, "In science, ideology tends to corrupt; absolute ideology, absolutely."

In the late 1970s, when I was a young fellow in electrophysiology training, I attended a presentation by Dr. Mirowski. He showed a short movie of a dog experiment in which a coronary artery was occluded, and the dog went into ventricular fibrillation, seized, and began agonal breathing, with slow near-death respiration. But the dog had an ICD implanted in its abdominal wall and connected to its heart. The device sensed the lethal rhythm and delivered a shock terminating it. The dog woke up but in the process had a bowel movement, which was shown on the film. The audience burst out in laughter, and many then walked out of the hall, signaling that the idea would amount to nothing but…

Dr. Mirowski and the group at Intec Inc. further refined the prototype to make it suitable for human implantation and eventually received approval from the FDA for clinical trials.

The first patient to have the ICD was a 57-year-old woman who had flown from California for the procedure. She had a previous heart attack and recurrent loss of consciousness with documented ventricular fibrillation. She was prepared for surgery on February 4, 1980, at Johns Hopkins University Hospital in Baltimore. Dr. Levi Watkins was the heart surgeon and Dr. Philip Reed the cardiac electrophysiologist. Initially, events didn't go smoothly in the operating room. When the surgeon requested the device, the circulating nurse accidentally dropped it on the floor. The ICD was damaged and unusable. Luckily, a spare one was available on standby.

The first defibrillator model was a success. However, it weighed 225 grams or half a pound, required a thoracotomy (surgical incision into the chest) to expose the heart, and could only do defibrillation (Fig. 14.2a). In the years that followed, a host of advances took place, including the development of synchronized cardioversion[1] for ventricular tachycardia. In the late 1980s, medical device companies developed a model using catheters, so that physicians could implant the defibrillator without cracking the chest (Fig. 14.3). This was indeed Mirowski's original vision.

I invited Dr. Mirowski to speak at our Grand Rounds in Cardiology around this time. He was very grateful for the invitation, particularly since Dr. Lown's editorial had appeared when Dr. Charles Friedberg, chief of Cardiology at the Mount Sinai Hospital, was its chief editor. Reminiscing the past opposition to his vision, Mirowski was simply elated to deliver his lecture at our institution.

The ICD changed the outlook of survivors of cardiac arrest. Although Mirowski was strongly convinced that the defibrillator saved lives, cardiovascular societies and the Centers for Medicare & Medicaid Services requested prospective, multicenter randomized trials.

Then the landslide of evidence began.

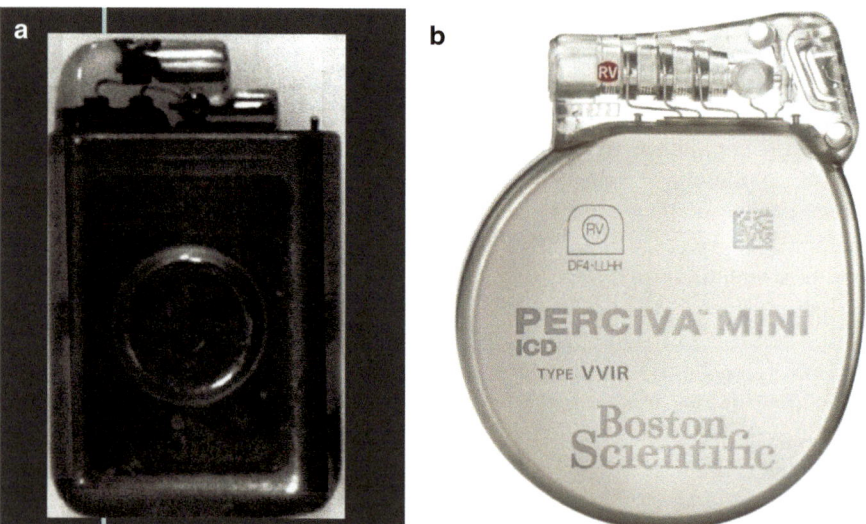

Fig. 14.2 The original ICD (left) and the current ICD (right). Legend: The original (left) and the current (right) ICD. (Courtesy of Boston Scientific Inc.)

---

[1]An electrical shock, synchronized to the QRS complex of the ECG, to restore the heart to normal rhythm

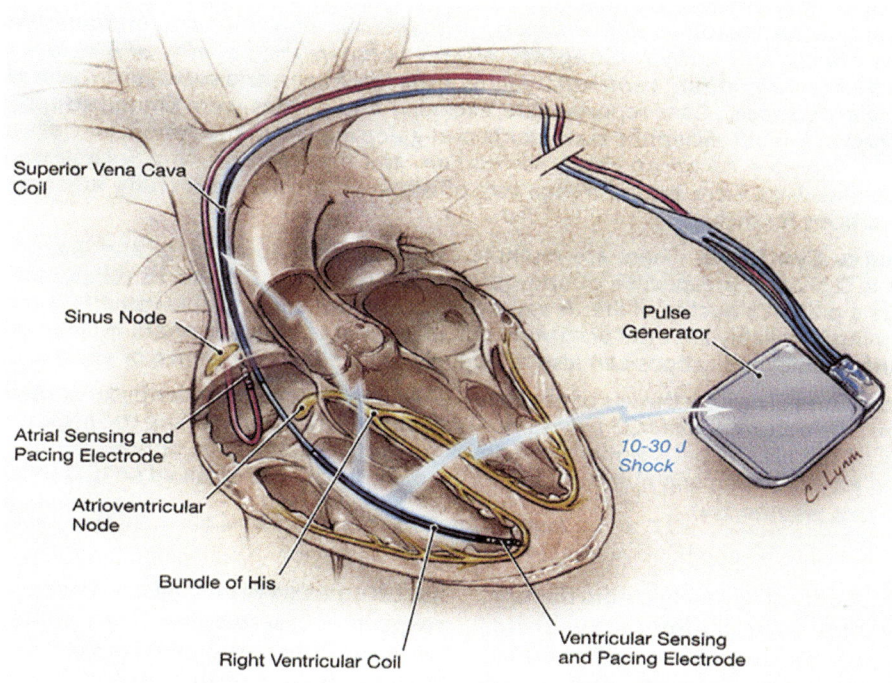

Fig. 14.3 The transvenous ICD system. Legend: The implantable cardioverter-defibrillator (ICD) showing leads in the right ventricle and right atrium attached to the pulse generator and the shock being delivered between the can and the RV lead. (Reprinted with permission from Gehi AK, Mehta D, Gomes JA: Evaluation and Management of patients after Implantable Cardioverter-Defibrillator Shock, *JAMA*, 2006; 296:1839–2847)

As useful as the ICD is for patients who had already suffered SCD, it could save far more lives by terminating an attack should one occur in the future in people at risk. We call this tactic "primary prevention," as opposed to "secondary prevention" of post-SCD patients. Hence, several trials of primary prevention also took place and showed that the ICD saves lives. They provided the scientific basis for guidelines for defibrillator therapy sponsored by the Heart Rhythm Society, the American Heart Association, the American College of Cardiology, and the European Society of Cardiology. These organizations recommended the ICD as class I indication for patients at high risk for SCD. In medicine, an "indication" means there is a valid reason to use a strategy, and "class I" is the top level, the green light for physicians to implant the device.

Modern devices are much smaller than Dr. Mirowski's half-pound prototype. The newest models weigh as little as 90 grams or 3 ounces and are less than a centimeter thick (Fig. 14.2b).

Recently, a "subcutaneous defibrillator" with no parts inside the heart or blood vessels was developed and is currently in use. Its single lead lies inside the skin next to the breastbone—completely outside the chest cavity. It is ideal for young survivors of SCD and high-risk patients who have diseases of their ion channels.[2]

Today, the ICD is used worldwide, and in the United States alone, there are approximately 120,000 implanted every year at a cost of around 5 billion dollars. Over 70% of these implants are for the primary prevention of SCD.

Dr. Mirowski lived to see the fruits of his labor, but not long enough. He died of multiple myeloma at age 66 in 1990, before the large-scale trials. His greatest legacy was the attention he drew to SCD and the invention of the ICD—a lifesaver, a gift bestowed despite years of ridicule, an idea realized through vision, will, and technological and engineering prowess. Recently, I learned that he had a few aphorisms that guided his life work. The two that I found most appropriate were the following: (1) *The bumps in the road are not bumps. They are the road.* (2) *Do not give up, do not give in, and beat the bastards.* The latter obviously reflects his scorn for those who ridiculed his vision.

The ICD probably could have saved Ann and Jeff. It has been chipping away slowly at the dominion of the Prince of Darkness, enabling patients to have longer, more productive lives. However, patients with poor heart function ultimately do succumb and die of heart failure.

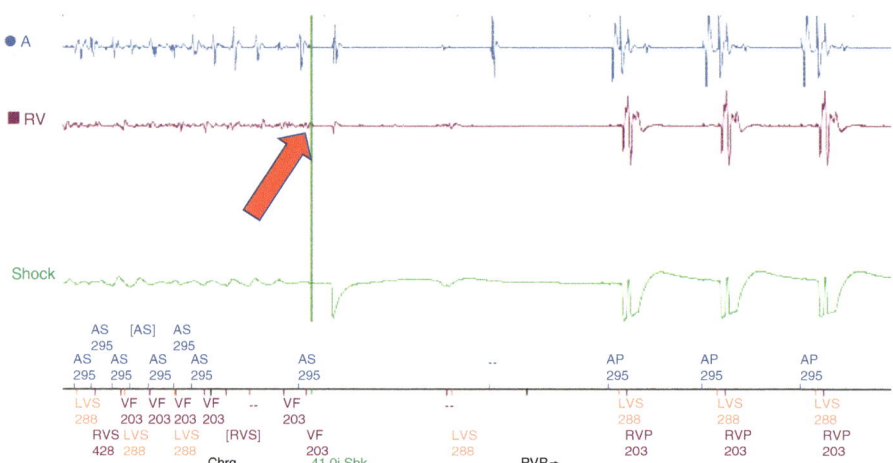

Fig. 14.4 Ventricular fibrillation terminated by an ICD shock. Legend: From top to bottom—electrograms from the atrial (A, blue) lead, right ventricular (V lead, red), shock lead (green), and timelines AS and VF showing rate. Note that the RV and shock leads show tiny wiggles denoting VF. Note that an ICD shock (red arrow) terminates VF, and clear A and V electrograms appear in sinus rhythm. (Courtesy of Boston Scientific Inc.)

---

[2]Called "channelopathies," these ailments may be congenital or may result from an autoimmune attack on the ion channels. In addition to heart impairments, they have been implicated in epilepsy, diabetes, migraine, irritable bowel syndrome, cancer, and other diseases.

Although the ICD is a lifesaver (Fig. 14.4), its use should not be taken lightly, particularly for primary prevention of SCD. From long-term follow-up studies, we have come to recognize a host of problems associated with it, including failure and recall of leads, risk of infection, and *inappropriate shocks* for atrial fibrillation that are psychologically devastating, degrading the quality of life and increasing overall cardiac mortality.

Yet its benefits have been as plain as the sun in the sky.

The Boy from Colombia

José was a 12-year-old Colombian boy who had a blackout spell while playing soccer for his school team in Bogotá, Colombia. A year or so later, he presumably suffered a cardiac arrest and was lucky to have survived. He turned out to have hypertrophic cardiomyopathy, a marked thickening of the heart muscle which can block blood flow, weaken valves, and shrink chamber size. We did not know then that this disease is due to a genetic abnormality in the actin-myosin protein element of the heart. (Actin forms thin, lighter filaments of the heart muscle and myosin thicker, darker ones.) In some of these patients, also possibly for genetic reasons, there is a high incidence of SCD. As a matter of fact, hypertrophic cardiomyopathy is the commonest cause of sudden death in young athletes like that of college basketball star Hank Gathers.

José's doctor in Colombia told his mother about the ICD. He also said the device was very expensive and was available only in the United States. His mother contacted the National Institutes of Health in Bethesda, Maryland. They confirmed the diagnosis, but since they did not implant the device themselves, they gave his mother a few names of the institutions in the United States where the device was implanted at the time. She contacted us.

I met with this young boy and his mother the day after they arrived in New York from Bogotá. They were staying with Colombian immigrant contacts in the city. I was impressed with the young boy's appearance and his mother's total dedication. "He is my only son," she said. "Doctor, please, you have to save his life." And she began crying. I reassured her that I would do my best.

We knew very little in those days about his condition and its relationship to SCD. Besides, there were no records available to show that he actually had ventricular fibrillation. I decided to do an electrophysiologic stimulation study but was concerned about a tragic outcome. What if he went into ventricular fibrillation on the table and I could not get him out of it? In those days, there was very little information if any in the literature about this entity. The next few days I agonized about this young boy and developed stress-related gastroesophageal reflux. I spoke to his mother, explaining the procedure in some detail, as well as the potential complications including the possibility of death. I could see in her face the trust she had placed in me. And trust heightens the responsibility. I had a lengthy discussion with Dr. Manuel Estioko, our cardiothoracic implant surgeon, requesting him to stand by with the pump team ready for any untoward eventuality. This cautious action helped to calm my nerves.

On the day of the procedure as I traveled from Staten Island to Manhattan, I went over the entire procedure in my own mind, a habit I had acquired during my car commute of an hour or more. We stimulated this young boy's heart, and not surprisingly, he went into ventricular tachycardia that lasted for about 40 seconds, and right before we were about to shock him out of it, the tachycardia stopped on its own.

"He needs a defibrillator." I said to the surgeon.

But saying was one thing and executing was another. The family had neither insurance nor money to pay for the device. But Mount Sinai Medical Center agreed to waive the payments, and so did I and Dr. Estioko, our surgeon. We did such things in those days. We had a mission and certainly the mission of a doctor, and a medical institution is to attend to the needy. Today, however, I'm sad to say that this would likely be impossible.

But what about the cost of the implantable defibrillator? The price was exorbitant. We spoke to our representative from Cardiac Pacemakers, Incorporated, the only company that made the device in those days. He called his headquarters. They agreed to donate the device for free.

The day of the procedure was set. Implanting a defibrillator in those days was not a simple matter as it is today. We had to crack the chest, suture the sensing leads and the defibrillation patches to the surface of the heart, and place the pulse generator in the abdominal wall after tunneling the electrical connections. Rather disconcerting and alarming was the fact that we then had to test the device. We had to induce the terminal rhythm, ventricular fibrillation, several times to gauge what is referred to as the "defibrillation threshold," the minimum energy needed to defibrillate the heart in this young boy.[3] What if the defibrillation threshold was high and we could not get him out of the terminal rhythm? I spent sleepless nights thinking of this very possibility. However, I showed no signs of panic either to the surgeon or to my associate Dr. Winters. In my own mind, I had to go ahead if I wanted to save this young boy's life. The responsibility was enormous.

The procedure went well. He was the youngest person to have the ICD in the United States at the time. I felt relieved and gratified.

He came back two more times from Colombia to have a new device once the battery was depleted, and Dr. Jorge Camuñas, our pacemaker and defibrillator surgeon, performed the procedure both times. Subsequently, our young friend graduated from college and began working for the same device company, now Boston Scientific, after it opened offices in South America and the implantable defibrillator went global.

---

[3] After the defibrillation threshold (DF) was determined, we would set the energy level for the first shock at 10 joules above the DF.

At the time of this writing, José is 38 years old. It seems that for him, everything fell into its rightful place.

Kathy's Blackout Spell

Kathy was 23 when I first saw her. She suffered from anorexia and was treated with the drug Adderall. She had lived a fast-paced life and had tried cocaine and ephedra and used laxatives for bulimia. But all seemed well until she was admitted to a hospital for pneumonia. After treatment with antibiotics, she was discharged. She was readmitted to the hospital because of a blackout spell while eating breakfast and lost control of her urine. She was transferred to our CCU for further workup and management.

Her heart monitor showed frequent extra beats, the VPCs, and the echo of the heart showed that her heart function was a dismal 17%. Because she urinated during the blackout spell, a seizure disorder was considered, but the electroencephalogram (EEG) was negative. I felt that she had a cardiomyopathy and that she had blacked out because of a self-terminating rapid VT. The side effects of Adderall were entertained and could not be excluded. Several of the doctors who saw her in the hospital argued that she might be suffering from a viral infection of her heart and that she could recover completely.

And so, the million-dollar question at the time was whether she should receive an ICD. The guidelines recommended waiting 9 months to see whether the patient would recover. But Kathy had fainted. Some of the physicians argued that her fainting episode was due to volume depletion rather than VT because she was anorexic and rather abusive of laxatives. All this was possible. But if she had another blackout from a VT, it could be her last.

I took a contrary stance and recommended that she get an ICD. Given my experience in the field, the other doctors deferred to my judgment. When I told Kathy that she needed minor surgery for a defibrillator, she was devastated. Her despair was palpable in her downcast expression. She asked no questions about her heart condition, its treatment, or its prognosis. She wanted to know when she could go home.

"The day after you have the defibrillator," I said, as I placed my hand on her shoulder.

She began to sob. Her heart skipped a beat, and then it skipped another and another, and the bedside alarm went off. I could see panic settling in. Her face contorted as if in intense pain, as her eyes moved rapidly from side to side. I called the nurse for a sedative and sat beside her. After she had calmed down, I reassured her that the defibrillator would be there to protect her if things went wrong.

"What about the lump from the defibrillator? The bulge would show, wouldn't it?" she asked.

I promised her that I would insert it deep under the muscle and would ask a plastic surgeon to assist in suturing the skin. I visited her later that evening and found her calmer and receptive. But when I went home and to bed, doubts crossed my mind. Was I doing the right thing by implanting a defibrillator in this young woman for a mere faint? Should I have waited a few months? I rapidly dismissed the thoughts. It would be worse if she had a cardiac arrest and died. Three weeks later, I received a call from her.

"Doc," she said. "I had a shock in my sleep. It was like a bomb explosion in my chest. It not only woke me up. It propped me up." I asked her to come to the hospital right away. My nurse, Elena Pe, and I interrogated the device. She had had a rapid VT that degenerated into ventricular fibrillation. The defibrillator had shocked her out of the lethal rhythm. Without it, she would have been found dead in bed.

As I write, it is over 8 years since she had the ICD. She has moved away to California where she works. Her heart function has shown considerable improvement and is near normal. I called her recently to find out how she was doing. She told me that her illness had devastated her in the beginning.

"I pushed my boyfriend away. I was upset and angry with myself and the world. Why me? But gradually and over time, I coped and adjusted and went on living," she said. "I have a boyfriend now, and my mum is here with me. I don't pray to a God. But I'm spiritual. Without the ICD, I wouldn't be here."

Friedrich Nietzsche said, "Some die too young, some die too old; the precept sounds strange, but die at the right age." This philosophical rumination is easier said! Dying is usually not our decision to make. More often than not, we are at the mercy of our genes and the environment we grow in. At other times, we can acquire illnesses, bacteria, and viruses we know not from where, and then some are lucky to have met the right doctors who made the right decisions for them.

♥

Chapter 15
To Freeze and Not to Fry

*The same water that will kill you, drown you, give you
hypothermia is the same water that will help you survive.*

—Joe Teti

Ajay, meaning unconquerable, invincible, and lovable person, was a 78-year-old engineer who came to the United States from India more than 30 years ago. He worked for the City of New York, Department of Environmental Protection. While returning home from work, after he got off the subway, he collapsed on Church Street in Manhattan and was in full-blown cardiac arrest for about 4 minutes before paramedics shocked him with an automatic external defibrillator.

They took Ajay to a downtown hospital where he lay in a coma with dilated pupils. The physician called his son, who was an infectious diseases doctor, and related the dire prognosis. The son apparently called the family's Hindu priest and discussed a cremation ceremony. He also called his brother-in-law Dr. Umesh Gidwani, the director of the CCU at Mount Sinai Hospital, who arranged an immediate transfer to our institution.

Ajay was placed on a hypothermic protocol with an Arctic Sun medical device that lowers temperature by circulating chilled water in pads next to the skin and transferred him over to us.

In our CCU, Ajay was unresponsive and comatose. He was continued on the Arctic Sun machine to maintain a temperature of 33 °C (91.4 °F) for 24 hours, after which he was gradually rewarmed over a 12-hour period. He awoke and began following simple commands. He underwent a heart catheterization which showed that all but one of the coronary bypass grafts he had in 1992 after a heart attack was still open. In 2 days, his heart function improved to near normal, and an MRI showed that he had previous heart attacks. Since Ajay had sustained cardiac arrest, my colleague Dr. Marc Miller implanted an ICD.

As I write, Ajay is 82 years old and fully functional. When I spoke to him, he excitedly told me his story, a story of survival right from his childhood years and his

© The Author(s), under exclusive license to Springer Nature
Switzerland AG 2021
J. A. Gomes, *Rhythms of Broken Hearts*,
https://doi.org/10.1007/978-3-030-77382-3_15

recent cardiac arrest. He was very proud that he is one of the oldest individuals to have come out of a coma with intact mental function.

We've known about the intriguing effects of lowering the body temperature (hypothermia) in medicine for a long time. The Edwin Smith Papyrus, from around 1600 BCE in ancient Egypt, described its use in traumatic brain injuries, and by the fifth and fourth centuries BCE, the Greeks were cooling whole bodies when treating tetanus. By 1803, the Russians were covering people with snow as they tried to resuscitate them. In 1812, Napoleon's surgeon-general Baron Dominique-Jean Larrey (1766–1842), who struggled back with the French army on its catastrophic retreat from Russia, found to his surprise that soldiers with frozen hands who stayed away from the campfire were more likely to survive than those who huddled close to a campfire and rewarmed.

On September 28, 1957, a 38-year-old man arrived in the ER of Johns Hopkins University Hospital. He had been stabbed in the chest and he was unconscious and breathing, but he had no pulse. Two minutes after admission, he stopped breathing. Doctors G. Rainey Williams, Jr. and Frank Spencer cracked his chest and found the heart in total arrest. They massaged the heart and quickly restored its rhythm. Then they sewed the chest wall together and closed him up. The procedure had taken 5 minutes. But he remained unconscious. They at once cooled him to 32–33 °C (89–91 °F) After 20 hours, he was able to respond to voice, and after 48 hours, he was completely alert. He showed no signs of brain damage, and there were no abnormalities a month after his release. Williams and Spencer reported these results and similar ones on three other patients in 1958. The value of hypothermia after cardiac arrest lay in reducing brain swelling, they felt and noted: "Similar patients treated without hypothermia have rarely survived."

Despite these findings, hypothermia did not gain general traction.

In 1964, Dr. Peter J. Safar (1924–2003), the father of CPR and the mind behind acute critical care medicine, recommended hypothermia as a key step in his influential ABCs of resuscitation (airway, breathing, circulation). However, in the 1960s, we still knew too little about it, and excesses began to cause complications and deaths in patients. Doctors grew wary and the technique fell out of favor for decades.

Meanwhile, the press occasionally reported startling cases. For instance, in May 1999, a 29-year-old Swedish radiologist named Dr. Anna Bågenholm was skiing when she slipped, slid downhill, and went headfirst into an icy stream. Her two friends called for help on their mobiles and tried to pull her out, but her gear grew wet and heavy, and the swollen spring current pulled her further under a 7-inch layer of ice. She became trapped between rocks, face up to the ice. She had found a pocket of air, but her body temperature was plunging. After 40 minutes, she suffered cardiac arrest and ceased moving. After an hour and 20 minutes, she was pulled out, finally. By one report, she was frozen solid.

A helicopter airlifted her to a hospital, and she arrived 2.5 hours after she'd fallen in, by which time her brain and core body temperature was 13.7 °C (56.7 °F)— lower than any temperature ever recorded in a living person. *If at all she was living.*

Her ECG was a flat line. "She has completely dilated pupils. She is ashen, flaxen white. She's wet. She's ice cold when I touch her skin, and she looks absolutely dead," the head of the emergency medical department said.

But doctors didn't give up. They connected her to a bypass machine and slowly began removing her blood, rewarming it, and pumping it back in. Some 4 hours after the accident, her heart began pumping on its own. Twelve days later, she opened her eyes. Rehabilitation took 6 years, but Ms. Bågenholm completely recovered and took a job at the hospital that saved her life.

This extraordinary incident was widely reported in the press and described in the British medical journal *The Lancet*, which recommended that physicians pay more attention to therapeutic hypothermia, and it may have helped change minds.

The pendulum finally swung in favor of hypothermia for preservation of brain function. In 2002, two large studies in Europe and Australia compared mild hypothermia (32–34 °C, 89–93 °F) to normal temperature in comatose survivors of cardiac arrest. The findings, which appeared in *The New England Journal of Medicine*, showed that the hypothermic group had better neurological function and possibly improved survival.

Progress followed. In 2003, the Advanced Life Support Task Force of the International Liaison Committee on Resuscitation recommended that unconscious patients who recover circulation after out-of-hospital cardiac arrest should be cooled to 32–34 °C (89–93 °F) for 12–24 hours. In 2005, the American Heart Association confirmed that hypothermia improves outcomes after cardiac arrest and recommended its use in these patients.

However, by 2007, only 225 of the 5700 total hospitals in the United States had machines for hypothermia induction. The July 23, 2007, issue of *Newsweek* in its cover featured a man in his swimming pool with a caption that read: "This Man Was Dead. He Isn't Anymore. How Science Is Bringing More Heart-Attack Victims Back to Life." After 2008, the number of hospitals using hypothermia rose sharply, so that today most ambulances carry equipment to start hypothermia right at the site of resuscitation.

International resuscitation guidelines now recommend therapeutic hypothermia, and its use has been extended to in-hospital cardiac arrest, including cardiac arrest from abnormal heart rhythms.

Today, most institutions follow a standardized treatment in unconscious patients, which consists of (1) rapidly bringing the temperature to 32–34 °C by surface and core cooling; (2) maintenance of hypothermia at goal temperature of 33 °C for 12–24 hours, with suppression of shivering; and (3) rewarming. This is the critical stage. The goal is to reach normal body temperature over 12–24 hours and to stop all sedation when normal body temperature is achieved.

♥

Chapter 16
Of Scintillating Lights, Tunnels, and Astral Encounters

I am incapable of conceiving infinity, and yet I do not accept
finity. I want this adventure that is the context of my life to
go on without end.

—Simone de Beauvoir.

I depart as air—I shake my white locks at the runaway sun,
I effuse my flesh in eddies, and drift it in lacy jags. I
bequeath myself to the dirt to grow from the grass I love.

—Walt Whitman

As previously narrated, some of my patients who survived an episode of cardiac arrest volunteered information seeing their long-gone ancestors, perceiving detachment from their own bodies, passing through a tunnel into another universe of scintillating lights, and subsequently being pulled back into their bodies as a result of successful resuscitation. These vivid, yet unusual and baffling perceptions have been more widely recognized since the 1970s, when physician and psychologist Raymond Moody published his book, *Life after Life—a study of subjects with near-death experiences* (NDEs).

The concept of afterlife goes far back to the ancient Egyptians and Mesopotamians. But the first description of NDEs is by Plato as far back as the fourth century BC, who wrote in his famed treatise the Republic, the "Myth of Er," where he relates the story of a soldier named Er who died on the battlefield and awoke on the funeral pyre to relate his sojourn in the afterlife. In the early sixteenth century, famous Dutch painter Hieronymus Bosch (1450–1516) executed a painting entitled *Ascent of the Blessed* (Fig. 16.1) that hangs in the Doge's palace in Venice. In the painting, he depicts souls ascending through a tunnel toward a shining light, akin to the description of NDEs. Whether this rendering reflects artistic imagination or insight into some experience remains unknown. In the nineteenth century, the accounts of the survivors of a Swiss mountaineering accident and the 1976 account of survivors of the Tangshan earthquake further confirm the occurrence of NDEs.

© The Author(s), under exclusive license to Springer Nature
Switzerland AG 2021
J. A. Gomes, *Rhythms of Broken Hearts*,
https://doi.org/10.1007/978-3-030-77382-3_16

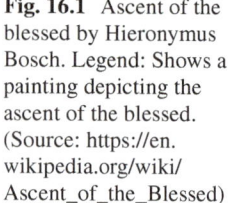

Fig. 16.1 Ascent of the blessed by Hieronymus Bosch. Legend: Shows a painting depicting the ascent of the blessed. (Source: https://en.wikipedia.org/wiki/Ascent_of_the_Blessed)

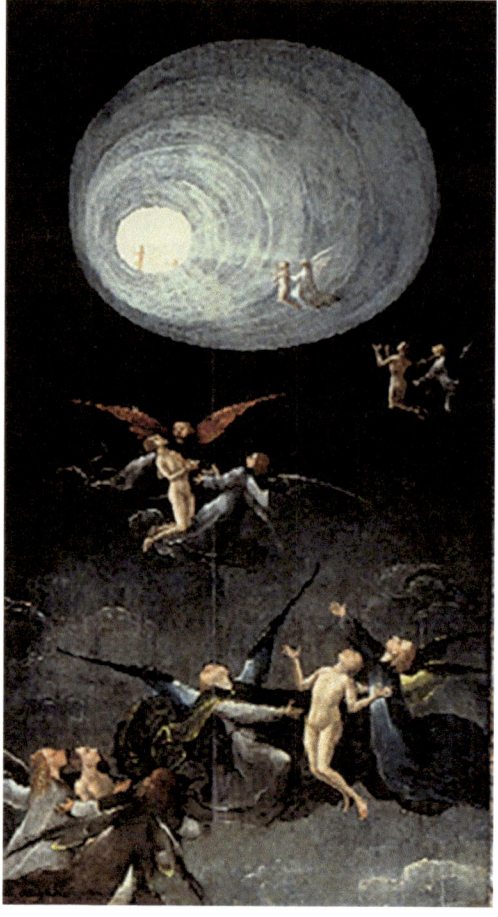

Retrospective analysis (looking back) in the 1970s reported a high incidence of NDEs particularly in children and young adults; however, more recent prospective studies that involved a standardized questionnaire of survivors found an incidence of 9–23%. In one study, of 42 patients undergoing electrophysiologic studies, 14% reported NDEs during induced hemodynamically unstable ventricular arrhythmia. However, another study failed to elicit NDEs in induced cardiac arrest during testing of internal defibrillators. This negative study might be related to a very brief duration of the induced cardiac arrest, the amnestic effects of pre-procedure sedatives, and the preoperative reassurances of no risk of dying from the procedure. The post-1970 literature abounds with several anecdotal, yet fascinating cases of NDEs. One captivating case that Greyson mentions is of a 55-year-old man who was admitted to a hospital with irregular heartbeats. During diagnostic angiography, he suffered a coronary occlusion and had to undergo emergency quadruple bypass surgery. Following the surgery, he reported having had an out-of-body experience. He was able to observe the operating room from above, accurately describing the behavior of the heart surgeon during the operation. He also described following a brilliant light through a tunnel to a region of warmth, love, and peace. Here, he encountered his dead relatives, who communicated to him that he should return back to his body.

In a prospective study done in the Netherlands and published by Pim van Lommel, in the British medical journal *Lancet*, a nurse caring for a patient describes a most intriguing case. "During a night shift, an ambulance brings in a 44-year-old cyanotic, comatose man into the coronary care unit. He had been found about an hour before in a meadow by (a) passers-by. After admission, he receives artificial respiration without intubation, while heart massage and defibrillation are also applied. When we went to intubate the patient, he turns out to have dentures in his mouth. I remove these upper dentures and put them onto the 'crash car' (cart). Meanwhile, we continue extensive CPR. After about an hour and a half the patient has sufficient heart rhythm and blood pressure, but he is still ventilated and intubated, and he is still comatose. He is transferred to the intensive care unit to continue the necessary artificial respiration. Only after more than a week do I meet again with the patient, who is by now back on the cardiac ward. I distribute his medication. The moment he sees me he says: 'Oh, that nurse knows where my dentures are'. I am very surprised. Then he elucidates: 'Yes, you were there when I was brought into hospital and you took my dentures out of my mouth and put them onto that car (cart), it had all these bottles on it and there was this sliding drawer underneath and there you put my teeth.' I was especially amazed because I remembered this happening while the man was in deep coma and in the process of CPR. When I asked further, it appeared the man had seen himself lying in bed, that he had perceived from above how nurses and doctors had been busy with CPR. He was also able to describe correctly and in detail the small room in which he had been resuscitated as well as the appearance of those present like myself. At the time that he observed the situation he had been very much afraid that we would stop CPR and that he would die. And it is true that we had been very negative about the patient's prognosis due to his very poor medical condition when admitted. The patient tells me that he desperately and unsuccessfully tried to make it clear to us that he was still alive and that we should continue CPR. He is deeply impressed by his experience and says he is no longer afraid of death. Four weeks later he left (the) hospital as a healthy man."

An international prospective study, AWARE (AWAreness during Resuscitation) reported by Parnia and coworkers in 2014, accessed the presence of NDEs in a total of 140 survivors of cardiac arrest, by using an interview system. In their study, 46% had memories with major cognitive themes that included fear, bright light, violence, deja vu, family, and recalling events, while 9% had NDEs, and 2% described awareness of seeing and hearing actual events during the resuscitation process. Several studies have now established that NDEs occur more often in young people, but it remains unclear whether the perceptions occur just before or during loss of consciousness. Of interest, a Dutch prospective study showed that those who had NDEs had an increase in the belief in an afterlife and a decrease in the fear of death during long-term follow-up in contrast to those who did not experience NDEs.

Obviously, we do not have clear scientific explanations for these perceptions. Parnia and coworkers argue that in their patients, perceptions were not hallucinatory or illusory since the recollections corresponded to actual verified events. Whether these perceptions occur from activity at some cortical level due to secretion of neurohormones remains unclear. On the other hand, whether they reflect the detachment of the living "soul" or "energy" from the body is tempting to consider but remains speculative as well.

Is There a Biological Explanation for NDEs?

Recent elegant studies by Dr. Benjamin Scherlag in a unicellular organism *Stentor coeruleus* revealed some fascinating observations. When the dwarf cells were placed in a toxic environment, they showed evidence of cell death. What was totally unexpected was the finding that within minutes, a morphological replicate of the cell separated (Fig. 16.2) and subsequently faded. They speculated on the possibility that the replicates of the dead or dying *Stentor coeruleus* cells represent an out-of-body experience—a persistence of life at a cellular level. It is noteworthy that the origin of the replicate did not arise from a protrusion of the cell membrane but as a transparent cell image unattached to the physical cell. Similar observations have been reported by Sun and Montell. Scherlag and his team went even further. They applied a magnetic field, and over the course of 20 minutes, the ghost-like replicates appeared to progressively retract back into the moribund *Stentor coeruleus* cells. Over a period of 24–48 hours, the cells showed mobility. This cellular restoration has been called "anastasis" which comes from the Greek word meaning "rising to life."

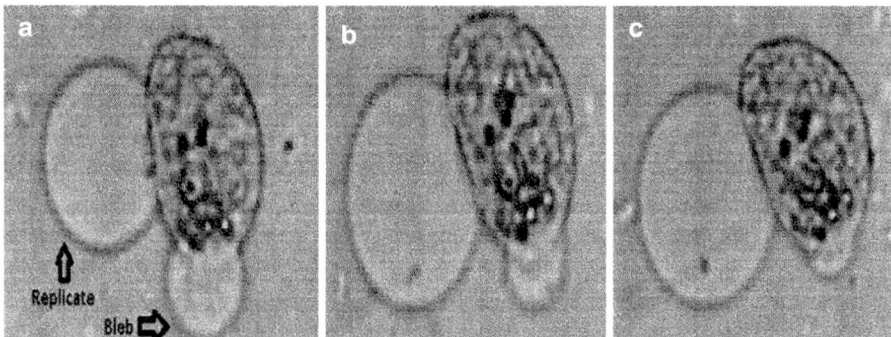

Fig. 16.2 *Stentor coeruleus* showing cell death and the appearance of a morphological replicate. Legend: Simultaneous development of Bleb and replicate from A to C, with retraction of the Bleb, but continuation of the replicate. For further explanation, see text. (Courtesy of Dr. Benjamin Scherlag)

One important question that is difficult to explain is how these vivid perceptions can occur during cardiac arrest when both circulation and brain activity cease.

Electroencephalographic (EEG) studies that register brain activity have been recorded during blackout spells (vasovagal syncope) induced by head-up tilt testing, where the bed is held at a 70- or 80-degree angle for 20–30 minutes. In one study reported by Dr. Fabrizio Ammirati and coworkers, 27 out of 63 patients blacked out during the test. The 16 patients who lost consciousness due to a fall in blood pressure demonstrated a slowing of EEG activity at onset of the spells. In the 11 patients who blacked out because of temporary cessation of heart rhythm (asystole), a similar slowing pattern in the theta range occurred at the onset, *followed by a sudden disappearance of brain wave activity*. That is, a flat EEG and its duration were between 1 and 46 seconds. The EEG normalized immediately after recovery. This study obviously proves that loss of consciousness due to heart stoppage even over a short time span is accompanied by loss of brain activity.

Drs. Jonathan Moss and Mark Rockoff reported on a 62-year-old woman who had simultaneous EEG and ECG during emergent carotid artery surgery. While the surgeon was closing the incision, the patient developed cardiac arrest. There was loss of EEG activity within 15 seconds of heart stoppage, and it returned almost instantly after resuscitation. In animal models of cardiac arrest produced by rapid injection of potassium chloride or ventricular fibrillation (the rhythm usually associated with cardiac arrest), a flat EEG occurred within 25 seconds of cardiac standstill.

Sabon mentions the compelling case of a young American woman who had complication during surgery for a cerebral aneurysm. The EEG of her cortex and brain stem had become totally flat. After the operation, however, she related having an out-of-body experience, which was subsequently verified to occur during the flat EEG.

These observations showed that the occurrence of cardiac arrest with resultant loss of blood flow to the brain was associated with a loss of brain electrical activity. Does this then imply that extrasensory perceptions during cardiac arrest are not related to brain activity, but rather to the *release of another form of energy from the body?* Although the answer to this question might be considered highly speculative, from the evidence provided, it almost seems so.

The Concept of Mass/Energy Applied to the Afterlife

One of the fundamentals of physics is that energy does not die, that it cannot be created or destroyed—*it simply gets converted into other forms of energy*.

In death, all the physical, biochemical, and mental energy within us, the very idea in our brains of who and what we are, is energy that dissipates slowly as the body cools down. Where does this energy disappear? On the other hand, one can plausibly argue that there is no such thing as a soul or spirit as separate entities; that the very soul or spirit resides in our brain as a conglomerated host of hormones, synapses, and neurotransmitters; and that its electrical and chemical interactions are what makes us feel and appreciate beauty, spirituality, a sense of transcendence. *And yet, any such interactions are, after all, a source of mass and energy.*

Could this energy pass on to another parallel universe?

As my friend and a pioneer in the field of cardiac electrophysiology, Dr. Benjamin Scherlag put it to me: "Just like the stars whose light (electromagnetic energy) goes on forever, our electromagnetic soul (energy) is immortal."

Undoubtedly, science has come a long way in understanding the physical nature of the human body, but our understanding of the human brain, the thinking process, such lofty and abstract attributes like spirituality, clairvoyance, the soul, and the presence or recognition of alternate parallel universes is deeply lacking. It is possible that life continues as forms of energy in a parallel universe!

♥

Part V
The Break Down

Chapter 17
The Broken Heart

*For my part, I prefer my heart to be broken. It is so lovely,
dawn-kaleidoscopic within the crack.*

—D. H. Lawrence

If I can stop one heart from breaking, I shall not live in vain.

—Emily Dickinson

Recently, I saw Dorothy, a middle-aged woman who within 6 months had her husband and her only daughter die, the latter from breast cancer. Dorothy told me that she was devastated and suffered bouts of anxiety and depression. She spent sleepless nights interrupted by sudden paroxysms of crying. She felt alone in the world, abandoned by man and God. A few weeks after her daughter's death, she was beset with chest discomfort and shortness of breath. She thought it was indigestion and took a couple of antacids and a sleeping pill. A few days later, while having breakfast, she passed out. An ambulance carried her to the emergency room of a neighboring hospital where she again passed out.

After she was transferred to our hospital for specialized care, she said to me, "As I was sinking to the floor, I felt I was going to die. I saw my husband and daughter in the distance. I was happy that I was going to join them. As I was running in an illuminated tunnel towards them, it was as if I was woken up by a searing blow to my chest."

That blow was an electrical shock to her chest administered by the paramedics in the ER. She was in ventricular tachycardia, and the shock saved her life. Cardiac catheterization showed that the arteries to the heart were entirely normal, but Dorothy's heart function was down.

What had happened to Dorothy?

We have known less about the heart's reaction to emotions like depression and bereavement. Even so, we all have come across cases personally or through the media where people have died of a *broken heart*, a common metaphor for the pain and suffering one feels for the loss of a loved one through romantic rejection,

J. A. Gomes, *Rhythms of Broken Hearts*,
https://doi.org/10.1007/978-3-030-77382-3_17

betrayal, breakup, separation, divorce, or death. A relative of mine died 24 hours after the death of her husband, and they had a joint funeral. This had happened before I was born—the story was told to me by my mother. It was said that she died of a broken heart, way before the "broken heart syndrome" was described. Similarly, my maternal uncle, who suffered from benign high blood pressure, died of malignant hypertension and intracerebral bleeding. It was precipitated by bereavement stress only a few days after the death of his mother. One wonders if Debbie Reynolds died of a broken heart a day after the death of her daughter Carrie Fisher.

The broken heart, not surprisingly, has been the subject of poets, songwriters, and playwrights for centuries. Doctors, however, have wondered at such events and at the very significance of the broken heart. How does a broken heart seem to break physiologically?

Voodoo and the Octopus Pot

I came across an unusual and most interesting case in 1980 at the Kings County Medical Center in Brooklyn. I was told the story of Jean Pierre, a Haitian immigrant in his late 40s who appeared in the ER. The triage nurse placed him on a cardiac bed because he said he was going to die of a heart attack. When the ER doctor saw him, he found him profoundly anxious. He was sweating profusely and constantly moving his arms and legs. He was unable to lie quietly. "I'm going to die of a heart attack," Jean Pierre kept repeating, turning his face to the wall. He denied any chest pain or shortness of breath. There were no abnormalities in his physical examination, his ECG, or the level of enzymes released when one is having a heart attack. He became upset and agitated when told that there was nothing wrong with his heart, and he might as well go home. Finally, he confessed to the psychiatrist that he was informed in Brooklyn, where he lived, that there was a voodoo ceremony in Port-Au-Prince, Haiti, during which a curse was laid on him for an affair he had had with his neighbor's wife on a recent visit. He was ultimately admitted to the psychiatry ward for observation.

Jean Pierre was found dead in bed the following day. The autopsy revealed no cardiac abnormality.

When I contemplated his case in 1980, I found it perplexing and mysterious and hard to believe. But today, we have a reasonably good idea what killed him. Fear alone can cause an outpouring of adrenaline and noradrenaline—an adrenergic storm—that leads to a lethal heart rhythm like ventricular fibrillation and sudden cardiac death.

In 1990, Dr. Hikaru Sato and colleagues in Japan first described "stress-related cardiomyopathy." This condition can produce symptoms very much like a heart attack, with chest discomfort, shortness of breath, a blackout spell, and even a rapid lethal heart arrhythmia followed by asystole or flatline. Dr. Sato called it

Fig. 17.1 The octopus pot or *takotsubo*. (Source: https://ispub.com/ IJANP/10/2/6269)

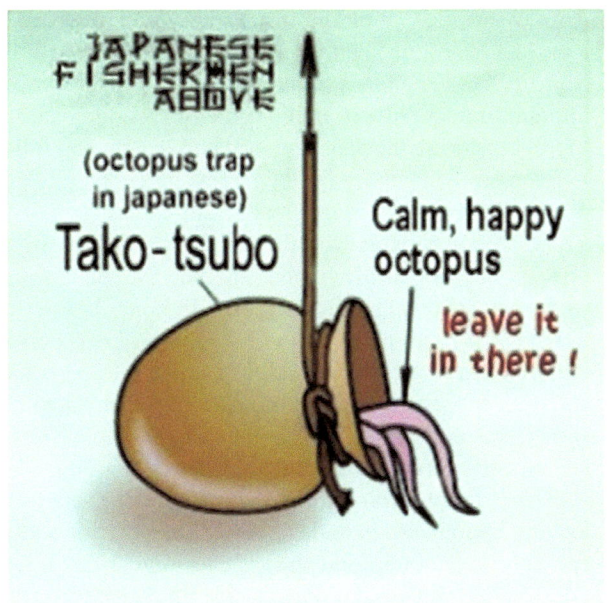

"takotsubo-like left ventricular dysfunction." In Japanese, a *takotsubo* is an "octopus pot"—a jar with a small neck and a balloon-like base used for catching octopus (Fig. 17.1). Fishermen lower it on a rope into the water, the octopus slips in for shelter, and in the morning, they pull the pot up onto the boat. The heart in patients with this affliction resembles a *takotsubo*, since it temporarily weakens and swells the cardiac muscle, and indeed, Dorothy's heart looked like one of these pots. This condition is now well recognized universally.

Takotsubo heart tends to occur after emotional stress like the death or a severe injury of a close family member. However, almost any severe stress can bring it on. It can happen after an earthquake, financial reverse, receipt of bad news, bad arguments, car accidents, a surprise reunion, a court appearance, a sudden big gambling loss, or public speaking. Sometimes there is no discernible trigger.

What killed Jean Pierre? He was frightened, certainly, but possibly he felt grief too. "Witch doctors" all over the world have exercised voodoo-like powers, and as anthropologist Walter B. Cannon observed in a classic 1942 paper, the hexed targets commonly lose all social support and often actually mourned before their deaths. Jean Pierre lived far away from Haiti and might have felt heartbreak at being cut off from emotional sustenance from those in his homeland. At the same time, since he believed he might die, he plainly felt enormous stress that probably resulted in an *adrenergic storm* and a sudden lethal heart rhythm abnormality like ventricular fibrillation that caused sudden cardiac death. Whether he harbored a genetic abnormality in the heart's electrical system (discussed in a previous chapter), we will never know.

In cases like that of Dorothy and my two relatives, people have literally "died of a broken heart" or been "scared to death," like Jean Pierre. But usually, *takotsubo* heart has an excellent prognosis. It is most often reversible, as with Dorothy. In a literature review of 816 published cases, sudden cardiac death occurred in 9 of the 816 cases during the acute episode and in 4 during follow-up, weeks to months later.

Women make up by far the largest percentage of sufferers. In a 2011 study conducted at seven tertiary medical health-care centers in Europe and North America in a total of 256 patients with this condition, the investigators found that 81% of them were postmenopausal women, another 8% were women under 50, and only 11% were men. The study cited triggers 48 hours before the event that were both emotional (30%) and physical (41%). Death of a relative or friend accounted for the majority of emotional events followed by interpersonal conflict, while stress before and after surgery accounted for most of the physical factors. As the name *takotsubo* shows, this condition changes the heart's shape. The study showed that in addition to echocardiography, magnetic resonance imaging (MRI) can identify the condition.

The pathophysiology of *takotsubo* heart remains uncertain. However, the two leading hypotheses include (1) excess adrenaline and noradrenaline (also known as epinephrine and norepinephrine) causing cardiac injury and (2) spasm of the heart arteries. Of the two, there is considerable evidence for the first and less for the second. Emotional stresses of many kinds can cause a spike in the two hormones that harms the heart muscle and precipitates rhythm abnormalities. In 2005, Dr. Ilan S. Wittstein and coworkers showed that such patients had elevated plasma levels of these hormones on initial examination. These levels in fact exceeded those seen in acute myocardial infraction and left ventricular failure.

Hence, when the situation is acute, doctors seek to mute the impact of the adrenaline and noradrenaline. They give patients beta-adrenergic blockers, which fill the receptor sites of these two hormones and keep them from acting on cells. The use of an implantable defibrillator requires consideration on a case-by-case basis.

When terrorists attacked the United States on September 11, 2001, Jennifer, a patient of mine, was in the North Tower of the World Trade Center. She received several defibrillator shocks as she was coming down the stairs and survived the disaster as well as the shocks from the defibrillator. After the attack, it was reported that many patients who had defibrillators for prevention of arrhythmic death experienced shocks from the device for the first time. Their heightened anxiety probably resulted in a high output of adrenaline, triggering fast heart rhythms that the defibrillator appropriately stopped. Studies in patients with defibrillators have also shown that abnormal, lethal rhythms can arise during emotional stresses such as anger and frustration. One can categorically state that stress is not good for the heart and that in some individuals stress can even be fatal.

The appearance of COVID-19 in the United States and throughout the world has seen death on a massive scale: over 400,000 in the United States and over a million worldwide. My friend the actress Linda Thorson wrote to me: "Hearts have been broken thousands of times more often in these past months either directly or indirectly due to COVID-19. Loss of loved ones, loss of potential lovers or existing lovers, loss of touch, of being held, loss of taste and smell, loss of work, of motivation, of freedoms and even of a raison d'etre. The idea that one heart must bear so much and yet maintain a rhythm sufficient to keep one alive is almost heart stopping in itself. Such a great demand on a thing the size of a fist."

The heart is not the seat of love or other emotions as we understand it today. However, the heart can be affected by physical as well as emotional stresses, inclusive of loss of a loved one, and fear and fright, with severe and even tragic consequences.

♥

Part VI
The Slow Down

Chapter 18
The Ubiquitous Faint

*He felt the whole vision turn to darkness and his very feet give
way. His head went round; he was going; he had gone.*

—Henry James, The Jolly Corner

*I tended to faint when I saw accident victims in the emergency
ward, during surgery, or while drawing blood.*

—Michael Crichton

Faint, swoon, passing out, blackout spell, syncope—these are all different names for
the same condition, one that has plagued and astonished human beings throughout
history (Fig. 18.1). In ancient times, one who fainted might have woken up to find
aromatic potions on the body and strange elixirs in receptacles tilted up to the nose.

The word "syncope" comes from the Greek words *syn* ("with") and *kopto* ("I
cut" or "I interrupt"). As we've seen, a host of rhythm disorders can cause syncope.
And there is the "common faint" or vasovagal syncope, the subject of this chapter.

A sudden decrease in heart rate is common in these faints, and perhaps the first
association of syncope and slow pulse came from Italian anatomist Geronimo
Mercuriale (1530–1606). In 1580, he said, in the scholarly Latin of the time: *Ubi
pulsus sit rarus semper expectanda est syncope* or "When the pulse comes seldom,
a faint is always to be expected." He made this observation almost 200 years before
Giovanni Battista Morgagni (1682–1771)—"the father of anatomical pathology"—
who described syncope as "epilepsy with a slow pulse" in 1761.

In "vasovagal" syncope, there is heightened activity of the vagus nerve on the
heart rate and blood vessels with an abrupt cutting off of consciousness and loss of
postural tone—usually collapse—with spontaneous recovery. It lasts from a few
seconds to minutes followed by complete wakefulness. These episodes can possibly
occur once in a while throughout one's lifetime. Also known in medical jargon as
"neurocardiogenic syncope," it usually happens in the absence of heart disease in
the young and the old. If the episode is prolonged and results in heart stoppage
(asystole) for several seconds, jerky movements of the limbs like those in an

© The Author(s), under exclusive license to Springer Nature
Switzerland AG 2021
J. A. Gomes, *Rhythms of Broken Hearts*,
https://doi.org/10.1007/978-3-030-77382-3_18

Fig. 18.1 A painting by
Pietro Longhi called
"Fainting". (Source:
https://en.wikipedia.org/
wiki/Pietro_Longhi)

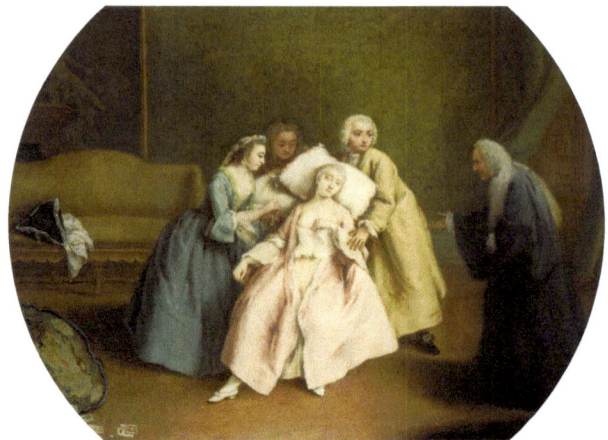

epileptic seizure can appear, and rarely loss of urine or bowel control. Not uncommonly, when the individual tries to get up after an episode, the faint can repeat itself within minutes.

Classically, it results from prolonged standing, often in a hot and crowded place. At other times, people faint while sitting, walking, eating, and less often exercising. The individual may feel nauseous and have profuse sweating, a "rush feeling," and dizziness before loss of consciousness. At other times, there is no warning. The faint may occur during or after a hot shower, during or just after urination particularly at night ("micturition syncope"), not uncommonly after heavy drinking the previous evening, and less commonly during defecation. It can occur with great pain or a blow to the belly, as well as during severe vomiting and coughing spell or after frequent bowel movements as a result of diarrhea. Powerful emotion can trigger it, such as the news of a relative's death, and in Samuel Richardson's novel *Clarissa* (1748), the heroine often swoons. Yet, it can also occur when a person awakes and then faints in bed or on standing up. Famously, the sight of blood or blood drawing can cause a faint, as it did with Michael Crichton. In *As You Like It*, Rosalind faints after reading a letter from Orlando and seeing a bloody cloth, and Oliver says, "Many will swoon when they do look on blood." In hundreds of cases I've encountered, syncope rather rarely occurs after sex or while driving.

In people with a predisposition, a fainting spell can arise from a decrease in the body's fluid volume—due to dehydration, profuse sweating, fever, or infection such as a flu-like syndrome or pneumonia.

Some situational syncope seems triggered by the distension of hollow organs, such as the rectum and bladder. In rare cases, swallowing can cause a faint, by stretching the esophagus.

The Impact of Syncope

Fainting is indeed a common problem and a costly one. It accounts for one million patients in the United States and more than 500,000 new patients per year. Nearly 170,000 people have recurrent syncope, while around 70,000 have infrequent and unexplained syncope. It results in 3% of emergency room visits per year of which around 30% to 40% are admitted to the hospital for further investigation at an annual cost of nearly $2.4 billion according to the Medicare database. The frequency of syncope varies with age group: 15% of patients are under 18, 20–25% are between 17 and 46, 16–19% are between 40 and 59, while 23% are over 70. But it's true incidence is hard to measure, partly because victims often don't report it.

Syncope has a significant impact on quality of life. Nearly 73% of victims suffer from anxiety or depression, 71% have to alter daily activity, 60% are restricted from driving, and around 37% have to change employment. In some, the episodes are recurrent and extremely bothersome, and in nearly half, they are associated with considerable injury. In my experience, patients over 60 are more likely to have substantial trauma to the face, head, and torso than those under 40.

Paradoxes of the Common Faint

The cause of the "common faint" is curious and paradoxical. Every time we stand up, 300–800 milliliters (0.3–0.85 quarts) of blood move from the chest to the legs. There is less blood in the chest and less blood is returning to the heart from the veins. The heart chambers don't fill completely, causing a drop in blood pressure. Therefore, the sympathetic system goes into action. It tries to maintain blood pressure by increasing adrenaline and noradrenaline. These quicken the heart rate, strengthen heart muscle contractions, and constrict the blood vessels. Normally this tactic works, but occasionally it backfires. Though less blood is filling the ventricles, sympathetic stimulation makes the partly empty left ventricle contract vigorously and stretch. The heart wall has receptors (mechanosensitive vagal cardiac afferent C-fibers), which sense this stretching and relay the information to the brain, which assumes the blood pressure is too high. The result? The deluded brain sends commands through the vagus nerve to reduce the pressure. The heart rate slows—as Mercuriale noticed long ago—and the blood vessels dilate, so blood pressure falls, and the person faints. These reactions become more pronounced if one is dehydrated to begin with.

In fright, there is releases of adrenaline and noradrenaline, which cause blood to flow out to the muscles, in preparation for possible attack. There is less blood in the heart, yet it is pumping faster, in an urgent effort to fuel the extremities. The heart wall stretches, receptors signal the brain, and it makes the same mistake: the vagus nerve slows the heart and causes a faint. A similar pattern occurs with other high emotions.

Some people faint more often than others. How do they differ physiologically from the rest? Do they have exaggerated cardiac reflexes or greater numbers of beta-receptors that make them more sensitive to adrenaline and noradrenaline? We don't know the answer. But whatever the cause, the physiology in such patients is usually a "temporary situation," rather than a permanent one since most will recover over time or the condition ameliorates.

The Tilt and the Monitor

Syncope can be a symptom of serious maladies, and it's important to rule out conditions such as long QT syndrome, WPW syndrome, and a previous heart attack, all conditions previously discussed. In my experience, the starting points in the evaluation are a good history, a physical examination, and an ECG. An echocardiogram is useful in establishing cardiac causes of syncope such as a prior heart attack, cardiomyopathy, and blockage of the aortic valve—all conditions with an ominous prognosis.

The absence of cardiac disease and recurrent bouts of fainting spells, often preceded by the warning signs noted above, point to vasovagal syncope, which is usually a benign condition.

The greatest fear is injury to the head, face, and torso.

The commonest test in the diagnosis of vasovagal syncope is the tilt table test (TTT). Since its description by Dr. Rose Anne Kenny of Trinity College, Dublin, in 1986, the TTT has been widely used in the diagnosis of the recurrent common faint. Kenny found that the test was positive in 67% of patients with unexplained syncope.

A TTT seeks to reproduce a faint in the clinical setting. The patient lies flat on his/her back on a special table, with straps to hold the body tight to the table. A nurse attaches an IV line and electrodes for the ECG, as well as an arm cuff to monitor the blood pressure. After baseline recordings of heart rate and blood pressure, the bed is tilted to a 70- to 80-degree angle (Fig. 18.2) for 20–30 minutes. Since the legs are strapped securely in, they can't move and consequently prevent the blood in the veins from returning to the heart as they normally do, and the stress on the sympathetic nervous system is maximized. If the test is negative after 20 minutes, the doctor may move to a second phase. Here, chemicals such as isoproterenol or nitroglycerine are administered to provoke an increase in heart rate or dilate the blood vessels, respectively. If the blood pressure or heart rate doesn't drop after another 10 minutes or so, the test is over.

Classically, most patients vulnerable to the common faint will drop their heart rate and blood pressure within 10–20 minutes into the test. In some, the blood pressure falls without a drop in heart rate, while others may initially show an increase followed by a marked slowing of heart rate to such an extent that there is cardiac

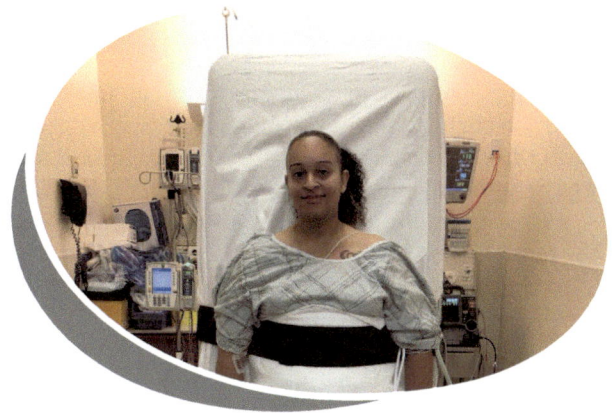

Fig. 18.2 A tilt table test. A patient undergoing a tilt table test

standstill lasting for over 6 seconds. Intriguingly, despite the heart having "stopped," I have never witnessed lethal ventricular fibrillation or death in this test. That is because vagal stimulation, despite its provocative mischief, is protective from developing lethal arrhythmia in contrast to sympathetic stimulation.

Tilting can also bring on sinus tachycardia (rather than bradycardia or slowing), with or without a drop in blood pressure. This condition is known as postural orthostatic tachycardia (POTS). Its causes are unclear, and 80% of POTS victims are women, mostly between 15 and 50 years of age. One of my patients, Mable—a 15-year-old student—began feeling week and dizzy as her heart kept racing when she stood up. She nearly fainted at school and was whisked to an ER and released with a diagnosis of dehydration. She couldn't partake in any activities. In the months that followed, she said, "I just didn't feel right. I was dizzy, my heart raced, and I felt very tired all the time."

She eventually had a TTT in our lab and received the diagnosis of POTS. By increasing her fluid intake, eating more salt including pretzels, tilt training (standing up for a progressive incremental time period), as well as a small dose of beta-blocker, she was able to attend school. But a quarter of POTS victims are unable to function for a variable length of time.

Less than 50% of people with syncope have a positive TTT; however, the positivity of the test varies substantially from patient to patient. That variance relates to a host of factors, including near-faints like dizziness vs. true faints, frequency of fainting, and time between the last episode and the test. Besides, the condition that triggered the episode may not be present during the test. In syncope triggered by situations, such as emotional events, micturition, and pain, the TTT is usually negative for the simple reason that tilting cannot replicate the "situation" causing the faint.

Treatment of Recurrent Fainting

The drug treatment of common recurrent faints has been rather disappointing. Lifestyle changes such as avoiding triggers, reducing alcohol intake, maintaining proper fluid and salt intake, as well as exercising moderately are often beneficial. They may be all one needs.

For instance, Rob was a 54-year-old male, a traveling salesman who began fainting rather recently. His episodes often occurred when he was on a plane, but also at other times when he was sitting or standing. Notably, because of his constant traveling, both his diet and fluid intake were erratic, so at times he would be dehydrated. He had no history of heart disease, and his physical, ECG, and echocardiogram were normal. Ten minutes into the tilt test, his heart rate dropped from 71 to 56 beats per minute, while his blood pressure held steady at 123/73. He complained of a cold sweat and a feeling of fainting, and then he passed out. His heart rate dropped to 20 beats per minute, and his blood pressure was unobtainable. As soon as we put him on his back, he recovered promptly, and both his heart rate and blood pressure normalized.

I suggested to Rob that he increase his fluid and salt intake to begin with. I also added a salt-retaining medication. He hid well on this conservative approach.

Beyond such lifestyle changes, small-scale studies have shown benefit from the use of beta-adrenergic blockers, as well as a chemical called fludrocortisone, which helps retain salt, and alpha agonists such as midodrine, which treats low blood pressure. Unfortunately, the large-scale, randomized studies have been disappointing. Nonetheless, I prefer to use an individual approach to treatment based on history, triggers, diet, salt and water intake, and results from the TTT.

Dr. Blair P. Grubb and coworkers proposed that selective serotonin reuptake inhibitors (SSRIs), used for depression, can reduce vasovagal syncope through effects on the synapses in the brain by reducing the response that slows the heart down and causes fainting. So far, there has been just one trial of the SSRI—paroxetine—and it did reduce the recurrence of vasovagal syncope significantly compared with the placebo during more than 2 years of follow-up. When other approaches fail, SSRIs may be tried.

Since vasovagal syncope can disappear on its own, assessing the effectiveness of a treatment can be difficult. For instance, the use of pacemakers has been controversial, since some studies show a positive response and others none at all. However, one study showed benefit in people who had significant slow heart rate and pauses.

Therefore, if the episodes are frequent and are associated with long pauses or asystole, a pacemaker maybe useful. If the heart rate falls first before a significant drop in blood pressure, pacing may abort the syncope, though not the dizzy feeling. It may also give the patient time to lie down.

I faced this decision with Anna, a 32-year-old nurse who complained of fainting spells. When she came to see me in the clinic, she had fainted three times in the previous month, twice at work and once at home. She was engaged to be married and was working hard, sometimes doing night shifts on her off days.

Ten minutes into the tilt test, her heart rate jumped from the 70s to the 80s.

"I'm not feeling well," she said. "I think it's coming on."

Hardly had I turned my head toward the monitor when she rolled her eyes and was out. Her blood pressure was not recordable, her heart rate had slowed into the 30s, and as we were bringing her down to the flat position, her heart stopped for more than 10 seconds, her eyes rolled, and her arms and legs began twitching. She was flat out. I thumped her on the chest several times, and gradually her heart rate picked up, and she awoke and began responding. It was a frightening experience, but it did not roil me. I knew she would be fine.

I told her what she had, reassured her that it was a benign condition, and said that she had to lie down immediately when she felt it coming on and that she shouldn't stay standing in one spot for longer than 10 minutes. I asked her to increase her fluid and salt intake and even eat a pretzel once a day to begin with. I also recommended that she have a pacemaker in view of her recurrent and prolonged heart stoppages that required chest compressions. Anna had a dual-chamber pacemaker, programmed to pace her heart if the heart rate drops down.

She has done well without any more fainting episodes.

♥

Chapter 19
The Stuttering Maestro: The Sick Sinus

And the maestro surely wielded the chairman's baton with extraordinary skill.

—Alan Blinder

You can't teach the old maestro a new tune.

—Jack Kerouac

After the discovery of the sinus node in 1906 by Keith and Flack, it generated intense scrutiny and study. My own interest in it peaked in the 1980s when I directed the electrophysiology laboratory and the coronary care unit at the Brooklyn Veterans Administration Hospital of the Downstate Medical Center, which had a substantial older population with disturbed sinus node function. Failure of the sinus node accounts for the majority of cardiac pacemaker insertions.

The sinus node has been called the "maestro" of the cardiac electrical system (Fig. 19.1). And like an orchestra conductor with a baton, it keeps the pace for the heart. It fires automatically, and the electrical system of the heart follows its timing. The term "heart rate" almost always corresponds to the activity of the sinus node. It triggers an average of 60–100 beats per minute, incessantly, every minute of every day throughout our lifetime.

It looks unprepossessing. It is tiny, pellet-shaped bit of tissue, about 0.6 by 0.2 by 0.08 inches (15 by 5 by 2 millimeters), just below the outer surface of the right atrium (see Chap. 2, Fig. 2.2). It has remarkable properties, and it is quite resistant to ischemia (insufficient blood supply). In the early 1980s, Dr. Winters and I encountered a female patient who had a rapid sinus rate for no identifiable reason, a condition referred to as "inappropriate sinus tachycardia." No medication worked, and because of her disabling symptoms, we recommended excision. The surgeon cut out her sinus node in the operating room and placed the little piece of tissue on the side table, and we were surprised to see it beat for some time with no blood supply whatsoever.

© The Author(s), under exclusive license to Springer Nature
Switzerland AG 2021
J. A. Gomes, *Rhythms of Broken Hearts*,
https://doi.org/10.1007/978-3-030-77382-3_19

Fig. 19.1 The maestro.
Legend: The cartoon
depicts the sinus node as
the maestro of the cardiac
electrical conducting
system

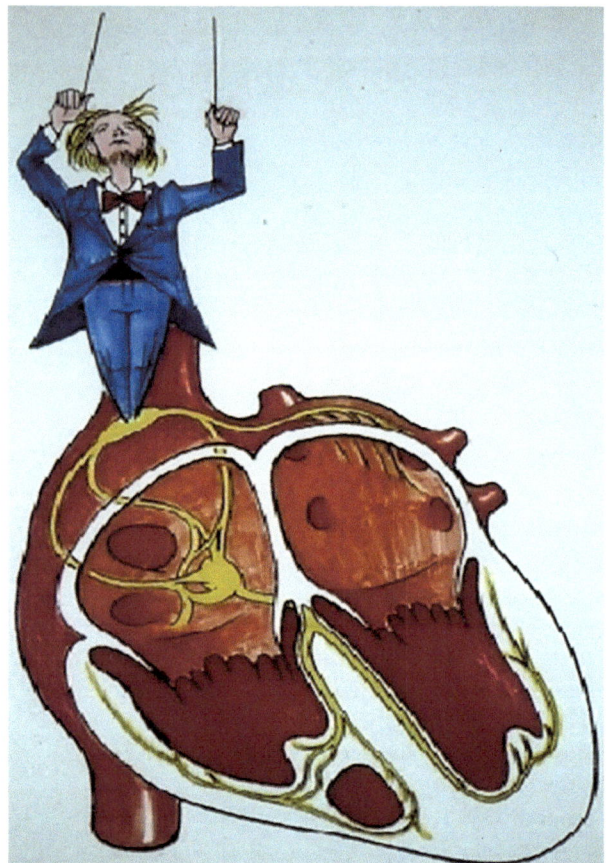

The Sick Sinus

As far back as 1961, the late Dr. Bernard Lown—an outstanding erudite Boston cardiologist, activist-humanitarian, and Nobel laureate—used a few provocative, poetic terms while delivering the Sir Thomas Lewis Lecture of the British Cardiac Society. He called delayed warm-up of the sinus node a "somnolent sinus." And he called a certain defect in sinus discharge or conduction the "sick sinus syndrome." Subsequently, in 1967, Dr. Irene Ferrer of Columbia University in New York popularized the term *sick sinus syndrome* (SSS). It is a basket term for a group of symptoms and ECG abnormalities that imply the sinus node isn't working properly. In SSS, the heart may be beating too fast or too slowly or have long pauses between sinus firing. One can also have paroxysms of tachycardia, such as atrial fibrillation or supraventricular tachycardia, followed by a long sinus pause or slowing. This speeding up and slowing down is called the "tachycardia-bradycardia syndrome" (Fig. 19.2), and it can result in dizziness, weakness, and syncope. Classically, the patient might complain of a sudden dizzy spell or a blackout spell due to slowing of

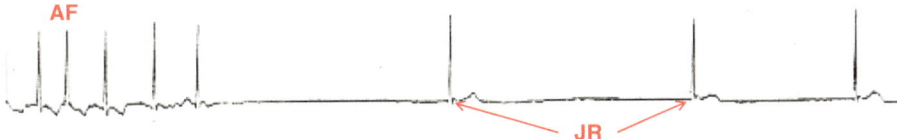

Fig. 19.2 The tachy-brady syndrome. Legend: The monitor strip shows atrial fibrillation (AF) in an elderly patient with SSS, after which there is a pause with a junctional pacemaker (red arrows) due to the failure of the sinus node to discharge resulting in near syncope

the heart rate or a long sinus pause following a run of rapid heartbeats. It has been postulated that the slow heart rates seen in the SSS are due to a reduction in their open funny channels. However, using direct recordings of the sinus node in patients with the SSS, we showed that the syndrome is more often due to failure in conduction in the tissue near the sinus node and less likely to failure in the automatic firing of the sinus itself.

The root cause of the SSS is unknown in most cases, but since we usually see it in elderly subjects, it is likely the result of age-related degenerative processes in the sinus node and/or the heart muscle around it. However, the syndrome can occur in young people as well, and a familial and congenital variety of the syndrome has been described of late.

One important source of the SSS that should not be ignored is iatrogenic, which is caused by medical treatment itself. Cardiac drugs, such as digitalis glycosides, beta-blockers, calcium channel blockers, and a host of antiarrhythmic drugs such as flecainide, amiodarone, and sotalol can bring it about. Therefore, drug history is of utmost importance in evaluating a patient with suspected SSS, and it can avoid a host of expensive, unnecessary tests and pacemakers. Other rare entities can also result in the SSS.[1]

Pathophysiology of the Sick Sinus

The heart rate results from a complex and delicately balanced interplay. The sinus sets the pace, the autonomic nervous system modifies it, and the conduction of its impulses into the atrial muscle can alter its downstream impact. Only in the last few decades have we recognized that the SSS is caused by (1) intrinsic abnormality in generating the sinus impulse, (2) extrinsic abnormality due to the autonomic nervous system, and (3) abnormalities in conduction near the node, that is, the failure of the impulse to exit this area. My own studies and that of other researchers showed that 38–60% of patients had the intrinsic variety, and around 40–62% had the

---

[1] They include ischemia and diseases such as amyloidosis, hemochromatosis, tumor, scleroderma, rheumatic fever, pericarditis, Chagas disease, diphtheria, cardiomyopathy, collagen vascular disease, surgical trauma, and muscular dystrophy.

extrinsic variety. Our observations revealed that patients with the extrinsic variety were younger and more athletic, with slow heart rates, whereas those with the intrinsic variety were older and had long pauses as well as paroxysmal atrial fibrillation. The extrinsic variety is likely related to excessive vagal tone and can be occasionally seen in long-distance runners. It is noteworthy that total failure of the sinus node took 7–29 years, with an average of 13 years.

A host of tests have been described to assess sinus node function. The one currently in use is long-term monitoring with an event monitor that can record an ECG and correlate symptoms with objective evidence of sinus slowing or arrest.

Before the advent of pacemakers, there was no treatment for the SSS, and patients suffered from shortness of breath, profound weakness, dizzy spells, and blackouts. Today, in symptomatic SSS, a pacemaker is recommended. Drug therapy to increase the heart rate is usually ineffective.

The Exhausted Student

Donald was a 20-year-old college student who was referred to me for evaluation of fatigue and lightheadedness. His symptoms started about 9 months earlier, when after working out he would feel exhausted. His quality of life and his social interactions plummeted over time. An extensive workup by his primary doctor only revealed a slow heart rate in the 40s. A few months later when in New Zealand as a visiting student, he felt worse and had to be admitted to a hospital where doctors found that his heart rate was in the 30s.

I diagnosed his condition as the extrinsic variety of SSS. I was not anxious to proceed at once to a pacemaker in this young man. I wanted to prove that my diagnosis was right, that the parasympathetic nervous system was slowing his heart rate, and thus I proceeded to do an invasive study. I blocked the autonomic system with drugs to assess how the sinus node functioned on its own. Not surprisingly, his sinus rate sprang back to normal for his age and weight. The diagnosis of the extrinsic SSS was confirmed.

We discussed at length the two options: a trial of medications to increase his heart rate, and if this approach did not work and the symptoms persisted, I would implant a pacemaker. A few months later, if anything, his symptoms got worse. An ECG showed that his heart rate was still in the 30s. I proceeded to implant a pacemaker and set it to a rate of 60 beats per minute with rate responsiveness should he need to increase his heartbeat during exercise. The effect was dramatic. After only 2 weeks, Donald was back to his original self, wide awake, chirpy, optimistic, fully enthralled with life and living.

♥

Chapter 20
Of Disconnected Highways: Heart Blocks

If the R is far from the P

Then you have a first degree.

Longer, longer, longer, drop!

Then you have a Wenckebach block.

If some P's just don't go through

Then you have a Mobitz II.

And if P's and Q's just don't agree

Then you have a third degree.

(Heart block poem, modified from the Princeton Surgical Group and Nurses Labs)

The Highway in the Heart

"Heart block" sounds very final, yet it comes in many forms.

You can think of the heart's electrical system as a highway with entrances and exits. Like the highway, it is insulated from the environment, and its traffic follows pathways, from the top of the heart down to every fiber. A signal runs from the sinus node to the A-V node, and after a pause, it flashes through the A-V junction, the His bundle, and the right and left bundle branches. Finally, it reaches the millions of Purkinje fibers—the exits—which activate the muscle mass. On a highway if a bad incident occurs, say, a landslide, vehicles can pass slowly or not at all. Similarly, blocks at different levels in the heart's electrical highway can slow or stop electrical impulses. Just as on a highway, heart block may be temporary or permanent. And depending on its degree and location, it may cause serious problems.

The ultimate result of heart block is a slow heart rate. The term "block" goes back to Darwin's close friend George J. Romanes (1848–1894), an amateur

© The Author(s), under exclusive license to Springer Nature
Switzerland AG 2021
J. A. Gomes, *Rhythms of Broken Hearts*,
https://doi.org/10.1007/978-3-030-77382-3_20

biologist who coined the term for obstacles in signals to the muscle of the medusa jellyfish. Renowned English physiologist Walter Gaskell (1847–1914) after removing a piece of tortoise atrium slowly increased the obstruction level and observed the result. "If the block is more severe," he noted, "then, instead of every contraction passing the blocking point, only every second contraction is able to pass." He had distinguished partial block from complete block.

So blocks can be of different degrees and significance. The customary classification is first degree, second degree types I and II, high degree, and third degree or complete heart block. They have a wide range of meaning and prognosis.

First Degree: "If the R Is Far from P"

On the ECG, the PR interval is the period from the start of the P wave, when the atria first contract, to the start of the QRS complex, when the ventricles begin to pump (see Chap. 4, Fig. 4.2). The delay in conduction at the A-V node accounts for most of this interval, but it also includes the time the current races through the A-V junction, His bundle, and bundle branches.

Normally, the PR interval lasts between 0.12 and 0.2 seconds. In first-degree A-V block, the PR interval exceeds this period (Fig. 20.1A), but the signals from the

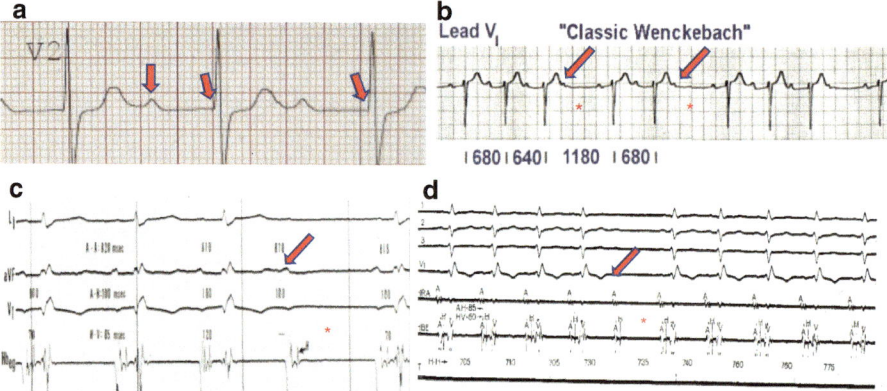

Fig. 20.1 First- and second-degree A-V blocks. Legend: **Panel A** shows a first-degree A-V block, Note the prolonged PR interval of nearly 0.4 seconds. **Panel B** shows ECG lead showing a blocked P wave (arrow, red star) showing a classical Wenckebach block (4:3), followed by 3:2 periodicity. **Panel C** shows ECG leads 1, avF and V1, and intracardiac His bundle recording (Hbeg). Note that the QRS complex shows right bundle branch block (RBBB). Note that the Wenckebach block occurs after the His bundle (red star). Note also the progressive prolongation of the HV interval before the blocked P wave (red arrow). Panel D shows sudden block of P wave (red arrow, red star). The block is below the His as noted on the Hb recording. Note that there is no PR or AH or HV prolongation before the block unlike in **Panel C**

sinus node still go through. There are no dropped beats. In this regard, the term first-degree heart block is a misnomer since there is no block.

First-degree block is usually benign. It often occurs as a result of medications such as beta-adrenergic blockers, calcium channel blockers, digitalis glycosides, sotalol, and amiodarone. One can determine its location by assessing the QRS complex. If it is narrow, shorter than 0.12 seconds, the delay is usually in the A-V node and very rarely in the His bundle itself. If it is longer than 0.12 seconds or if there is bundle branch block,[1] the conduction delay can be lower down in the His-Purkinje system. In any case, usually, no treatment is needed.

Second Degree Type I: "Longer, Longer, Longer, Drop!"

Dr. Karel Wenckebach (1864–1940, Fig. 20.2), whose contributions to VPCs I noted earlier, was a modest, contented, path-breaking physician, one of many brilliant Dutch cardiologists who have advanced our knowledge of the heart. He was born in

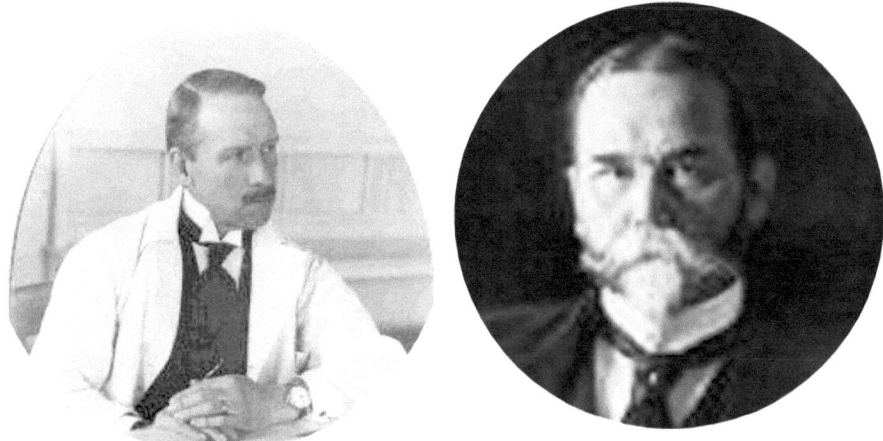

Fig. 20.2 Karel Wenckebach and Waldemar Mobitz. Legend: On the left is Karel Wenckebach and on the right is Waldemar Mobitz. (Source for Karel Wenckebach: https://en.wikipedia.org/wiki/Karel_Frederik_Wenckebach#/media/File:Karel_Frederik_Wenckebach.jpg; Source for Waldemar Mobitz: Reprinted from Charles B. Upshaw, Jr., MD, and Mark E. Silverman, MD∗ Woldemar Mobitz: early twentieth century expert on atrioventricular block. *Clin Cardiol.* 32(11): E75–E77 (2009))

---

[1] Bundle branch block can be of two types. In both, the QRS duration is 0.12 or greater. Right bundle branch block (RBBB) is defined by a secondary R wave (Ri) in the right precordial leads (V1-3) and a wide slurred S wave in lateral leads due to delay in activating the right ventricle. There can be associated ST and T-wave changes in the right precordial leads. Left bundle branch block is defined by broad monomorphic R waves in I and V6 with no Q waves due to delay in activating the left ventricle.

The Hague, studied medicine in Utrecht, and became a professor of medicine at the University of Groningen in 1901. Later, he moved to the University of Strasbourg and subsequently to the University of Vienna in Austria.

In a book entitled *Die Unregelmassige Hertztatigkeit* (*Arhythmia of the Heart*) published in 1904, he first described second-degree block that bears his name. His elegant clinical observations are worth remembering. Of his first second-degree block case, he wrote that the patient was "a female, aged forty years, of nervous temperament, who had long observed that her pulse did not beat regularly. She had a weak circulation but exhibited no other lesions of the heart than slight dilation. She was delicate and anemic ... her pulse was small, soft, and showed a continual intermission after every three or at most six beats, usually after every four or five. The heart sounds were weak, but pure."

In second-degree block, some signals from the sinus node don't get through. In Wenckebach block, there is a signature pattern. The PR interval increases progressively—that "longer, longer, longer" in the poem above—until there is a missed heartbeat (Fig. 20.1B). On the ECG, we see a flat line where the dramatic QRS complex should be. Then the cycle starts over again. It is as if the system grows more and more tired, gives up, and then finds its energy restored after the failed heartbeat.

The pattern tends to be regular, and we see a single ratio of P waves to QRS complexes. For instance, the ventricles may contract two times for every three atrial contractions, a ratio of 3:2. In this group of beats, there are two P waves or atrial contractions, each followed by a QRS, but after the third P wave, there is no QRS till the next cycle. Other common ratios are 4:3 and 5:4. And in some patients, the patterns can shift (Fig. 20.1B), as they did with Wenckebach's first patient.

What is of considerable fascination to this day is that Wenckebach identified this block with no help from the ECG. He described it in 1899, 2 years before Willem Einthoven constructed the ECG machine. He accomplished this feat by analyzing the pulse of the jugular vein in the neck with superb precision. The 1893 experiments by Italian neuroscientist Luigi Luciani (1840–1919) in the frog heart aided his efforts. Giving due credit to Luciani, Wenckebach called this form of beating "Luciani periods." In 1906, now aided by the ECG, Wenckebach documented that the PR interval progressively increased before the missed heartbeat. His ladder diagrams depicting this type of block are to be marveled at, to this day.

Where is the obstruction in Wenckebach block? In the early days, cardiologists felt it lay in the A-V node. However, we now know that block could occur anywhere in the cable system: in the A-V node, but also the His bundle, below the His (Fig. 20.1C), and in the bundle branches. With more precise intracardiac recordings in man—those from inside the heart, which show us electrical activity in parts of it rather than in the whole organ as ECGs do, Dr. Damato and his associates revealed an interesting complexity. In one study, 72% of these cases originated in the A-V node, 7% in the His bundle, and 21% below it (Fig. 20.1C).

Their work also revealed that if the QRS complex is narrow, the problem lies in the A-V node, just as it does in first-degree block. Most of such cases are typically benign. If the QRS complex shows right or left bundle branch block or bifascicular block[2]—block of the right bundle branch plus one of the two left fascicles, leaving just one fascicle to carry current to the Purkinje fibers—the prognosis is grave even if the patient is asymptomatic. If the remaining fascicle becomes blocked, the person suffers complete heart block.

Second Degree Type II: "If Some P's Just Don't Go Through"

Another medical giant of those days was Woldemar Mobitz (1889–1951, Fig. 20.2), and to this day, his name, like Wenckebach, is uttered many times on a daily basis in the lecture halls and corridors of medicine throughout the world.

He was born in St. Petersburg, Russia, the son of a prominent surgeon who died at an early age. His family migrated to Tübingen in Germany, and he attended the Gymnasium at Meiningen, Saxony. He studied medicine at the University of Freiburg and subsequently at the University of Munich, where he graduated in 1914. He was a scholarly individual plagued by chronic illness. An outstanding clinician and investigator with a mathematical mind, he applied astutely in the study of arrhythmias. Indeed, it has become rather clear that heart rhythm disorders and the study of electrophysiology require a logical, mathematical mindset even to this day.

Like Wenckebach, he left a rich legacy. While working as a lecturer at the University of Munich, he devised a classification we still use to this day. In July of 1923, Mobitz delivered a lecture at the meeting of the Association of Munich Specialists in Internal Medicine identifying two types of second-degree heart block. In 1924, he authored the seminal article on these types that still bear his name: Mobitz I and Mobitz II.

Mobitz I is basically Wenckebach block. But in Mobitz II, the PR interval remains constant (Fig. 20.1D). There is a sudden unexpected block of the P wave's progress to the QRS. That is, "some P's just don't get through" and the heartbeats you'd expect don't occur. The ratios here may follow a pattern such as 3:1, 4:1, and 5:1. In other words, one of three, one of four, one of five, or more ineffective P waves can occur before a heartbeat. However, often there is no regular pattern.

Mobitz II is far more likely than Wenckebach block to lead to third-degree block and even sudden cardiac death. It is usually due to block within the His bundle or below the His (Fig. 20.1D) and rarely if ever in the A-V node. Hence, if the QRS complex is narrow, Mobitz II is rarely the diagnosis.[3] It also differs from Wenckebach block in that its cause is commonly tissue fibrosis.

---

[2] The experimental studies of Dr. Mauricio Rosenbaum, with Marcelo Elizari established guidelines for the presence of block in the anterior fascicle of the left bundle when there was a left axis shift of ≥ -30 degrees and block in the posterior fascicle of the left bundle when there was an axis shift to the right of $\geq +120$ degrees.

[3] Often it is related to a pseudo-Mobitz II pattern when there is an increase in the P-P interval before the block, suggesting an increase in vagal tone.

Mobitz classification of A-V block earned him an invitation in 1928 from Dr. Hans Eppinger, Jr. to join the Faculty of the University of Freiburg, where he remained for 15 years. In March of 1934, he came up for promotion to senior assistant physician. Dr. Siegfried Josef Thannhauser, his senior by 4 years, opposed his promotion, on the grounds that his laryngeal tuberculosis made him a health risk. It was decided that his illness was not a threat, Thannhauser was dismissed, and Mobitz took the position. And yet, 10 days later, he was replaced by Dr. Otto Bickenbach, likely for political reasons. Bickenbach was a professor at the University of Strasbourg who had joined the Nazi Party on May 1, 1933, 3 months after Hitler became chancellor of Germany.

Meanwhile, Mobitz left the University of Freiburg to become director of the State Medical Clinic in Magdeburg. He stayed there until 1945 when American, British, and Soviet forces occupied Germany. He then returned to Freiburg where he worked until his death in 1951 at the age of 61 years.

Third Degree: "If P's and Q's Just Don't Agree"

In third degree or complete heart block (CHB), there is total interruption of conduction from the upper chambers to the lower chambers. It is noteworthy that high-degree heart block (usually 2:1) may precede the occurrence of CHB (Fig. 20.3A).

In 1827, Irish physician Robert Adams (1791–1875) described a patient with a heart rate of around 30 beats per minute who had spells of dizziness and blackouts. Notably for his time, he stated that the cause of such patients' blackouts lay in the heart and not the brain, as contemporaries believed. In 1861, he became both surgeon in ordinary to Queen Victoria and a professor of surgery at Trinity College.

Third-degree block or CHB (Fig. 20.3B) can result in what is known as the Stokes-Adams syndrome, particularly when it is paroxysmal and occurs suddenly (Fig. 20.3C). Another Irish physician, William Stokes (1804–1878), described two cases similar to Adams's, observing that "the pulsation of veins is of a kind which we have never before witnessed." This syndrome became known as the Stokes-Adams syndrome.

However, Stokes and Adams were hardly the first to describe this syndrome. That honor goes to Marcus Gerbezius (Marko Gerbec, 1658–1718), who published a description posthumously in 1719. He was a physician of Slovenian descent, who grew up in a poor family and graduated in 1684 from the University of Bologna. He subsequently practiced medicine in Ljubljana, where a bust of him stands today, and became a member of the renowned German Academy of Natural Scientists in Halle. Forty-two years later, in 1761, Italian Giovanni Battista Morgagni also described the syndrome in his esteemed work *De Sedibus et Causis Morborum per Anatomen Indagatis* (*On the Seats and Causes of Diseases as Investigated by Anatomy*). And so, it should rightly be called the Gerbezius-Morgagni-Stokes-Adams syndrome.

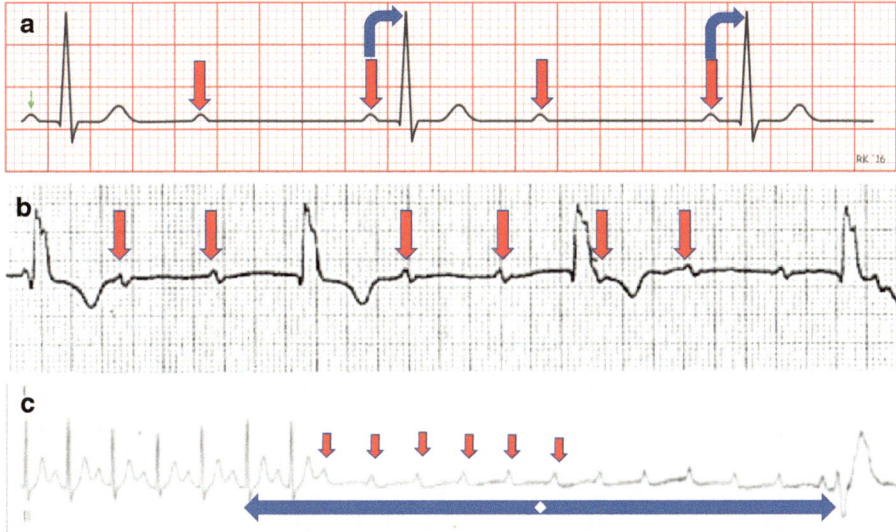

Fig. 20.3 High-degree, complete, and paroxysmal heart block. Legend: **Panel A** shows high degree (2:1) with a narrow escape pacemaker from the A-V junction. **Panel B** shows complete heart block with an escape pacemaker from the His-Purkinje axis with a right bundle branch block configuration. Some of the P waves are marked by red arrows. The third P wave is not marked since it falls within the QRS complex. Note the lack of relationship between the P waves and the QRS complexes that occur independent of each other. **Panel C** shows sudden appearance of complete heart block with a long pause causing syncope and Stokes-Adams syndrome. Some of the P waves are marked with red arrows

In complete heart block (Fig. 20.3B, C), there is total interruption of conduction from the atrium to the ventricles. As a result, the lower chambers must supply the beat on their own, and this backup system is markedly slower.

The electrical system of the heart in addition to being akin to a highway also has a power hierarchy, akin to the military. Its chain of command reaches from the top of the heart down to every fiber. In case of heart block, nature has bestowed safety mechanisms known as "escape pacemakers," at places below the level of block. They keep the heart beating. But none of these pacemakers are as efficient as the sinus node, and their rate depends on their location. The lower an escape pacemaker is in this system, the slower the heart rate. Or as Walter Gaskell put it long ago, "The power of independent rhythmical contraction decreases regularly as we pass from the sinus to the ventricle." If the sinus node stops firing, the A-V node takes control, and the heart will beat around 40 to 60 beats per minute. If the block is far down (i.e., below the His Bundle) and the Purkinje fibers have to take control, the heart will beat a sluggish 20–40 times a minute.

The lower the pacemaker, the less reliable and more prone to failure!

I still remember the case of an elderly man who appeared in the ER when I was a resident in 1972. He had a Stokes-Adams attack, and his ECG showed heart block with a rate of 40 beats per minute. He requested the nurse that he needed to make a phone call, and the nurse allowed him to use the phone booth. He collapsed in the booth and died instantaneously!

In a Stokes-Adams attack, the slower unstable escape pacemakers take over, and that's why a person suffers dizziness, fatigue, and blackout spells. Typically, such an attack occurs without warning, leading to sudden loss of consciousness lasting about 30 seconds or more, and it may be accompanied by twitching or a seizure due to a lack of blood supply to the brain. At times, the block may be associated with a ventricular tachycardia of the *torsade des pointes* variety and will urgently need pacing of the heart. Other features associated with complete heart block include poor exercise tolerance, heart failure, and death. As with Dr. Rabin, (see below) these patients typically need artificial pacemakers. Before the advent of cardiac pacing, CHB was a dreaded entity treated with ephedrine or sublingual isoproterenol, administered every 2 hours.

Causes of Heart Blocks

Heart blocks are usually seen in the elderly population and are thought to be due to age-related fibrosis or scarification of the conducting system. Nonetheless, congenital heart blocks can be seen in a young population due to maternal systemic lupus and genetic mutations. Lyme disease and sarcoidosis should be suspected when A-V blocks appear de novo particularly in individual less than 60 years of age. An acute heart attack is another important cause of heart blocks and is usually transient in patients with inferior myocardial infarction, whereas in patients with anterior myocardial infraction with bundle branch block the occurrence of heart block is usually associated with higher mortality.

A Case of Stokes-Adams Syndrome

Dr. Rabin was a 78-year-old general practitioner who was considering retirement after a long career in internal medicine. He had been well all his life and was extremely active, taking long walks and biking. One morning, he woke up and blacked out when he went to the bathroom. He thought it was a common faint, but when he went to the kitchen, he blacked out again with some seizure activity. His wife, who witnessed the episode in the kitchen, rushed him to a clinic where he saw a young doctor who told him that his heart rate was very slow. An ECG showed complete heart block. Rabin told the young doctor: "I felt I was having Stokes-Adams attacks."

"What's that?" the young doctor asked. "You are having syncopal episodes due to heart block. I think you need a pacemaker. I'm going to transfer you to Mount Sinai Hospital."

I met him in the ER with my fellows and residents in training. I concurred that he was having Stokes-Adams attacks and explained to my young doctors in training what these attacks meant. Of course, Dr. Rabin was pleased that he had met a doctor who knew the names of Stokes and Adams.

On the computer, I accessed his previous cardiograms. They showed the presence of right bundle branch block with left axis deviation (the axis is the net direction of current in the heart), commonly known as bifascicular block. I thought of the pioneer Dr. Mauricio Rosenbaum who proposed the bifascicular and trifascicular concept of the conducting system, an Argentinian cardiologist I knew very well. The Lasser brothers from the Mount Sinai Hospital, both of whom I also knew very well, had shown that 59 percent of patients with CHB had right bundle branch block with marked left axis deviation preceding CHB. It was as if I saw the reincarnation of these giants of the past in front of me—they had passed away years ago. I felt a sense of déjà vu perhaps because I had spoken often with these men and had interacted with them. I continued lecturing the young doctors on the history and the personalities behind the diagnosis and mechanism of heart block. I arranged for Dr. Rabin to have a pacemaker by one of my colleagues. He was discharged home the following day rather happy with the outcome.

♥

Part VII
A Brand-New Rhythm: A Brand-New Heart

Chapter 21
The Artificial Pacemaker: A Life-Giver

That's one small step for man, one giant leap for mankind.

—Neil Armstrong

At some point in every person's life, you will need an assisted medical device - whether it's your glasses, your contacts, or as you age and you have a hip replacement or a knee replacement or a pacemaker. The prosthetic generation is all around us.

—Aimee Mullins

By the 1900s, the medical community was aware that electric current made the heartbeat. Physicians understood that breakdown in electrical transmission between the atria and ventricles caused heart block. The Stokes-Adams syndrome was described in 1890, and its lethal association with heart block was well established. Doctors knew that if they could control the heart rate, they could save countless lives. But pacing the cardiac electrical system was a farfetched dream.

The Evolution of the Cardiac Pacemaker (Fig. 21.1)

In 1952, Paul Zoll (Fig. 21.2) published the use of a pacemaker capable of electrically stimulating the chest wall in *The New England Journal of Medicine*. In 1956, he developed the Electrodyne PM-65 pacemaker that comprised an ECG monitor and an electric pulse generator. In 1958, Earl Bakken (Figs. 21.1 and 21.2) created a portable wearable pacemaker the 5800 in the then garage company Medtronic Inc. Bakken's device was not just the first wearable pacemaker, but the first successful application of transistor technology to pacemakers. Today, Medtronic Inc. is one of the largest device companies in the world, with annual revenue of over $20 billion.

However, the pacemaker system with exterior wires had several disadvantages, namely:

1. The risk of carrying infection to the heart.
2. In many patients, heart block reappeared causing several deaths.

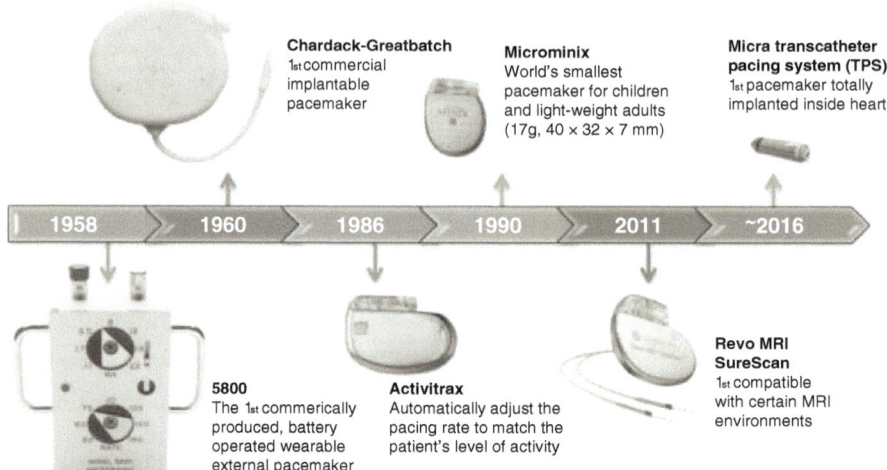

Fig. 21.1 The evolution of the cardiac pacemaker. Legend: Shows the years in the middle from 1958 to 2018. 1958, the wearable pacemaker; 1960, the Chardack-Greatbatch pacemaker; 1986, the Activitrax (activity sensing); 2011, the Revo MRI (MRI compatible); 2016, the Micra Transcather pacing system. (Reprinted from Wen Ko, Peng Wang, Shem Lachhman: Chap. 6 - System integration and packaging. ScienceDirect articles. *Implantable Biomedical Microsystems* 2015, 113–136)

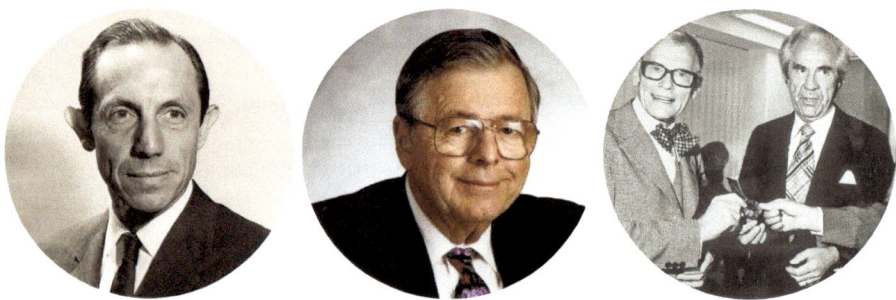

Fig. 21.2 Paul Zoll, Earle Backen, Rune Elmqvist, and Åke Senning. Legend: Dr. Paul Zoll (left), Earle Backen (center), Rune Elmqvist, and Dr. Åke Senning. (Paul Zoll, Source: https://www.zoll.com/about-zoll/dr-paul-zoll. Earle Backen, Source: Courtesy of Medtronic Inc. https://www.massdevice.com/medtronic-founder-bakken-backs-covidien-buy/. Rune Elmqvist and Åke Senning, Source: http://www.medicinhistoriskasyd.se/SMHS_bilder/displayimage.php?album=11&pid=3152)

It was apparent that many patients including children and adults required a permanent pacemaker.

The Implantable Pacemaker

Nineteen fifty-eight was the Year of the Dog in the Chinese calendar. It was also the year when a BOAC Britannia flew London to New York in a record of 7 hours and 57 minutes and Dmitri Shostakovich's Second Piano Concert premiered in New York. *The Bridge on the River Kwai* won the Academy Award for Best Picture, the hula hoop appeared, and a little-known vocal group called The Quarrymen had to pay 17 shillings 6 pence for their first recording (they were later renamed The Beatles).

In medicine, it was the year when the first implantable pacemaker made the news.

At the Karolinska Hospital in Stockholm, Swedish surgeon Åke Senning (1915–2000) and physician-inventor Rune Elmqvist (1906–1996) (Fig. 21.2) developed an implantable pacemaker, one that could reside wholly in the body. The first patient to receive the pacemaker was Arne Larson who suffered from heart block and Stokes-Adams attacks over a 6-month period. Apparently medical treatment consisting of a host of stimulants that included ephedrine, pentymal, atropine, isoprenaline, caffeine, digoxin, and even whisky was tried and failed. Throughout his life, Larsson would have his pacemaker replaced 26 times. He outlived the two physicians who saved him and died of skin cancer on December 28, 2001, at the ripe age of 86.

Undoubtedly the implanted pacemaker was a great accomplishment. Patients wouldn't just wear it, but make it part of their anatomy, and it would greatly reduce the number of infections that an external pacemaker was prone to.

In 1960, 2 years after the operation on Larsson, Dr. Chardack reported the first implant of a permanent pacemaker developed by engineer Wilson Greatbatch (Fig. 21.1) in a 77-year-old man with complete heart block, and in 1961, they reported on a series of 15 patients. Greatbatch later invented the long-life corrosion-free lithium-iodine battery that is used to this day.

In subsequent years, substantial and significant developments occurred in pacemakers. These developments occurred in leads (i.e., wires); battery life; the introduction of steroid-eluting leads, which reduced the risk of inflammation; the use of sensors to detect body movement and accordingly adjust the heart rate up or down (Fig. 21.1); miniaturized, microprocessor-driven pacemakers able to detect and store events using complex algorithms; and MRI compatibility. Home monitoring of pacemakers became possible, and the information could be automatically uploaded to a server via the Internet. Today's pacemakers are way smaller than before, and physicians replace the battery in a brief operation under local anesthesia. Whereas in the past the task of pacemaker insertion and follow-up was the domain of the cardiothoracic surgeon, this function is now entirely that of the heart rhythm expert.

The Future of the Cardiac Pacemaker

Approximately 200,000 pacemakers are implanted yearly in the United States and over 1 million worldwide. In view of an increase in life span and people living longer with cardiovascular diseases, a substantial increase in pacemaker utilization in the future, both in the United States and globally is assured. Indeed, the pacemaker has been a life-giver by dramatically improving the quality of life and survival of patients with heart block, sick sinus syndrome, slow heart rate, and heart failure.

Despite the huge advances in pacemaker technology, over the short and long term, pacemaker-related adverse events occur in nearly one out of ten patients. These untoward complications are related to:

1. Dislodgement, fracture, and insulation brake of leads that are inserted through the venous system. Furthermore, occasionally the leads can perforate the heart and cause venous obstruction.
2. Infection, pocket hematomas due to collection of clotted blood, and skin erosion.

To avoid the abovementioned complications of conventional pacemakers recently, pacemakers without leads called leadless pacemakers (Figs. 21.1 and 21.3) that are inserted directly into the heart chamber have been developed. These pacemakers are very small, just 1 cubic centimeter in volume, and cardiac electrophysiologist places them in the right ventricle through the femoral vein, using a steerable sheath, without any chest incision. At this time, the leadless pacemaker is a single-chamber pacemaker, but research on a dual-chamber system is ongoing. Undoubtedly, the long-term reliability of the leadless pacemaker remains to be determined;

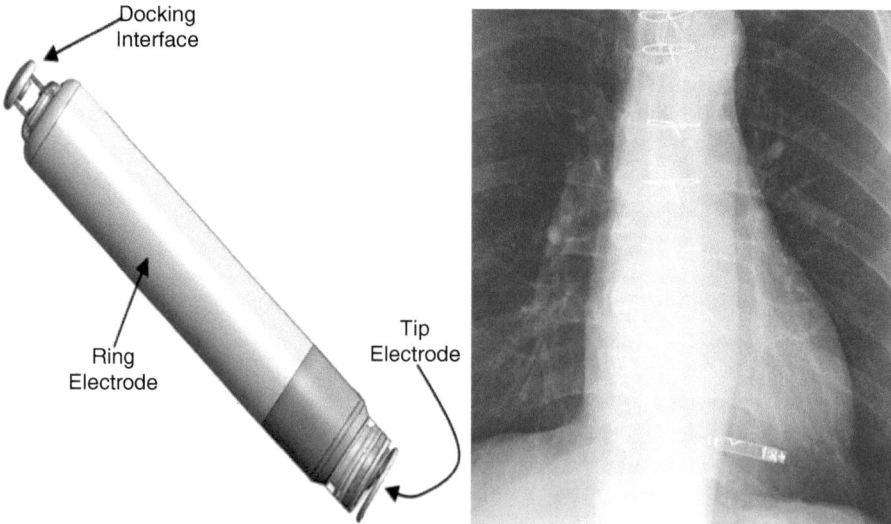

Fig. 21.3 The leadless pacemaker. Legend: The leadless pacemaker (left hand panel) and its position on an X-ray (right hand panel). (Courtesy of Dr. Vivek Y. Reddy)

nonetheless, the leadless pacemaker is a major advance and possibly the future of pacemaker technology.

The Biventricular Pacemaker for Cardiac Resynchronization Therapy (CRT)

There are about five million people who suffer from heart failure in the United States and 26 million worldwide. Half of these people will die within 5 years of diagnosis. Of these five million, approximately 800,000 people have severe heart failure. In most patients, heart failure results from previous heart attacks, cardiomyopathy, disease of the heart valve, and other causes. About one-third of these patients have a blockage in one of the electrical conducting pathways (i.e., the left bundle branch). This blockage results in out-of-sync activation of heart chambers and consequently uncoordinated movement of the right and left chambers resulting in worsening heart failure. In the past, experts in heart failure administered drugs to increase the contractility of the *beaten heart—akin to whipping a donkey carrying an overloaded cart up a hill*—but to no avail. Sophisticated pacemakers, known as biventricular pacemakers capable of simultaneously pacing both chambers of the heart providing synchrony in contraction developed in recent years, have had a dramatic impact in some patients with severe heart failure. However, for a variety of reasons, approximately 1/3 of patients do not respond adequately to CRT. *Patients who are in sinus rhythm and have left bundle branch block with depressed heart function (ejection fraction of less than or equal to 35%), with a QRS duration of ≥150 msec., and with New York functional classes II and III or ambulatory class IV symptoms on optimal medical therapy are ideal candidates for CRT.* Novel methods such as His bundle pacing, left bundle pacing, epicardial and endocardial pacing, and ultrasound-mediated energy transfer utilizing a novel technology—the wise wireless technology for left ventricular pacing—are all under investigation to further improve the results of CRT in heart failure.

Treating Larry

There is no magic cure, no making it all go away forever. There are only small steps upward; an easier day, an unexpected laugh, a mirror that doesn't matter anymore.

—Laurie Halse Anderson, *Wintergirls*

I encountered Larry at a time when CRT had just come in the armamentarium of the heart rhythm expert. He was a young IT engineer who was referred for heart failure. When I examined him, he had some crackles in his lungs and some leg swelling despite being on heart failure medications. I listened to his heart with a stethoscope and heard a soft murmur suggesting that he had a leaky valve due to an enlarged left ventricle.

Fig. 21.4 Diagram of the heart showing lead position for biventricular pacing. Legend: Position 1, pacemaker; position 2, lead in the right atrial appendage; position 3, lead in the right ventricle, and position 4, lead in the lateral branch of the coronary sinus for left ventricular pacing. (Reprinted with permission from Srinivas Iyengar, William T. Abraham; Cardiac Resynchronization Therapy: A Better and Longer Life for Patients With Advanced Heart Failure. Circulation 2005;112:e236-e237)

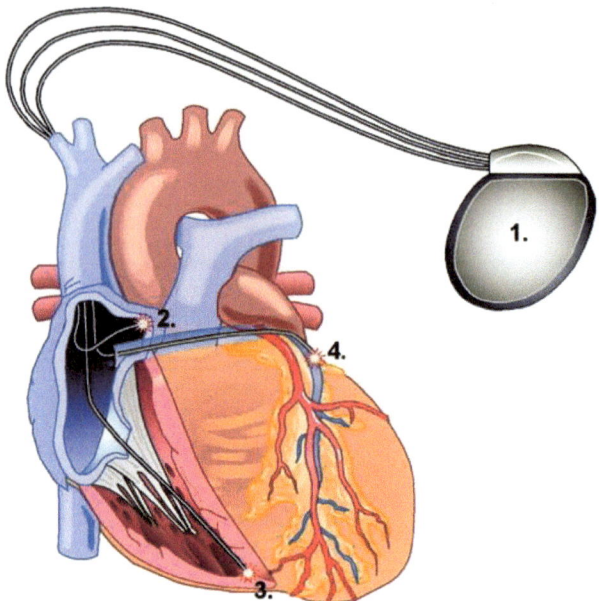

His ECG was most revealing. He had left bundle branch block with a long QRS duration—176 milliseconds—that had recently appeared with the relapse back into heart failure. I explained to him and his wife the two options. One was CRT with a defibrillator (CRT-D). The defibrillator would be there to treat sudden death if it occurred. The other was evaluation for a heart transplant. I stressed that I would proceed with a CRT-D and if there was no significant improvement only then I would refer him to one of my transplant colleagues. They seemed reassured.

A week later, we took him to the lab and inserted a CRT-D (Fig. 21.4). The next day, Larry peed torrentially, so much so that his blood pressure dropped and the swelling in his legs went down. I had to stop the diuretic and give him fluids. In a month or so, Larry's heart function improved to 40%, and within 6 months, it had gone up to 50%.

Larry and Cindy and their two kids have their lives back. CRT had a life-changing impact.

To array a man's will against his sickness is the supreme art of medicine.

—Henry Ward Beecher

♥

Chapter 22
When All Is Said and Done: Waiting for a Heart Transplant

For a dying man it is not a difficult decision to agree to become the world's first heart transplant ... because he knows he is at the end. If a lion chases you to the bank of a river filled with crocodiles, you will leap into the water convinced you have a chance to swim to the other side. But you would not accept such odds if there were no lion.

—Christiaan Barnard

If a man will begin with certainties, he shall end in doubts; but if he will be content to begin with doubts, he shall end in certainties.

—Francis Bacon

The dramatic words on the logic of choice by Dr. Christiaan Barnard (1922–2001), the South African surgeon who performed the first heart transplant on grocer Louis Washkansky in December 1967, resonated deep inside me when I was a medical student. I was stupefied, fascinated, and above all inspired by such a medical feat. At the time, I felt that only man's landing on the moon could equal Dr. Barnard's accomplishment. And like the mysterious moon and its romantic glow that inspired poets and lovers alike over the centuries, the heart, the presumed seat of love, was likewise conquered and replaced. *Newsweek* hailed the Cape Town effort as "the opening of a new era in medicine…an era as significant as the age of the atom."

However, the medical community, particularly in the United States, felt that this achievement was not quite as earth-shattering as the press did. The road to heart transplants had been laid by the pioneering work of French Nobel laureate Alexis Carrel (1873–1944), Frank Mann (1887–1962) and his coworkers, and especially Norman Shumway (1923–2006), Richard Lower (1929–2008), and their associates at Stanford University. Indeed, Dr. Barnard had learned the heart transplant technique while studying with the Stanford group.

Washkansky's fate after the operation attracted voracious media attention. He was a stubborn man who had been dying of heart failure, but he told his wife that he

© The Author(s), under exclusive license to Springer Nature Switzerland AG 2021
J. A. Gomes, *Rhythms of Broken Hearts*,
https://doi.org/10.1007/978-3-030-77382-3_22

was all right even as his condition kept getting worse. He had a good early recovery after the transplant, as reporters closely watched his progress and reported it to the world. He died of pneumonia 18 days later.

The second heart transplant was performed on an infant just 3 days after the first by Dr. Adrian Kantrowitz (1918–2008) and his associates at Maimonides Medical Center in Brooklyn, New York. The child died 6.5 hours later of cardiac arrest. After a second failed attempt, Dr. Kantrowitz left the field. "I'm a surgeon and surgery is what I know," he said. "The problems involved in making this work on a broad basis are not surgical problems, they're immunological problems. I do not bring any special talent to solving those problems."

The third heart transplant patient, Philip Blaiberg, a South African dentist, promptly left the hospital marveling to his wife in the car, "Look, the leaves are so green. The sky is so blue—isn't it beautiful?" He lived 592 days, dying of hepatitis and organ rejection.

The medical world soon realized the perils after the transplant: rejection, opportunistic infections, and damage to the interior walls of the blood vessels resulting in coronary artery disease that could lead to graft failure and death. These complications had a devastating effect on the survival of these patients. We could transplant a heart, which was the easy part. We couldn't keep it beating.

The Story of Cyclosporine

In 1969, Dr. Hans-Peter Frey and his wife took a vacation in Norway. He worked for the pharmaceutical company Sandoz, based in Basel, Switzerland. They rented a car and drove from Oslo toward Bergen, through beautiful Hardangervidda National Park. There, he often stopped to photograph the scenery, and when he did, he scooped soil into a small plastic bag. Sandoz employees often did that when they went on business trips or holidays, since these samples could contain several thousand microorganisms worthy of study. He returned to work with 50 bags.

In one of them, Sandoz found a fungus called *Tolypocladium inflatum*. It is a white mold normally in its asexual state in the ground, but in its sexual state, it becomes a parasite of the scarab beetle. At the microbiology department at Basel, in Z. L. Kis' laboratory, its main metabolite, cyclosporine, was isolated. Ultimately, this discovery would take transplant surgery into the mainstream of medical practice. However, the road to approval proved long and arduous. Until 1976, only the scientists at Sandoz knew about the drug. Finally, in that year, Jean-François Borel and coworkers described it to the outside world in a publication entitled "Biological Effects of Cyclosporin A: A New Antilymphocytic Agent." Cyclosporine, he wrote, not only helps keep the immune system from rejecting foreign transplanted tissue, but it inhibits the chronic inflammation from immune reactions. It might make transplants work.

Dr. Borel described the effects of cyclosporine in person at the April 1976 meeting of the British Society for Immunology. It so happened that in the audience was

Dr. David White from Cambridge, who worked with Sir Roy Y. Calne, who in turn had done transplant research in the early 1960s. Dr. White immediately expressed interest, and Sandoz shipped a supply of the drug to Cambridge, where the first animal experiments outside Sandoz took place.

Meanwhile, company officials were growing wary. They foresaw a small market, since transplants were quite rare, and yet purification and marketing looked expensive. So they proposed to end production. Drs. Calne and White traveled to headquarters in Basel and urged executives not to. They were persuasive enough that the company decided to continue research on the drug, but mainly for the prestige value.

In June 1978, clinical studies were initiated by Dr. Beat von Graffenried from Sandoz with Dr. Calne at Addenbrooke's Hospital, Cambridge, and with Dr. Ray L. Powles, Royal Marsden Hospital, Sutton, in kidney and bone marrow transplant patients, respectively. Dr. Calne began using it for kidney recipients in 1979 but found that in higher doses it caused problems. However, it was discovered that adding prednisone made a much safer anti-immune cocktail. It significantly improved the outcome of heart transplant recipients.

In March 1981, surgeons at Stanford University faced a patient dying of both pulmonary hypertension (lung disease) and heart disease. Heart-lung transplants had occurred before, but nobody had ever lived longer than 23 days, and the FDA had not approved cyclosporine for such operations. The increasingly desperate patient, a former newspaper executive in Arizona, had to rely on her journalist colleagues to canvas political contacts in order to obtain special FDA approval before she died. It came through, and cyclosporine along with conventional immunosuppressive agents was used. She lived 5 more years and did not die from rejection of the tissue. It was the first successful heart-lung transplant.

In 1983, the FDA approved cyclosporine for heart, lung, and kidney transplants.

Not surprisingly, Sandoz officials were wrong about the sales of cyclosporine. For instance, from 1954 and 1973, 10,000 kidney transplants took place worldwide. But in the year 1986 alone, with cyclosporine, almost 9000 kidney transplants were performed just in the United States. By 1994, cyclosporine accounted for over 20% of the company's pharmaceutical sales and 40% of the profits.

Over the next two decades, physicians grew more and more skilled at donor and recipient selection and management of recipients after the transplant. And researchers discovered other immunosuppressive agents. Today, advances in such factors as organ preservation, monitoring of immunosuppressants, immunosuppressive regimens, and control of infections are leading to further improvement in quality of life and survival.

It has been over half a century since the first heart transplant and much has changed. Physicians are now considering older patients and a greater proportion of patients with congenital heart disease. There is also an increase in the number of patients who undergo mechanical circulatory support as a bridge to transplant, and more patients are having re-transplants.

Linda and the Wait

Linda was 47 years old when she suddenly blacked out. She was rushed by ambulance to a neighboring hospital. In the emergency room, she had repeated bouts of ventricular tachycardia for which she had painful electrical shocks delivered to her chest. She was immediately transferred to our institution.

Since she was going in and out of this lethal twister, I started her on intravenous medications, placed her on a respirator, and knocked her out with an anesthetic, after which she stabilized. But that was only the beginning of her tribulations. Just as in patients with cancer, the sword of Damocles hangs over the heads of people with significant heart disease and ventricular tachycardia. An MRI showed that the walls of her heart were infiltrated by sarcoidosis.[1]

My associate, Dr. Winters, and I had previously reported that involvement of the heart by sarcoidosis could be the initial manifestation of the disease and result in sudden cardiac death due to a ventricular tachycardia. In 1991, in an original article in the *Journal of the American College of Cardiology*, we highlighted for the first time the lethal nature of this entity and recommended an implantable defibrillator in such patients. Accordingly, Linda had a defibrillator implanted.

Two years later, she received a "lifesaver shock," for ventricular tachycardia. She told me that it was painful and frightening, and yet the defibrillator gave her confidence. She realized it would be there for her if she had the death-twister again.

Linda had an only daughter who was 12 years old. It affected the girl profoundly. She feared for her mother having witnessed her black out and the terror when the defibrillator shocked her mother who was right in front of her. I understood this fear, had experienced it in my 6-year-old daughter when her mother was sick with cancer. In the case of my daughter, she had asked me one morning, when her mother was sleeping, "Dad, is mummy going to die?" I reassured her that mummy was not going to die. I had not lied to her. My wife had Hodgkin's disease, and I believed that she would be cured. She died a few months later of complications of chemotherapy. The image of my daughter asking me that question has never left me, and I have always wondered whether children in their innocence often have a better perception than adults.

A few months later, Linda was admitted with heart failure. I inserted a special pacemaker that would pace both chambers of the heart, so they would contract at the same time providing synchrony. She felt better with the pacemaker, but I wondered how long she would carry on with a heart that had fallen apart. It was time to

---

[1] Sarcoidosis is a granulomatous disease, that is, one with flattish granular layers atop tissue. Though Jonathan Hutchinson (1828–1913) noted the first case of sarcoid involving the skin, it was Cæsar Boeck (1845–1917), a Norwegian dermatologist, who in 1899 described nodular skin lesions that resembled sarcoma cells, thus the name "sarcoid." Mitchell Bernstein and his team were the first to recognize involvement of the heart in 1929 in a patient with systemic sarcoidosis. In 1952, Warfield Longcope and David Freiman found that the heart was involved in 20% of 92 autopsied sarcoid cases. It most commonly affects the lung, but it can develop in the lymph nodes, eyes, brain, musculoskeletal, renal, and endocrine systems. Its cause remains unknown.

evaluate her for a transplant. She was young, and it could be months or years before she got a heart. As predicted, her heart function would get progressively worse until she was almost bedridden and admitted to the hospital for intravenous medications and placed in the highest category for transplantation.

She waited anxiously. She was one of the lucky ones. After 6 months, she received a new heart.

At the time of penning this chapter, I met her when she had signs of rejection and had been hospitalized for change in medications and a heart biopsy. I asked her what had kept her going.

"I am of the Baptist faith," she said. "I believe that God kept me going. I have a lot of faith in my doctors. I pray for them every day." For a doctor, it is wonderful to hear that one has made a difference in someone's life. It is much more than money can buy. Linda is a happy story, at least for now. The future, no one can tell. But there are many others who were not as lucky; they died suddenly while waiting for a heart, especially before the defibrillator was available. Still others waited for agonizing years and passed away of heart failure.

Transplants Today

Since 1993, the paucity of donor hearts has spurred considerable research into the use of nonhuman hearts. It is now possible to transplant a heart from another species—called a "xenograft"—or implant a man-made heart. However, the outcome of these two options has been less successful than the far more common allografts, from one human to another. Additionally, today we have mechanical devices like the HeartMate III, which will take over the pumping action of the heart. It can provide blood flow to all the vital organs of the body and keep a person alive until a heart is available for transplant or simply maintain the patient for several years. Perhaps, no patient exemplifies its use better than former Vice President Dick Cheney who received one in 2010, when he was near death, with an ejection fraction around 10%. He has readily exhibited the hardware on TV while promoting one of his books, and he wore the device until he received a transplant in 2012.

The prognosis for heart transplant patients after the procedure has risen greatly over the past 20 years. From January 1982 to June 2013, the estimated median survival was 11 years, and the median survival after getting past the first year was 13 years. Because the death rate declines significantly after the first year following a transplant, the survival rate after 1 year gives patients a more realistic expectation.

Carol and the Tetralogy

Unlike cancer, heart disease can be a lifelong challenge, particularly in people born with cardiac abnormalities. Many of them have now survived, and some have lived a rather limited, yet robust life. One such person, named Carol, is 55 years old at this writing, and she has been under my care for almost 29 years. I first saw her when her pediatric cardiologist, Dr. Leonard Steinfeld, the former chief of Pediatric Cardiology, asked me to take over her care when she was admitted with ventricular tachycardia and heart block that had produced shortness of breath and near fainting episodes for which she required a pacemaker.

Carol was born with the heart defect known as tetralogy of Fallot.[2] This is the most common cause of blue baby syndrome. It occurs due to faulty development of the fetal heart during the first 8 weeks of pregnancy.

The condition was described by French physician Etienne-Louis Arthur Fallot (1850–1911) as the "maladie bleue" in a classic 1888 paper, and though he fully acknowledged his predecessors, his name became attached to it. Fallot himself died, as a friend said, "after a period of purifying loneliness," and since he forbade any eulogy of himself, we know relatively little of his life.

With the arrival of X-rays, it became much easier to diagnose this disease, since the heart's boot-like appearance (*coeur en sabot*) stands out clearly. Nowadays, we diagnose congenital heart defects with echocardiography, which is quick and very specific, involves no radiation, and can be done prenatally.

The tetralogy was thought untreatable until 1944, when surgeon Alfred Blalock (1899–1964), cardiologist Helen B. Taussig (1898–1986), and surgical technician Vivien Thomas (1910–1985) at Johns Hopkins University Hospital developed a palliative surgical procedure. Intriguingly, Thomas was an African American in a prestigious institution in an era when the only other blacks were janitors, and he attracted startled looks as he strode the halls in his white lab coat.

Tetralogy of Fallot is a complex defect, and it resisted total repair until 1954, when a team led by the brilliant and flamboyant Dr. Walton Lillehei (1918–1999) achieved it in an 11-year-old boy. At first the operation had a high mortality rate, but from 1981 on, total repair in infants has had success, with a comparatively low mortality.

Carol had her initial surgery at the age of 6 months by Dr. Robert Litwak (1925–2013), a rather gregarious, verbose, but courteous surgeon and then chief of Cardiothoracic Surgery at the Mount Sinai Hospital. He established the heart surgery program at the hospital. He was also an accomplished jazz drummer who once played in the Benny Goodman Band. I knew him well and often took care of his

---

[2]It classically involves four abnormalities, hence "tetralogy. These include (1) ventricular septal defect, that is, a hole in the wall between the ventricles; (2) a narrowing of the right ventricular outflow tract just below the valve, which reduces blood flow to the lungs; (3) an "overriding aorta," in which the main artery sits right above the hole in the wall and takes unoxygenated blood straight from the right ventricle; and, because of the first three, (4) hypertrophy or thickening of the walls of the right ventricle of the heart. Notably, of the four abnormalities, only three are always present.

musician friends with heart rhythm problems. I distinctly remember Christmas holiday parties where he performed with his jazz troupe.

It so happened that little Carol suffered a cardiac arrest after the palliative surgery and was lucky to have survived. Dr. Litwak did corrective surgery again when she was 5, but she apparently remained weak, short of breath, in need of oxygen, and mostly wheelchair-bound. She says that she remained hospitalized for 7 years. She was allowed to go home on some weekends and for Christmas. This is rather amazing and in today's day and age virtually unbelievable. But in those days, patients with heart attacks were hospitalized for weeks, as well as those with cardiomyopathy due to alcoholism or a virus for a 6-month stretch. I wonder what the bill was for a 7-year hospitalization and who paid it.

I called Dr. Steinfeld, who I knew very well and who had retired recently after an exceptional career. "I thought she was going to die," said Dr. Steinfeld. "It is amazing that she's still alive and well."

Surprisingly her life changed for the better after she went home. She was admitted to third grade in a public school. She played volleyball, jumped rope, and even ran track. She met her husband-to-be when she was 15, married at 20, and had three children. But in her third pregnancy, she developed syncope due to heart block and ventricular tachycardia. Subsequently, her course was downhill: she developed heart failure.

I decided to ask my colleague to evaluate her for a transplant about 8 years ago when she was 46. During Carol's evaluation for a heart transplant, mammography revealed a breast tumor which turned out to be malignant, though without any metastasis. She had a mastectomy and has remained free of cancer. Recently, Carol was operated upon for a pulmonary valve replacement, after which her heart function improved substantially. She remains in compensated heart failure on the transplant list for now. She and her doctors know that her condition will not stay stable for the rest of her life.

"I'm at peace with myself. Let God do his work," she said. "I don't want to be lingering on machines, in pain, my family suffering. I try to be pleasant."

I asked her what has kept her going for all these years. She has lived with disease all her life since birth. Her answer was simple: her faith. Despite her limitations, she is very involved in church activities, which include feeding the homeless, caring for the sick, and providing advice for her community. Despite her bad luck at birth, she's fortunate to have a supportive husband of 35 years. And she had advice to give: "One needs something to smile or laugh about, irrespective. That's half the battle."

I saluted her: *Namaste*!

I remembered a wonderful passage I read many years ago in *The Snow Leopard* by Peter Matthiessen, who, while travelling in the Himalayas after the death of his wife from cancer, saw a child crawling up a hill dragging bent useless legs. She pulled herself up like a broken cricket, her nose to the stones, with cow dung, and muddy trickles. "I long to give her something—a new life?—yet I'm afraid to temper with such dignity," he writes. "And so I smile as best I can, and say: *Namaste!*" "Good morning!" How absurd. And her voice follows as we go away, a small clear smiling voice,—"*Namaste!*"—a Sanskrit word for greeting and parting, which means, "I salute you!"

One feels a sense of pity and utter helplessness for the deformed child that Peter Matthiessen encountered on the rugged snow-capped slopes of the Himalayas and for Carol, I encountered in the clinic, notwithstanding their exemplary dignity and will to survive.

♥

Part VIII
The Quest to Overcome Heart Attacks

Chapter 23
Of Bypasses and Clot Busters

> *What is wanted is not the will to believe, but the will to find out, which is the exact opposite.*
>
> —Bertrand Russell

> *Scientists have become the bearers of the torch of discovery in our quest for knowledge.*
>
> —Stephen Hawking

You might wonder why I'm writing about coronary artery disease (CAD) and heart attacks when the book is mostly about heart rhythm disorders. The answer is that most lethal ventricular arrhythmias and sudden cardiac death (SCD) are the result of CAD and its consequences: heart attacks, diminished heart function, and heart failure.

"Atherosclerosis" comes from the Greek words *athera* or "porridge" and *sklerosis* or "hardening." It is a condition wherein fat is deposited in the arteries, causing CAD and peripheral vascular disease (PVD). It can affect the arterial system throughout the body including that of the brain and kidneys. The critical biochemical event in atherosclerosis is the deposition of apolipoprotein-B (apoB) containing lipoproteins within the wall of an artery. This process leads to local responses that result in an accumulation of macrophages[1] that consume the retained lipoproteins. Unfortunately, these macrophages fail to emigrate from the site and are intricately involved in the formation of atheromatous plaques. These plaques can ultimately lead to heart attacks. But the workings of this process have long been elusive. And yet, the quest to save people from heart attacks has been rather dramatic.

---

[1] A large mobile white blood cell that is capable of locating microscopic foreign bodies, cellular debris, microbes, cancer cells, etc. and to engulf and digest them by a process of phagocytosis.

© The Author(s), under exclusive license to Springer Nature Switzerland AG 2021
J. A. Gomes, *Rhythms of Broken Hearts*,
https://doi.org/10.1007/978-3-030-77382-3_23

The Heart Surgeon and the Bypass

What could doctors do when the heart vessels get blocked? If a landslide blocks a road, you can create a detour around it, or if the situation is bad, just create a new road. Heart surgeons tried the same approach. It is called "revascularization," essentially "re-vesseling" the heart. The first attempt at revascularization in patients with CAD and angina was performed as early as 1945 by Dr. Arthur M. Vineberg (1903–1988) of Canada, whose own father had died of CAD. He sutured the artery that normally supplies the left front chest wall and breast, called the "left internal mammary artery," into the heart muscle itself. This relief-from-elsewhere strategy became known as the Vineberg procedure. It kept one of his first patients alive for another 10 years and seemed to have promise. However, it did not gain wide acceptance. Dr. Charles Friedberg, chief of the Division of Cardiology at the Mount Sinai Hospital in New York City and the editor of the prestigious *Circulation*, the journal of the American Heart Association—whose office I would occupy in 1984—opposed heart surgery. He was the author of the one and only American textbook of cardiology of the times and a much sought-after consultant, whose opinion was greatly valued. He depicted heart surgeons as knife-happy: "If the heart has a hole in it, they want to close it, if the heart doesn't have a hole they make one." As a result of such opposition, Vineberg's technique remained largely confined to his own institution, though it slowly grew more common over time. Dr. Charles Friedberg died in 1972, after he met with a car accident as he was returning after a consultation in Upstate, New York.

The next advancement came from a man who lived through the horror of the 872-day Siege of Leningrad, where one million Russians died. Dr. Vasilii I. Kolesov (1904–1992) almost perished in the blockade. He lived in a room in the hospital basement and did elective surgery at night, and during one operation, a bomb fragment barely missed his head. After the war, he focused on the heart. He knew that Dr. Vineberg had sutured the mammary artery into the heart muscle itself, the part that contracts. But it would clearly be better to feed it straight into the coronary artery, and in 1964, he linked the blood vessel in the first successful coronary artery bypass graft. Some have heralded this moment as the dawn of modern coronary surgery. Yet, in 1967, when he first published his results in English, the journal prefaced his article with this caution: "The opinions concerning the management and surgical treatment of angina pectoris as expressed in this paper by Professor V.I. Kolesov are at variance with the concepts of many surgeons in the United States." His work did not gain wide acceptance in either the USSR or the United States, until Dr. René Favaloro (1923–2000, Fig. 23.1) burst into the scene.

Dr. Favaloro was an Argentinian who had spent many years as a country surgeon in the Pampas. He came to the United States, and after some creative research in the animal laboratory, in May 1967, he introduced the bypass grafting procedure in humans, at the Cleveland Clinic, in Cleveland, Ohio. His new technique used a saphenous vein—the longest vein in the body, running the whole length of the leg.

Fig. 23.1 Dr. Rene
Favaloro. (https://en.
wikipedia.org/wiki/
René_Favaloro)

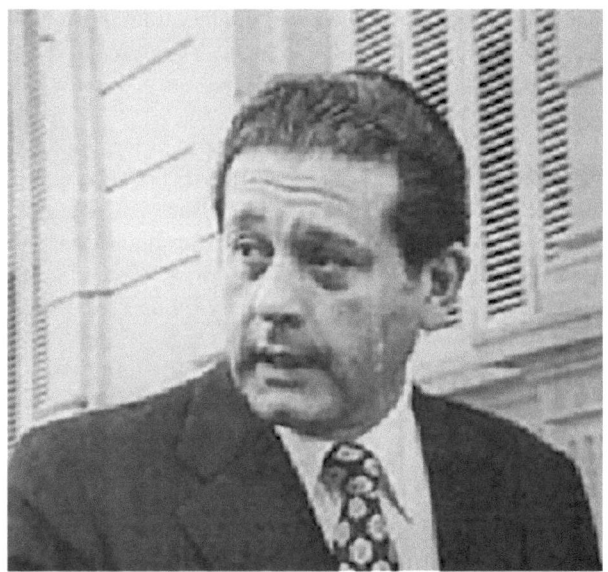

He took a segment of this vessel and used it to replace a partly blocked segment of
the right coronary artery. If a water pipe becomes obstructed, one strategy is simply
to replace the clogged section of pipe with a new one, and that's essentially what he
did. But you can also build a detour around the block: a bypass. Later, Dr. Favaloro
successfully used the leg vein to bypass a partly obstructed coronary artery, and that
has become the typical coronary artery bypass graft (CABG, pronounced "cab-
bage") technique.

I met Dr. Favaloro when I visited Argentina in 1988 to lecture at their Federation
of Cardiology National Meeting in Salta, at the foothills of the Andes, about
3780 feet above sea level. One evening, before our excursion to the Andean mountain range, the Argentinian hosts took us to a Flamenco restaurant frequented by
gauchos, the famed Argentine cowboys. At our table sat Dr. Favaloro and by his side
a gaucho who was totally charmed by my name and flabbergasted to learn that having been born in India I could speak Spanish. He was at a loss when I told him that
I came from Goa, a Portuguese colony for 451 years. He seemed to have heard of
Gandhi and kept on calling me Gomes-Gandhi. He offered me his knife, which he
carried on his belt. I politely told him that he did not have to part with his knife, but
that was not his intention. Dr. Favaloro explained to me that the gauchos carry their
own knives to carve their steaks, and he had offered his knife for me to carve mine.
René also told me that it was an honor to be offered a knife by a gaucho. And so, I
carved my succulent Pampas steak with the sharp gaucho knife.

I felt privileged to meet Favaloro, a tall, distinctive man with a flamboyant
personality and an assertive tone of voice. This pioneer of heart surgery had
rejected several highly lucrative positions and returned to Argentina to steamroll

his pet project, the Favaloro Foundation in Buenos Aires, committed to basic research, education, and excellence in the practice of cardiovascular medicine. He was an acknowledged legend not only in South and North America but also universally.

Unfortunately, he met a tragic end. In December of 1999, Argentina's economy collapsed (a not uncommon event in this country), and the president-elect, Fernando de la Rúa, promised to save the nation with massive spending cuts. The Favaloro Foundation, which depended on government grants, fell in debt of millions of dollars. Favaloro sought relief but all doors were closed. This heart surgeon, who had performed coronary bypass surgery on nearly 15,000 patients, said that he felt like a beggar in his own country.

He closed his bathroom door and rather dramatically shot himself in the heart on July 29, 2000. When his suicide note was released many years later, it was reported that his death was not just a response to his debts, but also an act of protest against corruption in Argentina's medical system. In a letter, he wrote before his death, he stated that the Foundation had a commitment to provide care to hundreds of poor patients free of charge. He lamented that now, at his age, he couldn't discard the ethical principles that distinguished him throughout his life. "I can't change, I would rather disappear," he wrote. When I look back at my encounter with Favaloro on that night in the Flamenco restaurant, together with my wife Marina and my daughter Tanya, where we chatted and ate and drank and danced the night away, he came across as a passionate man who strongly believed in his lofty ideals. Fortunately, his nephew now runs the Foundation, and it is again a viable and successful entity.

Soon after Dr. Favaloro's pioneering work with saphenous veins, others made further advances. Dr. Dudley Johnson extended the bypass to include left coronary arterial systems, while New York heart surgeon Dr. George Green figured that an artery would work better than a vein for artery bypasses and successfully used the internal mammary artery akin to what Russian surgeon Kolesov had done. However, these innovative and breathtaking procedures were limited to a few major centers and were not as popular as today. Like Charles Friedberg, Dr. George Burch—New Orleans cardiologist and editor of the *American Heart Journal*—disliked innovation and growled, "If you were offered an anti-anginal pill that cost $10,000 and had a 5% chance of killing you, would you take it? Of course not. Well, that's bypass surgery."

And so, in medicine as in technology and science, the breakthrough is a glorious moment and the spread to general use is a much slower, subtler, and a more pedestrian process. But it happened, and the consequences were enormous. In 1996, surgeons in the United States performed some 600,000 bypass operations, though by 2012, the number had fallen to around 300,000.

The Discovery of Thrombosis in Acute Myocardial Infarction

In the 1970s, most if not all cardiologists believed that progressive narrowing (stenosis) of the coronary artery, causing symptoms of angina pectoris,[2] would ultimately result in an acute myocardial infarction.[3] British physician Dr. William Heberden (1710–1801) first named the condition as "angina pectoris" and described the entity as far back as 1772: "They who are afflicted with it, are seized while they are walking, (more especially if it be up hill, and soon after eating) with a painful and most disagreeable sensation in the breast, which seems as if it would extinguish life, if it were to increase or continue; but the moment they stand still, all this uneasiness vanishes." He added: "The seat of it, and sense of strangling, and anxiety with which it is attended, may make it not improperly be called angina pectoris."

That "most disagreeable sensation" is due to insufficient blood reaching the heart muscle, and cardiologists in the 1970s believed the cause was progressive narrowing (stenosis) of the coronary artery. Hence, they thought angina would ultimately result in a heart attack, called more precisely an acute myocardial infarction (AMI). (An "infarction" is a blockage, from the Latin verb *farcire*, to stuff. So, AMI = "urgent heart muscle blockage.") Although autopsy studies and coronary bypass surgery often revealed a clot—a thrombus—in the coronary artery, everyone thought thrombosis was a secondary factor, one that appeared after the heart attack.

In a groundbreaking study, Dr. Marcus DeWood and his associates published an article in 1980 in *The New England Journal of Medicine* refuting this concept. They demonstrated that AMI was due to the formation of a blood clot or thrombosis that was found in 87% of their patients with heart attacks. Subsequently, in 1988, Dr. John Ambrose and his coworkers from our institution showed that AMI often occurred from previous non-severe blockage of an artery.

These observations were revolutionary and would change the management of heart attacks for years to come. The demonstration that acute thrombosis was the cause of heart attacks saw a monumental shift—from the narrowed coronary artery, our attention shifted to the thrombus (i.e., blood clot).

It has been demonstrated that there is a *vulnerable soft plaque*, which when it ruptures sets up a cascading blood clotting process that results in thrombosis and myocardial infarction. Indeed, the reader might have heard and even encountered an individual who only a couple of weeks back had been given a clean bill of health by his cardiologist after his exercise test was negative for CAD. Three weeks later, the individual dropped dead from a heart attack. The man, possibly, had a nonsignificant narrowing of his coronary artery that would not show a "demand/supply" ischemia" during an exercise test. However, his left anterior descending coronary artery likely had a soft, ulcerated plaque, which ruptured and set up a process of

---

[2] Chest pain due to a lack of blood supply to the heart muscle. The pain is often described as dull, pressure-like, or squeezing. It occurs on exertion but can occur at rest. It can be relieved with rest and nitroglycerine.

[3] Heart attack.

thrombosis (akin to what happens when we cut ourselves accidentally), that resulted in a total occlusion of the artery, resulting in a heart attack, that was followed within minutes by ventricular fibrillation and death—a rather tragic event in an otherwise healthy individual.

The Clot Busters

Until the late 1970s, the treatment of AMI was mostly palliative. The introduction of coronary care units (CCU) in 1961 brought down the early mortality rate; however, a more effective method to treat AMI directed at its root cause was needed. The demonstration that acute thrombosis was the cause of heart attacks saw a monumental shift in management. "Dissolve the clot" was the call to action!

The Bug and the Clot Buster

Dr. William Smith Tillett (1892–1974) was a man who believed that chance plays a big role in our lives. It had in his own, giving him pleasant breaks throughout his career, and it would smile on him again at the critical moment of his professional life. Indeed, his discovery occurred through sheer serendipity not unlike the discovery of penicillin and a host of other drugs in medicine. Louis Pasteur's famous saying readily applied to Tillett: "Chance favors the prepared mind."

In 1933, he observed that the bacteria streptococci dissolved clots. At the time he was Director of the Biological Division at Johns Hopkins University. He reasoned that the bacteria had to be making something that dissolved the clots. We call such dissolution "lysis," a term echoed in the household cleaner Lysol. In the same year, he and R.L. Garner isolated the critical chemical in stable form and showed that it was an enzyme. They called it fibrinolysin, a reasonable enough name, except that this substance did not actually dissolve clots. It woke up a second, slumbering enzyme, which then performed the task. Hence, in 1945, Drs. L.R. Christensen and Colin MacLeod renamed it streptokinase. "Strepto" is a nod to the bug and "kinase" refers to its enzyme family.

Over the next decade, Drs. William Smith Tillett and Sol Sherry undertook trials of streptokinase on patients with various illnesses. In 1955, Tillett's group showed that clot lysis or dissolution was possible in patients who received intravenous streptokinase. Later, Sherry's group performed studies of intravenous streptokinase for the treatment of AMI patients. The infusion of the drug for prolonged periods after AMI resulted in significant lower mortality in patients who had received the drug, in comparison with other modalities of treatments. Except for the development of hemorrhage in a few patients and pyrogenic[4] reactions, there were no significant complications. This proved that streptokinase infusion via the intravenous route was a promising therapeutic approach in AMI. After the success of Sherry and coworkers, the idea of using fibrinolytic agents in the treatment of coronary thrombosis assumed importance especially since there was no drug available that could actually improve the prognosis after AMI.

In 1959, Ruegsegger and colleagues, with the use of serial coronary arteriography, showed dissolution of intracoronary clots for the first time in isolated segments of coronary artery in animals following administration of streptokinase. Another significant finding was that *the heart muscle could not be saved from death if more than a few hours passed between clotting and lysis but the area of infarction was comparatively smaller than that in the control animals.*

Despite these initial successes, in 1960, Lederle Laboratories abandoned further production of streptokinase because the company had failed to produce preparations that had a low incidence of pyrogenic reactions. However, European pharmaceutical firms rescued the drug. As American cardiologists focused their attention on another clot buster, urokinase, further research into streptokinase passed into the hands of scientists in Europe and Australia.

In 1979, the *European Cooperative Study Group for Streptokinase Treatment in Acute Myocardial Infarction* published results of a trial involving 2388 patients. Within 6 months of streptokinase therapy after AMI, the all-cause mortality rate was 15.6% in the streptokinase group and 30.6% in the control group. Twice as many people were dying without the drug. Still, these results did not lead to practice guidelines.

In the mid-1980s, a large number of small clinical trials reported that when physicians infused streptokinase within 1.5 to 3 hours of AMI, they achieved 90% rates of vessel clearing and refilling (reperfusion). Finally, in 1986, a large multicenter landmark Italian trial called GISSI (*Gruppo Italiano per la Sperimentazione della Streptochinasi nell'Infarto Miocardico*) of 11,806 patients in 176 CCUs solidly established the role of streptokinase therapy in AMI.

But by then, the drug had competition.

The Story of Tissue Plasminogen Activator (t-PA—Activase)

Physicians had already begun searching for a drug with fewer reactions. In Belgium, in the late 1970s, Dr. Désiré Collen using cells from human melanoma cancers purified an agent, tissue plasminogen activator (t-PA), that could dissolve clots. Genentech, a startup company at the time in South San Francisco, collaborated with Dr. Collen's group and subsequently ended up manufacturing the drug

---

[4] Drug-induced fever.

after successfully cloning the gene that expressed t-PA. Using cells derived from a Chinese hamster ovary in 1982, they managed to manufacture commercial quantities of the drug, and by 1987, the drug received FDA approval. Genentech called the drug Activase, though physicians also refer to it as t-PA for "tissue plasminogen activator."

Large multicenter trials such as GUSTO (*Global Utilization of Streptokinase and Tissue Plasminogen Activator for Occluded Coronary Arteries*), GISSI -2 (*Gruppo Italiano per lo Studio della Sopravvivenza nell'Infarto Miocardico*), and ISIS-3 (*Third International Study of Infarct Survival Collaborative Group*) compared the efficacy of t-PA with that of streptokinase. They found no significant difference in mortality rates after 30–60 days between the two drugs; however, GUSTO showed a better 1-year survival for t-PA as compared to streptokinase. An American consensus developed that t-PA was probably better in patients who were younger, presented earlier, had anterior infarctions, or had received streptokinase for a previous AMI.

A controversy soon raged between European and American cardiologists as to which drug was better, streptokinase or t-PA. The Europeans preferred streptokinase, while the Americans favored t-PA, though it was ten times more expensive.

The use of clot-dissolving drugs, called "clot busters," in lay terminology had a tremendous impact in patients with AMI. Whereas, prior to the widespread use of thrombolysis, we were busy managing patients with massive infarcts with recurrent ventricular tachycardia, heart block, and cardiogenic shock in our CCUs, gradually these challenging and lethal complications of AMI slowly but surely began to decrease in frequency, and the slogan "Save the myocardium" had come full circle. But that was not the end of the story!

♥

Chapter 24
A Riveting New Era: The Birth of Interventional Cardiology

Discovery is seeing what everybody else has seen and thinking what nobody else has thought.

—Albert Szent-Gyorgyi

Imagination is more important than knowledge. Knowledge is limited. Imagination encircles the world.

—Albert Einstein

Hardly had cardiologists begun to administer clot-dissolving drugs to patients with AMI when the field took an abrupt turn. A new field of balloon angioplasty of the coronary arteries appeared on the horizon pioneered by Dr. Andreas Roland Grüntzig.

Balloons in the Bloodstream

Andreas Roland Grüntzig was born on June 25, 1939, in Dresden, Germany, the "Florence of the North," a city on the River Elbe renowned for its beautiful Gothic cathedrals, opera house, and palaces—a city of high culture. Wary of the looming war, his family moved to Rochlitz, a small town about 60 miles away. His father, Dr. Willmar Grüntzig, served as a meteorologist in the Luftwaffe and went missing in action. At the end of the war, the village escaped the massive British and American bombardment of Dresden that killed 25,000 people, destroyed 75,000 homes, and turned the city into rubble.

On April 14, 1945, the 6th Armored Division of the US Army led by General George Patton approached the bridge to Rochlitz. The house where the Grüntzigs lived was occupied by the American regimental brass and became the headquarters of the American occupation of Rochlitz.

J. A. Gomes, *Rhythms of Broken Hearts*, https://doi.org/10.1007/978-3-030-77382-3_24

Young Andreas, his brother Johannes, and his mother Charlotta, a teacher and a pianist, moved to Leipzig and struggled to survive, sometimes scouting for mushrooms in the forest for food. In 1950, Charlotta with her two sons moved to Argentina, to the home of an uncle, but homesick for the cultural past of Leipzig, and concerned about her children's education, she returned to East Germany with her two boys in 1952. Andreas enrolled in the Thomas Gymnasium in Leipzig, where he excelled. Founded in 1212, it was the oldest classical high school in Germany, a place where Johann Sebastian Bach had directed its now world-famous St. Thomas Boys Choir.

In 1958, Andreas and his brother fled the repressive communist regime and settled in Heidelberg in West Germany. He obtained his medical degree in 1964 from Heidelberg University and specialized in radiology. In 1969, he started working as a clinical fellow at a hospital in Darmstadt, Germany, that specialized in vascular medicine. It was here that a patient asked him whether it was possible to clean his obstructed arteries the way a plumber cleans tubes with wires and brushes. Grüntzig found this idea fascinating. At that moment, he later said, he began to develop his theories about intervening directly on the blood vessels.

Dr. Robert Hegglin (1907–1969) soon recruited Grüntzig to join the Medical Polyclinic at the Kantonsspital of the University of Zurich, Switzerland. There, he heard of Oregon physician Charles Dotter (1920–1985), the father of interventional radiology. Dr. Dotter was a compelling speaker willing to try new solutions and so dismissive of convention that some called him "Crazy Charlie." He had devised his own "trademark," a crossed pipe and wrench, because "if a plumber can do it to pipes, we can do it to blood vessels." And in that spirit, he developed a method of opening blocked peripheral arteries with a catheter.

Intrigued, Grüntzig went to Nuremberg to learn "Dottering," and back in Zurich, he performed Dotter's angioplasty in several patients. He used a catheter to ram open the artery that caused calf pain known as claudication, as well as to help leg gangrene. However, the technique had hazards. It risked dislodging plaques and debris that could block vessels distally.

Dotter had also conceived of another technique. What if you put a balloon on the tip of a catheter, push it into the narrowed artery, inflate it, and press the obstruction back into the wall? That approach wouldn't dislodge anything. He attempted it, but couldn't find a balloon rigid enough to work. For him, it was a dead end.

Grüntzig thought otherwise. He obsessed about it and went to work at night on his kitchen table with his assistant Maria Schlumpf—whom his biographer called his muse—and he also included her husband, as well as his own wife, Michaela, in his quest. His daughter Sonja, who ate meals at that table, joked that she was the "twin" of the device.

During this period in his life, Grüntzig worked hard and played hard, racing in his motor scooter at dizzying speeds from his home to the hospital. He loved speed and a fast-paced life. He learned to pilot aircraft, first a Piper Club and then a Cessna. He was mesmerized winging over the long expanse of Lake Zurich with the Alps in the background.

He persisted with the balloon, while others sneered and told him he was in essence trying to throw a rock to the moon. "He had the 'sacred fire,' as the French call it," recalled cardiac surgeon Marco Turina. "It was what he thought about constantly. I have never seen somebody so centered on a single idea like Andreas was. Never in my life. Everyone was telling him his idea would never work, and had been tried before, and that he was going to fail, that there were pitfalls at every turn. But the idea was consuming him all the time." Clearly, those who think outside the box, those who take risks, whether in the arts or the sciences, turn out to be the innovators and earth shakers.

In Zurich, while others laughed or ridiculed his ideas or thought them impossible to accomplish, the world-renown pioneering cardiac surgeon of Swedish origin, Åke Senning of pacemaker and open heart surgery fame, fully supported Andreas' research. When Andreas approached him one day and asked whether he could count on his support, Senning answered:

> Herr Grüntzig, Sie werden mir die Patienten wegnehmen, aber legen sie los!
> (Mr. Grüntzig, you will be taking away my patients, but get started right away!)

The critics were right that the balloon posed many challenges. It had to keep its shape under high pressure and deliver enough force to the vessel wall. Grüntzig tried a host of substances like latex and rubber attachment to the end of a catheter and was met with failure. He spent several years contacting a host of manufacturers until he met Professor Hopf, a retired chemist who introduced him to polyvinyl chloride (PVC) compounds. After many trials and failures in his kitchen laboratory, with the assistance of engineer Helmut Schmid, he finally came up with a double lumen balloon catheter that could retain its shape at high pressures, as well as deliver substantial force to the vessel wall. He rushed to the animal lab and conducted his experiments in dogs.

Gradually, he began experimenting with the balloon catheter in the coronary arteries of dogs. The balloon catheter worked. After much experimentation, he was ready for primetime, at least that's what he thought.

He came to the United States for the first time in 1976, for the 49th Scientific Sessions of the American Heart Association, held in Miami. I myself attended as a young fellow and presented my findings on heart function using the new field of cardiac ultrasound. I had a packed house as I showed that drugs which widen the blood vessels—vasodilators—improve the ejection fraction in heart failure patients. Dr. Harvey Feigenbaum, one of the pioneers of cardiac ultrasound, chaired the session. During the Q&A, he gave me a hard time for using single-plane echocardiography—the only method available at the time—but science moves forward through tough questioning, and at lunchtime, he came to my table and congratulated me on the presentation.

Dr. Grüntzig didn't give a presentation. He had just a poster display of his work on dogs. Unfortunately, I wasn't aware of his poster—cardiac catheterization was not my interest at the time—and I later heard that many cardiologists passed by his display with no interest whatsoever. However, Dr. Richard Myler from San Francisco was awed by the balloon technique and enthusiasm of the young German. Unlike others, he listened and realized the approach had a future.

Grüntzig wished to initially try the balloon on patients during open heart bypass surgery, and he approached several heart surgeons. Those in Zurich had politely declined. But Dr. Elias Hanna, who worked with Dr. Myler, agreed, and a year later, in May 1977 in San Francisco, Grüntzig successfully performed the first coronary angioplasty in a human during open heart coronary bypass surgery.

Back in Zurich, he was anxious to perform the procedure with a catheter. He just needed a suitable patient. After a lengthy search, in September 1977, he found Adolph Bachmann. Bachmann was a 37-year-old businessman with severe angina pectoris due to a critical obstruction of his left anterior descending coronary artery. He was recommended to undergo coronary bypass surgery. Dr. Bernhard Meier, who was caring for the patient, informed Grüntzig of this possible candidate, and the two approached Bachmann. Grüntzig told him that he would be the first man in the world to have the procedure without opening his chest and mentioned that emergent bypass surgery would be available if the procedure failed or a complication arose. Without hesitation, Bachmann agreed.

But nothing is as simple as it seems.

On September 16, 1977, orderlies wheeled the conscious but sedated Bachmann to the cath. lab. A dozen or so doctors were watching with fear and expectation. Heart surgeons stood ready to crack the chest if an emergency occurred. Outwardly, Grüntzig remained calm. First, he tested the balloon. It wouldn't inflate. He tore open another sterile package. The second one wouldn't inflate either. He saw his dream pale. Finally, the third balloon worked.

After infiltrating Bachmann's groin with an anesthetic, Grüntzig, with Maria Schlumpf by his side, punctured the femoral artery and slipped a wire up and through the aorta into the mouth of the diseased coronary artery. Over the wire, he slid his catheter. He injected dye to outline the artery and the large, partial blockage. Then he pushed the wire through the tiny opening at the obstruction site and advanced the catheter over the wire. He had put the balloon in place.

He was now in unknown territory. The tension in the lab was running high.

He inflated the balloon to two atmospheric pressures and then to five. He kept the balloon inflated for around 15 seconds. Blood flow in the vessel completely ceased.

Then he deflated the balloon. The coronary pressure beyond it rose, suggesting that much more blood was flowing through. He inflated the balloon a second time and released it.

The on-looking cardiologists, radiologists, and surgeons expected complications—a heart attack, ventricular fibrillation, cardiogenic shock—but nothing of the sort happened.

Injection of the dye showed that the artery stayed open. The procedure was an amazing success.

History was made!

"Every observer was impressed with the simplicity of the method," Grüntzig later recalled, "and I began to realize that my dream had become true."

Bachmann's angina disappeared, and he came off all medication. Twenty years later, he was still alive, and his coronary artery was fine. It was a monumental achievement. If not for the procedure, Bachmann would have required open heart surgery which meant that his chest would have to be cracked, his sternal bone cut with an electrical saw, his body put on cardiopulmonary bypass, his heart stopped, a vein harvested from his groin area for the bypass, and later his sternal bone put back with metallic stitches. He'd then need weeks and even months to recover. Not surprisingly, Bachmann was ecstatic.

After this success, Grüntzig enthusiastically improved the technique. When the time came for the 50th Scientific Sessions of the American Heart Association, he was invited to give a full presentation. He began describing his first few angioplasty patients. When he showed the slide of the fourth one successfully treated, the audience started applauding, and he almost couldn't proceed with the presentation. This was in sharp contrast to the reception that another pioneer, Dr. Michel Mirowski, received.

Soon, interest in angioplasty would overtake the United States. The first cases were performed simultaneously in March 1978 by Drs. Myler in San Francisco and Simon Stertzer in New York, a physician who in 2001 attracted news stories by purchasing a Las Vegas strip club to fund his research.

Grüntzig started a televised closed circuit course, the first of its kind, during which he demonstrated a series of cases. Twenty-eight physicians attended the first of these courses.

At the last course in Zurich in August 1980, Grüntzig invited Dotter, Mason Sones, and Melvin Judkins, the past pioneers of angioplasty and coronary angiography. They dined on a final spaghetti dinner high on a mountaintop above Lake Zurich, and after many glasses of wine, Grüntzig passed torches to everyone, first to the old pioneers and then to others. The lighting of the Olympic torch was an ancient Greek custom commemorating the theft of fire by Prometheus and the gift to humanity, and here it symbolized gifts for future generations.

Science knows no country, because knowledge belongs to humanity, and is the torch which illuminates the world.

—Louis Pasteur

Frustrated with the bureaucratic limitations on his career in Zurich, Grüntzig sought to move to the United States. After offers from a host of American institutions, including the renowned Cleveland Clinic, he joined the faculty of Emory University School in metropolitan Atlanta, then flush with a $105 million gift from Atlanta's Coca-Cola Co. He was made a full professor and director of Interventional Cardiovascular Medicine in late 1980, and classified as a "national treasure," he received automatic US citizenship in the same year. Even before his arrival in the United States, he had been instrumental in setting up the National Heart, Lung, and Blood Institute registry, soon joined by American investigators and industry.

The strikingly handsome, passionate, vibrant Andreas, described by one of his nurses, as an alchemist's version of Clark Gable, Errol Flynn, and Omar Sheriff, would become a sought- after celebrity, and with it came riches. He worked hard and began playing hard. According to his biographer, the wife of Dr. Spencer King who was instrumental in recruiting him to Emory said of Andreas: "Some women just threw their clothes off at the sight of him." Many of his acquaintances felt that Andreas' values changed after he came to America, the consequence of sudden wealth and celebrity status. His wife Michaela, a psychologist, did not thrive in Andreas' frantic social lifestyle, and not working in her native German undermined her self-confidence.

In 1981, the year after his arrival, a young, dashing Southern belle and medical student named Margaret Anne Thornton began to take her place. Michaela and daughter Sonja moved back to Germany. Grüntzig married Margaret in 1983. He bought a mansion where they threw lavish parties, a Porsche that he often drove recklessly at high speeds, an aircraft Beechcraft Baron that he piloted, and a weekend cottage on St. Simons Island off the Georgia coast. He had stepped into the American Dream, and indeed much more.

One Friday, in late October of 1985, after performing an angioplasty on a vascular surgeon, Grüntzig and his young wife with their two dogs took off for the weekend to the island, rather anxious to beat off the fast approaching hurricane Juan. Saturday morning he received a call that the coronary artery of the vascular surgeon he had opened was closing, and that his partners, Drs. King and Douglas, were taking the patient to the cath. lab. Grüntzig decided to take off for Atlanta with his wife and dogs in his Beechcraft Baron. As he approached Macon, Georgia, there was a rainstorm and dense fog. About 10 minutes into the flight, he turned Southeast instead of turning northwest, as instructed by the tower control, probably due to malfunction in the autopilot system.

Three minutes later, his plane disappeared from the radar.

The crash of the Beechcraft Baron would leave the world of cardiology shaken at its roots. Andreas Grüntzig, dead at just 46, would leave a rich legacy in the field of interventional cardiology that he pioneered.

Angioplasty developed swiftly throughout the 1980s, and it established a new specialty: intervention cardiology. The early interventionists were busy defining predictors of complications as well as restenosis. They were also busy training young fellows and attending teaching courses. However, nothing was honky-dory as it seemed on the surface. *With balloon angioplasty, rates of acute and chronic vessel closure were unacceptably high (≥ 30%).* The high incidence of restenosis was secondary to acute and chronic recoil and constrictive remodeling due to fibrosis.

The Cowboy Cardiologist

He was a young, brash, aggressive, booted, and hatted Midwesterner, a one-time bass guitarist, whose high school band performed throughout Indiana. He wore cowboy boots to work, liked fast cars and motorcycles, and carried angioplasty further into the unknown.

His name was Geoffrey Hartzler (1946–2012).

After Grüntzig performed the first human angioplasty in 1977 in Zurich, the Mayo Clinic developed a protocol: doctors had to perform peripheral artery angioplasty on 100 patients before they attempted coronary angioplasty. However, before Hartzler completed this protocol, he was asked to treat a patient with an isolated lesion of the left anterior descending artery. Only two balloon catheters were available at Mayo. Hartzler used the first catheter in a St. Bernard to learn the technique and manipulated it into the dog's left anterior descending artery. The dog died before he completed the procedure.

But in his hard-hitting cowboy style, the next day he went ahead with the patient, a water tower maintenance man. It was not a wise decision, since he had never even seen the procedure performed on a person. The chairman of Medicine, whom he had informed only moments before, stormed into the cath. lab with an army of angry heart surgeons. But it was too late to turn back. "I still get choked up about it," he recalled decades later, "because I realized then, and I do now, how close it came to my career being over. It's really true." He worked desperately for over 2 hours trying to pass the catheter through, but it wouldn't go. Finally, his superiors ordered him to stop. He pleaded for 5 more minutes, and they relented. "There were a lot of bad vibes in the room by now," he recalled, but suddenly by a stroke of luck, he managed to get the balloon to cross the lesion. He then inflated it. The angiogram showed a perfect result, to the relief of some who had been watching the procedure intensely, some with anxiety and others with outrage.

But he had succeeded. He was a hero. That's what he thought. At least for the moment.

His colleagues and superiors remained angry at his boldness in jumping in without adequate training and risking the life of the patient. Hartzler was not deterred. He performed a series of angioplasties in the next few months, but his aggressive nature did not fit in with the cautious Mayo Clinic. In his enthusiastic manner, he initially dabbled in invasive electrophysiology as well and was the first to attempt ablation of ventricular tachycardia in man. The powers at the Mayo Clinic finally decided that he was a trigger-happy cowboy, too much of a risk for their widely respected institution. They fired him.

Subsequently, he joined the Saint Luke's Mid America Heart Institute, in Kansas City, Missouri. There, he extended the use of angioplasty procedures to patients with multivessel disease, as equipment became more refined. He believed that in CAD, one, two, or three vessels could be safely opened during a single procedure. This idea was revolutionary for the times, particularly since Andreas Grüntzig believed that angioplasty should be reserved for single-vessel disease.

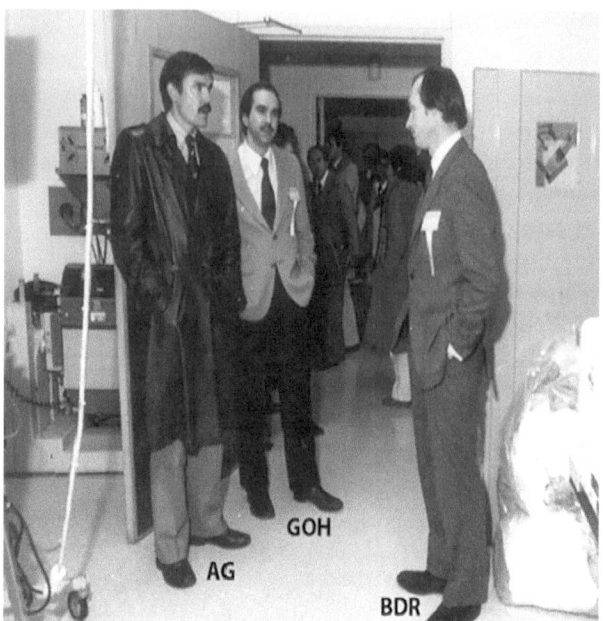

Fig. 24.1 Pictured from left to right, Dr. Andreas Grüntzig (AG), Dr. Geoffrey O. Hartzler (GOH), and Dr. Barry D. Rutherford (BDR) at Saint Luke's Mid America Heart Institute Catheterization Laboratory in 1984. (Reprinted with permission from Barry D. Rutherford, Joel K. Kahn, David Strelow, and David R. Holmes Jr: Geoffrey O. Hartzler, MD, A Tribute, *Circulation* 2012; 125 (23): 2958–2960. https://doi.org/10.1161/CIRCULATIONAHA.112.113274)

Hartzler and Grüntzig (Fig. 24.1) were at odds with each other. In academic cardiology circles, Hartzler was considered the "cowboy from the Midwest," while Grüntzig was the "thoughtful scientist." However, criticism did not dent Hartzler's enthusiasm; besides, he possessed enormous energy, intense concentration, and exceptional skill in the laboratory and thus the confidence. He described some of the first cases using two and three wires, "kissing balloons," "hugging balloons," removal of debris, and management of complications.

His audaciousness carried him further into unchartered territory. It so happened that he had a patient in the hospital with angina pectoris who was scheduled for angioplasty the following day. The next morning, the ward called the cath. lab to cancel the procedure, since the patient was having an acute myocardial infarction. But it didn't deter Hartzler who brought the patient to the lab and opened his closed right coronary artery with the balloon—an absolute no-no in those times—and a first. As soon as he opened the artery, the chest pain went away, the ST segment on the ECG came down, and signs of a heart attack disappeared. The patient was discharged from the hospital in a few days rather than the 2–3 weeks that was normal in those days.

It was another huge milestone. Hartzler had revolutionized the treatment of heart attacks by using a balloon to open a vessel instead of a drug. He subsequently developed a protocol for balloon angioplasty in heart attack patients and in 1983 reported his successful results in a large number of patients. It was highly controversial and demanding to treat heart attack victims with angioplasty at the time. Despite intense criticism, he continued refining and defending the procedure. And he was absolutely right. A few years later, several trials established that angioplasty yielded superior outcomes to clot dissolution when performed within 2 hours of a heart attack. Early mortality dropped from 20% to 30% to single digits. Hospital patients were discharged in 2–3 days and could return to an active and productive lifestyle. Finally, after 15 years, direct angioplasty was established as a class I recommendation by the American and European Cardiovascular Societies and the preferred standard of care.

The dynamic and bold Geoffrey Hartzler was a jack of many trades, and he performed superbly in all. In addition to ablative therapy for VT, multivessel angioplasty, and angioplasty in patients with heart attacks, he was also involved in the early development of defibrillators and cofounded Ventritex Inc., a defibrillator company, and Intraluminal Inc. Additionally, his Kansas City band, called Heart Rock, performed and recorded several CDs. Unfortunately, he gave up interventional cardiology after developing a bad back. He died of cancer in 2012 at the age of 65.

Tubes Within Tubes: The Stent Story

As worldwide experience accumulated, we learned to our dismay that balloon angioplasty was associated with high rates of re-blockage of the coronary arteries. Symptoms of angina reappeared. The problem was not re-accumulation of cholesterol, but recoil of the vessel wall and scar tissue formation. To deal with these problems, two French cardiologists, Dr. Ulrich Sigwart and Dr. Jacques Puel, independently conceived of implanting a hollow metal cylinder they called a "stent." Put a hard tube at the site, the thinking went, and it would keep the vessel wide permanently.

Jacques Puel implanted the first coronary stent in a patient in Toulouse, France, on March 28, 1986. Both he and Ulrich Sigwart reported in *The New England Journal of Medicine* on March 19, 1987, their experience in France and Switzerland in their landmark studies on the use of stents to prevent reocclusion after angioplasty. After their breathtaking feat, Dr. Julio Palmaz (Fig. 24.2), an Argentine-born interventional vascular radiologist working in the United States, invented the balloon-expandable stent. He received a patent filed in 1985, and this patent has appeared on the list of the ten most important inventions of all times.

In 2004, Dr. Palmaz gave an interview to Medscape, attributing his advance to sheer serendipity. At a conference in 1978, "Andreas Grüntzig described this amazing new technique of balloon angioplasty," he said. "It was exciting—a way to open

Fig. 24.2 Dr. Julio Palmaz
(https://alchetron.com/
Julio-Palmaz). (The Free
Social Encyclopedia of the
World) (https://ourstory.jnj.
com/
palmaz-schatz-balloon-
expandable-stent)

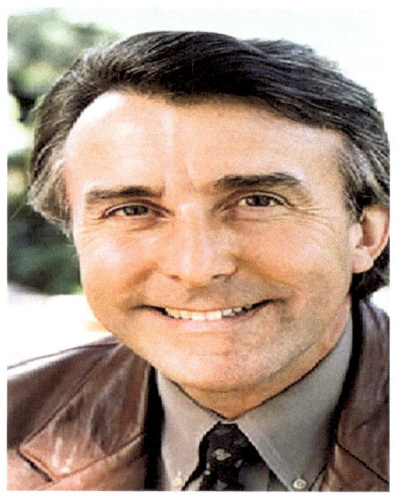

vessels through a catheter. He could have dazzled us with the novelty of the technique, but instead he actually dwelled on the limitations, showing us X-rays and microscopic images of how vessels could still occlude. I think it was his explanation that elicited in my mind the idea of why not put a scaffold in the vessel." He began doing balloon angioplasty, and afterward, he'd wash the balloons and take them home. "I was making my own nets there, playing with them, expanding them inside rubber tubes," he said. "I started having a feel for the mechanical problems that making a stent would impose."

At first, he toiled in his garage, and later he and Dr. Richard Schatz, a cardiologist from the Brooke Army Medical Center, worked together at the University of Texas Health Science Center in San Antonio. The stent for the coronaries was eventually called the Palmaz-Schatz stent.

In October 1987, Palmaz and Schatz placed the first peripheral stent in a patient at Freiburg University in West Germany. Later, that same year, they did their first coronary stent in Sao Paolo, Brazil. Both procedures were successful. The stent was licensed to Johnson & Johnson, and they designed the clinical trials. After several randomized studies between stents and balloon angioplasty, the FDA approved coronary stenting in 1994.

After that, according to Palmaz, "Johnson & Johnson had to scale up to the rapidly increasing use of stents, plus there was the enormous task of training everybody to use them. Then it hit us that the stent was going to have a far bigger role than we had anticipated. We thought that maybe 20% of all patients would receive stents, but then it was 30%, then 40%. Next, we knew it was 75% to 80%. It became really crazy."

The bare metal stents (BMS) cut the restenosis rate, but about one in five patients experienced a new form of damage, a thickening of the artery wall called neointimal hyperplasia. Stents coated with drugs, known as drug-eluting stents, were developed. "Elute" here means to exude drugs, and these stents slowly release them to prevent the growth of extra cells. They reduced the rate of restenosis further by half, down to less than one in ten patients.

Pedro Sanchez Today

You may remember my first patient in 1970, when I was an intern in one of New York's city hospitals. I gave his name as Pedro Sanchez, and he died a few hours after his massive heart attack. Let's revisit Pedro and see how he would fare today.

After his sudden death episode, the paramedics would immediately alert the ER, messaging with a live ECG recording that they were bringing a man with an AMI and sudden death. The ER would at once contact the catheterization staff. As soon as Pedro was stabilized, he would be rushed to the cath. lab. The intervention cardiologist on call would perform an angiogram and stent the culprit artery. Pedro would then go to the CCU.

This procedure would save the anterior wall of his heart from extensive damage. He would be out of danger, and in a few days, he would be sent home. He would be placed on a beta-blocker, aspirin, clopidogrel or ticagrelor, and statin drug to lower his cholesterol. He would receive detailed instructions on lifestyle changes and risk modifications. If Pedro had only single-vessel disease, took his medications, and was serious about risk modification—if he stopped smoking and lost weight—he might be alive to see his grandchildren graduate.

On the other hand, if Pedro's heart function was down (less than 35%), he would receive a LifeVest Wearable Defibrillator for a 3-month period for protection. If a repeat echo 3 months later shows no significant improvement in heart function, he would have an ICD to prevent SCD. And ultimately if he developed intractable heart failure, he would be evaluated for a heart transplant.

Stents or Bypasses or Conservative Medical Treatment?

A stent could have given Pedro a long life. However, we often see patients with symptomatic coronary artery disease who need either stenting or coronary artery bypass grafting (CABG) or just conservative medical management with drugs. It's a question of widening the tunnel or rerouting entirely or just treating with drugs referred to a guideline-directed optimal medical therapy. Potentially all three are capable of relieving symptoms, but which is better? This question has been controversial for some time.

For instance, recently I got a call from an acquaintance of mine—Dr. Ferrari, a retired surgeon, who recently developed angina pectoris. I asked him to email me his records, and reviewing the nuclear stress test, I suspected three-vessel coronary artery disease. He also had uncontrolled diabetes, and diabetes turns out to be a potent risk factor for stent occlusion, even with drug-eluting stents. I considered the possibility of open heart bypass surgery but refrained from mentioning it for fear of adding anxiety. I asked our renowned interventionalist, Dr. Samin Sharma, to do a coronary angiogram. It turned out that he indeed had three-vessel disease, and since he was a diabetic, Dr. Sharma recommended surgery. The heart surgeon came by immediately, but Dr. Ferrari, a surgeon himself, refused open heart surgery. Since his heart function was normal, I concurred with stenting. He'd had a stent placed about 10 years before, and both he and I requested Dr. Sharma to proceed with stenting. He was brought back to the laboratory late in the evening on the same day, and a stent was placed in his main artery. He came back 4 weeks later and had additional stents in his other arteries. He is now free of angina and he has done superbly well.

A 2007 trial called Clinical Outcomes Utilizing Revascularization and Aggressive Drug Evaluation (COURAGE) questioned the effectiveness of stents relative to drug therapy in people with stable CAD. There are approximately one million stents inserted in such patients. Many of them have repeated interventions and remain on the same drugs they were on before the stenting, in addition to anticlotting drugs. It has been shown that as many as 12% of drug-coated stents are unnecessary and an additional 38% are of uncertain benefit. Not surprisingly, despite the results of COURAGE,[1] many patients prefer stenting rather than undergo the trauma of open heart bypass surgery with its prolonged recovery and associated complications. This study showed that in patients with severe CAD and diabetes with or without decreased heart function and who require intervention, bypass grafting is associated with better survival than stents, and therefore, it should be considered as the initial approach.

In a recent trial[2] performed in patients with stable coronary disease and moderate or severe ischemia, there was no evidence that an initial invasive strategy, when compared with an initial conservative strategy with medications (guideline-based), reduced the risk of heart attacks or death over a median of 3.2 years. However, an invasive approach (stenting or coronary bypass strategy) does more effectively relieve symptoms of angina particularly in patients with frequent episodes.

---

[1] Clinical Outcomes Utilizing Revascularization and Aggressive Drug Evaluation.
[2] The ISCHEMIA trial in patients with stable ischemic heart disease.

Mortality Reduction in Coronary Artery Disease

Deaths from CAD overall peaked in the late 1960s and 1970s. Over the decades that followed, the age-adjusted death rate slowly decreased across much of the Western world. Today, the rate is about half that in 1968, and it dropped 25% alone in the United States between 2004 and 2014.

Why did this change occur? A team led by the University of Liverpool developed an international preventative policy model called IMPACT, now standard in the field, and it found that the decline in mortality stemmed from a multitude of factors working in concert. They included contributions from coronary artery bypass surgery, as well as angioplasty, lifesaving treatments, better care after heart attacks, control of blood pressure, greater physical activity, and less smoking. About half of the advancement came from better medical treatment and half from reduction in risk factors like smoking.

And so, we can see a host of avenues that may lead us to the goal of conquering CAD, but it's still out of sight. From clot busters to stents and bypasses and even the futuristic stem cells, we've seen strategies after the fact, when the patient is in dire need of an intervention. However, prevention is better than cure, and we can still achieve a lot by controlling risk factors such as high blood pressure, diabetes, cholesterol, obesity, and smoking.

♥

Part IX
Stories of Survival

Chapter 25
A Family Affair

When everything goes to hell, the people who stand by you
without flinching—they are your family.

—Jim Butcher

Death leaves a heartache no one can heal, love leaves a
memory no one can steal.

—From a Headstone in Ireland

Sudden death leaves sorrowing widowers and family members in its terrible path.
No one else is perhaps as devastated as the spouse. The pain is emotional, but also
social and often economic. There are many regrets, about not discussing family
finances, not keeping a will, and, above all, not expressing love. The longer people
are married, the more they can take each other for granted. And the spouse of a
person who *survives* cardiac arrest is elated at first, but fear and uncertainty follow,
which can linger for the rest of their lives together.

How does she handle the insecurity and fragility the event has wrought? Charles
survived sudden cardiac arrest, and I was so impressed with the love and caring and
gratitude of his wife that I feel compelled to give her perspective of the experience.

"Charles was fit as horse," Ruth said. "No illness whatsoever except for a flu after
an airplane flight!"

"Just before the cardiac arrest?" I asked.

"A week or so before."

"What exactly happened?"

"I was asleep. Luckily, I'm a light sleeper. He liked to work late. Burn the midnight lamp as they say."

"Did he complain to you at all? Shortness of breath? Chest pain? Dizziness?
Palpitations?"

"Nothing! He was fit as a fiddle."

Apparently, Charles had been sitting at his desk working. He liked to work late.
At about 2:30 am, he came to sleep. She heard a loud thud. She immediately got off

© The Author(s), under exclusive license to Springer Nature
Switzerland AG 2021
J. A. Gomes, *Rhythms of Broken Hearts*,
https://doi.org/10.1007/978-3-030-77382-3_25

the bed and found him on the floor seizing. She gave him CPR and called 911. He came out of the seizure by himself a minute or so later.

"To me it seemed a lifetime," she said. "I called my son who's a doctor."

The paramedics found him in atrial fibrillation. His heart was beating 120 times a minute. They took him to a Brooklyn hospital and in the ER he went into cardiac arrest.

"They worked on him for a long time and applied electrical shocks to his chest several times," she said. "Luckily, he didn't sustain any brain damage."

Their son requested transfer to the Mount Sinai Medical Center under the care of Dr. John Ambrose, then the head of Cardiac Catheterization. The angiogram of the coronary arteries showed no blockage, and the biopsy of the heart was normal. Spasm of the coronary arteries was ruled out. Since no one knew the cause of the cardiac arrest, his doctors did not know how to proceed. I was asked to consult.

I subjected him to an EPS. I was able to initiate only a few beats of a rapid ventricular rhythm, what we call non-sustained ventricular tachycardia. Studies had shown that induction of a non-sustained tachycardia is a nonspecific response, one that doesn't require treatment. We labeled his lethal rhythm an "idiopathic ventricular fibrillation." When doctors can't find a cause for an illness, they call it *idiopathic*. Did it warrant just a beta-blocker to reduce the sympathetic drive on the heart? Should I implant a defibrillator? I debated the issue with the resident physicians in the CCU. Implantation was not a simple undertaking in those days. We had to crack open the man's chest and attach the leads to the heart's surface. He could suffer infection, fracture of the leads, and inappropriate shocks from the defibrillator. Besides, after 3–5 years, the whole device needed replacement. But he had nearly died and what if the episode recurred? He might not be as lucky the next time around. Needless to say, in those times, we did not know what we know today. Currently, an ICD is indicated for patients surviving a cardiac arrest in the setting of "a normal heart."

When I explained to his wife that I simply had no idea whether he is at high risk of having another cardiac arrest, she began crying. I placed my arms around her, but there was no way I could console her.

"Do what you feel is right," Ruth said after she calmed down. "I'm placing his life in your hands, doctor."

When a patient or spouse says something like that, it is indeed a tall order. There was no literature at the time to back either form of treatment—implanting a defibrillator or just putting the patient on a beta-blocker and letting nature take its course—particularly since his heart function was entirely normal and his coronary arteries were clear. After much thought and considerable debate with myself and with my colleagues including Dr. Camunas, our implant surgeon, I decided to go ahead with the defibrillator. Only time would tell whether I had made the right decision.

The defibrillator implantation went well, and he was discharged. I saw him every 3 months or so and there were no events. He was working full time in a metal factory, leading a productive life. I saw in him a sturdy, stoic, and solid individual. His wife on the other hand was strong, but emotional and frightened of the future. She loved him dearly and was afraid of losing him.

More than a year passed since Charles had the cardiac arrest, and since he remained healthy and entirely free of symptoms, I wondered whether my recommendation to implant a defibrillator was overkill.

A year and a half passed, and all was well. Then one day I received a frantic call from Ruth saying that the defibrillator had gone off four times during one night. He had one of the first-generation devices that could not record the abnormal heart rhythm, so all I could surmise was that a problem had occurred. What was interesting and somewhat perplexing was the fact that the defibrillator had gone off in the early morning hours when he was sleeping. He'd had the first cardiac arrest in the early morning hours as well.

I told Ruth that I wanted him admitted to the hospital right away. He was placed in the telemetry unit for monitoring. Two days passed, and nothing happened. On the third morning at six o'clock, he suddenly and unexpectedly went into the lethal rhythm, ventricular fibrillation, (Fig. 25.1), and within a few seconds, the defibrillator did its job: it zapped him back into normal rhythm (Fig. 25.1). If not for the shock, Charles would have likely died. Indeed, Charles would have died in his sleep 3 days before.

I placed him on amiodarone, gradually decreasing its dose to 100 mg a day so that he wouldn't develop toxicity.

It has been around 29 years since his cardiac arrest, and he remains well and alive. I have absolutely no doubt that if we hadn't inserted the defibrillator, he would have died. When I last saw him and his wife, I asked her what had gone through her mind all these years.

"It was all so dramatic and traumatic," she said. "My husband is a very strong and confident man. He doesn't think about the problem at all, and just goes on with

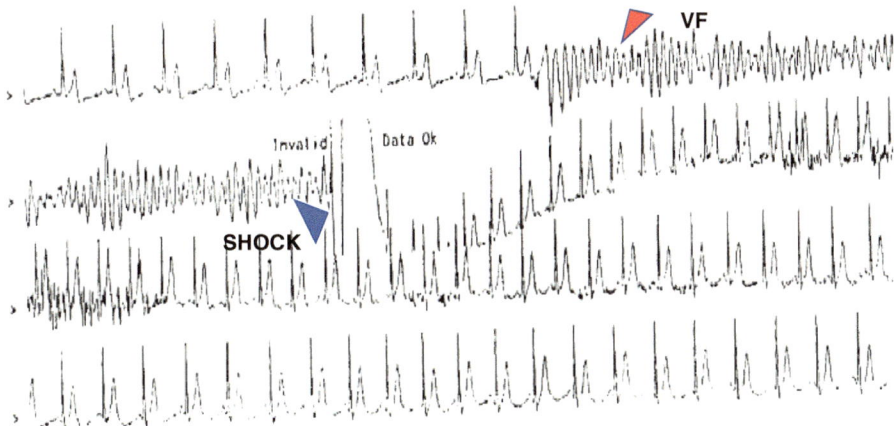

Fig. 25.1 Charles in-hospital VF terminated by an ICD shock. Legend: Real-time ECG strip (telemetry) shows ventricular fibrillation (VF) occurring early in the morning. It is quickly terminated by a lifesaving jolt from the defibrillator (ICD), as described in the text. The red arrow points to ventricular fibrillation (VF), the blue arrow points to the ICD shock that terminated the VF, and the patient goes back into normal rhythm

his life. Psychologically, he has handled it remarkably well and certainly better than I have. My son and my daughter-in-law cannot handle a phone call at night even to this day."

"Has the ICD given you and your husband more security?"

"Absolutely, it was like an insurance policy in the beginning. But when the device went off four times and once again in the hospital, it was a lifesaver! You saved his life, Doc. You gave him back to me."

I could see in her face, her eyes that she meant it. I could see love pouring out from her, from him. They were still in love with each other.

"God saved him through you," she said. "Perhaps my waking up at 2:30 in the morning might have been a divine act."

I was much moved. I couldn't resist the tears flooding in my eyes.

"I pray for you Doc," she said.

"Thanks," I said.

♥

Chapter 26
Cruising Through Complications of a Heart Attack

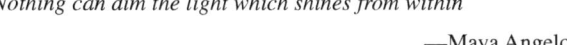

Nothing can dim the light which shines from within

—Maya Angelou

The weak overcome its menace, the strong overcomes itself.
What is there like fortitude! What sap went through that little
thread to make the cherry red!

—Marianne Moore

Cardiac disease can come at a most inopportune time: at the very prime of life and during the sunset years—a time of retirement, introspection, and relaxation. Most patients view this unexpected change in their lives as a fall from grace. They are suddenly at the mercy of mysterious, alarming elements, and they feel morose, insecure, and bewildered. Fears of disability, of suffering, of death itself are uppermost in their minds.

However, as everything else in life—whether hoping for a cure or dealing with a worsened ailment or even preparing for death—the ultimate goal should be adaptation. One needs to move forward while attaining an inner peace with oneself and with one's surroundings. As Confucius said: "Our greatest glory is not in never falling, but in rising every time we fall." But this is not an easy task.

This point is illustrated by the life and tribulations of a wonderful man, a patient of mine I shall call Paul. He was a corporate lawyer who worked for a large law firm. His beginnings were humble. He came from a blue-collar family, but earned a scholarship to Columbia University and worked hard until his retirement in 2000 at 62. He looked forward to traveling and doing many things he couldn't do before. Among other endeavors, he volunteered with the legal aid society, doing DNA matching in incarcerated criminals.

Unfortunately, he suffered a massive heart attack in 2005, when he was 67. He underwent coronary artery bypass surgery and a mitral valve repair. His course was complicated by the development of ventricular tachycardia and kidney failure. He

J. A. Gomes, *Rhythms of Broken Hearts*, https://doi.org/10.1007/978-3-030-77382-3_26

received an implantable defibrillator, and after a lengthy hospital course, he was discharged.

"The defibrillator gives me a sense of security that I will not drop dead suddenly," he said. "But now I have constant anxiety because I attribute almost every pain and discomfort to a worsening of my heart function."

A few years later, he developed atrial fibrillation and went into heart failure. He was unable to function. I got him back into normal rhythm after applying a shock to the chest, which markedly improved his functional capacity. Once normal rhythm was restored, he was back in action.

However, a year or so later, he came to see me utterly depressed. Now he could barely walk a block or so without getting out of breath. He had gone back into heart failure and his exercise tolerance had plunged. Moreover, his heart failure specialist felt he was nearing the end and wanted to insert a left ventricular assist device to help the pumping action of his heart. He was devastated.

I immediately sensed his dilemma. He could not deal with what was happening to him and was desperate for alternate choices. When I interrogated his device, I found that he was back in atrial fibrillation. Indeed, atrial fibrillation is present in 20–50% of patients presenting to the hospital with class IV heart failure, the most serious level. Conversely, when patients have atrial fibrillation, the prevalence of heart failure has been estimated at 42%. I suggested that his heart failure and exercise struggles were likely the outcome of his reverting back into atrial fibrillation. His face lit up. He saw some light at the end of the tunnel and readily took up my suggestion.

I again used the electrical shock and placed him on amiodarone to prevent him from going back into the abnormal rhythm. Fortunately, he showed marked improvement in his exercise tolerance, and he returned to his usual self with renewed hope. I warned him that he could go back into the abnormal rhythm, and if he did, I would consider an ablative procedure. A 2016 multicenter study[1] reported that patients who had ablation did better than those taking amiodarone on several important scores: recurrence of AF, improvement in heart function, hospitalization, and all-cause mortality over a 2-year period. However, when I saw Paul, ablation was not widely used for such sick patients. It was just a possible option.

Paul did reasonably well for a few more years, and then he regressed back into heart failure. I told him that I would use the shock again to get him back into normal rhythm but warned that we might not see significant improvement this time around. Over time, such patients are subject to remodeling of their heart, what we call "reverse remodeling"—not for the better, but for the worse. With the decline in his condition, his anxiety and insecurity returned.

In fact, Paul had done better than most. He had beaten the odds. I had a long conversation with him about acceptance, his struggles, his brave fight for survival, and his inspiring determination to pursue life no matter what.

---

[1] The Ablation vs. Amiodarone for Treatment of Atrial Fibrillation in Patients with Congestive Heart Failure and Implanted ICD/CRTD (AATAC-AF in Heart Failure) study.

I remembered the wise words of Joan Didion: "I'm not telling you to make the world better... (but) To look at it. To try to get the picture... To seize the moment. And if you ask me why you should bother to do that, I could tell you that the grave's a fine and private place, but none I think do there embrace. Nor do they sing there, or write, or argue, or see the tidal bore on the Amazon, or touch their children."

Over time, Paul came to terms with his condition and was content going whenever possible for dinner, a movie, a holiday in Florida, and the company of his grandchildren.

Gradually, as time passed, he came to realize that he was nearing the end. And yet, the last time I saw him, I was myself caught up with his optimism and hope for the future. He had kept abreast of the literature and, after needling his cardiologist, was being considered for stem cell therapy to regenerate his heart muscle.

"What has kept you going, all this time?" I asked.

"My strength is personal, inward," he said. "I'm not religious."

Unfortunately, the researcher abandoned the stem cell protocol and Paul gradually entered into terminal heart failure. He finally agreed to proceed with a left ventricular assist device but succumbed to complications and passed away.

The story of Paul is one of perseverance, self-reliance, and a constant struggle to find ways and means to get better, to heal his heart, and, perhaps if the time had been right, to mend his heart altogether with stem cells. I had always seen an inner struggle in this man and hope beyond hope to live on. He gathered this fire not from prayer, not from a religion or a God, but from the god within that is perhaps present in all of us, a god that we must struggle to find. As it turned out, he lived long enough, much longer than most patients with his condition, but not long enough for a cure.

♥

Chapter 27
A Missed Diagnosis: A Lifetime of Endurance

As any doctor can tell you, the most crucial step toward healing is having the right diagnosis. If the disease is precisely identified, a good resolution is far more likely. Conversely, a bad diagnosis usually means a bad outcome, no matter how skilled the physician.

—Andrew Weil

Every calamity is to be overcome by endurance.

—Virgil

All of us dread a missed or an incorrect diagnosis and its dire consequences. Despite the easy availability of a plethora of specialists and superspecialists in the United States, about 12 million Americans are misdiagnosed each year. Diagnostic errors are missed roads. They can cause severe harm, including disability and death. And they happen despite the fact that we do so many tests and procedures, many of which are redundant and some are not even indicated. Each year in the United States, we perform about seven billion diagnostic tests (such as blood, urine, saliva, and spinal fluid). That's about 22 for each man, woman, and child in the nation. We also do 100 million CT and MRI scans and 17 million nuclear medicine scans. In 2012, the number of CT scan growth was 8% per year, MRIs 10%, ultrasounds 4%, and PET scans 57%.

"You have a good chance of being misdiagnosed if you have a really rare disease or a really common disease which presents nonspecifically or in some atypical fashion," says Dr. Mark Garber, founder and president of the *Society to Improve Diagnosis in Medicine.*

Heart attacks remain one of the commonest misdiagnosed diseases, often mistaken for indigestion and anxiety.

Endurance, that word of steel that lets people overcome *the slings and arrows of outrageous fortune*, is nowhere better exemplified than in the mysterious and chilling story of Clara. I first met her in March 2005, when she was admitted to our

J. A. Gomes, *Rhythms of Broken Hearts*, https://doi.org/10.1007/978-3-030-77382-3_27

CCU. Despite treatment with a host of medications, she suffered from heart failure due to a cardiomyopathy, the cause of which remained unknown. I was consulted because she had atrial fibrillation. She had received the drug amiodarone at a local hospital, but unfortunately, she couldn't tolerate it. She had also gotten treatment with steroids and bronchodilators for bouts of asthma that kept recurring over several years. In view of her poor heart function and heart failure, she had an implantable defibrillator for the primary prevention of sudden cardiac death.

We were perplexed by her symptomatology and wondered whether her heart and lung conditions were somehow related. Indeed, her condition had long puzzled physicians.

It is hard enough to endure a chronic ailment as it swings back and forth from worse to better to worse; it is even more difficult and frustrating to go for so long without a diagnosis. This fact underscores the importance of getting a second opinion from doctors at a reputable institution such as a university hospital. This is not to belittle the physicians in private practice, but doctors at university teaching hospitals are bound to see more complex and unusual cases.

Earlier, in 1987, a well-known local pulmonologist had diagnosed her with asthma. He prescribed an inhalant and told her to come back for a checkup in about 3 months. But she never needed to use the inhalant and in fact never felt she had asthma the way other people do. Several years later, the problem came back. Her lungs would fill up with mucus and she couldn't breathe. "This was the beginning of my journey on prednisone," she said. "The doctor and I would refer to the mucus in my lungs as a 'flare-up', and he would prescribe prednisone which would provide immediate relief with my breathing. It also gave me the energy I needed for my daughter's care."

When Clara was 40 years old, she become pregnant. During her pregnancy, the flare-ups were coming monthly, and she had to stay on a high dose of the prednisone for her breathing. She was in a high-risk category, and she later wondered whether the prednisone had something to do with her daughters' development in her womb.

"It was a miracle when I conceived," she said, with a smile. "Marianne was born on June 27, 1999, with brown curly hair. She was God's gift to us."

But their joy quickly turned to worry when Marianne developed problems drinking her bottle. She wouldn't gain weight. Her pediatrician felt that she had reflux and recommended her to a gastroenterologist, who told to pursue DNA testing. Apparently, doctors felt she had a genetic syndrome because of her facial features. Marianne was also diagnosed as "failure to thrive," since she was unable to take any nourishment. She saw a host of pediatricians. None of them could link her to any known genetic syndrome. And so, the saga of Marianne went on, from one doctor to another. Ultimately, she had a "g" tube implanted to deliver food straight to her stomach. The weeks turned into months and nothing changed. Clara was both physically and mentally exhausted. While taking care of Marianne, Clara had to care for herself. Like Marianne's, her condition baffled physicians. Her doctor gave her various pills and inhalants to stop the asthma flare-ups, but none worked, and she ended up on the prednisone. He wrote in his report that she was noncompliant with medication..

While Marianne's tolerance to the food was causing problems, Clara's mother took a turn for the worse. She had diabetes and it was not under control requiring amputation of her legs.

To top it all, Marianne had gotten to the point where she barely tolerated the feedings, and the vomiting was worse. Clara was beside herself. She needed to talk to someone. She was raised a Catholic and attended Catholic elementary school, and she figured she could sit down with the priest, and he could shed some light on God's purpose, on what it all meant. She went to a rectory one morning and asked if she could speak with the priest. He asked why she had come. "At this point I was so filled with emotion I could barely talk," she said. "I didn't get very far with my story when he asked my name again. He kept looking through a list of names and informed me that my name was not on the parish list or the Sunday envelope collection list. I tried to explain what's been going on in my life for the last couple of years, but he informed me that I was not a member of that parish, and therefore, he couldn't help me.

"I left and just sat in my car crying. It left me totally confused about my beliefs. I didn't think I could go back to that church or any church for that matter. Now I felt totally alone with no one, not even God, to turn to. I just got through those days as best I could, taking care of Marianne by day and spending my evenings with my mom. I was like a zombie."

Her mom passed away on June 20, 2000

The Terrorist Attack

It turned out that Clara had worked as a senior computer network engineer in the South Tower of the World Trade Center when a truck bomb exploded under the North Tower in 1993. The work she did in the disaster recovery brought her not only a sizable pay increase but also promotion to assistant vice president of her company.

On September 11, 2001, she had taken Marianne to the babysitter's house when she saw the Twin Towers burning on the TV. Her own Tower and the floor that she worked on were billowing thick black smoke. She had been in the Network Support Department for over 15 years, and she knew everyone in the company.

"Everyone tells me that Marianne was my angel that day," she said. "I was late because I had a progress meeting with her therapists."

She lost a very close friend along with many more friends. Over the weeks and months that followed, there were many memorials and funerals to attend.

I related to what Clara was saying. I myself was near the World Trade Center at about 8:15 that morning to drop off my wife. She worked on the 56th floor of the South Tower. She was there when the first plane struck the North Tower. She had called to tell me that a plane struck the North Tower, but she didn't know what was going on. The phones stopped working after that, and it was sheer agony to wait and ponder the outcome. Luckily, she was coming down the stairs when her Tower was struck, and she escaped unharmed.

In March of 2002, Clara was laid off from her job after 25 years. It was very hard for her and extremely upsetting. She wondered how her family could survive on one salary. What kind of job could she get when she had to tend to Marianne. They had medical bills to pay off as well as other debts. They didn't know if they could keep their house.

The inability to diagnose her own, and Marianne's illness, was set to cause further havoc in their lives

And yet, she said, "I didn't realize it then, but everything happens for a reason. With the loss of my job, I was able to dedicate 100% of myself to Marianne. This layoff turned out to be a special blessing that I'll be forever grateful for."

Even so, in April of 2003, their hopes seemed near an end. Marianne was not tolerating the feeds anymore, and she wasn't getting nutrition. Then an ENT surgeon at New York University Hospital recommended a surgical procedure called a fundoplication. It would prevent reflux of food and let Marianne gain weight and grow. The surgery took place in May of 2003. As the days went by, they watched Marianne in amazement. She was tolerating her feeds and her weight was coming on fast.

In July 2003, they packed up for summer vacation and headed to Wildwood, New Jersey.

"I was so excited," she said. "Life was good, and I was ready to lay back and just enjoy everything and everybody. The worst was behind us."

On July 18, Marianne passed away suddenly while they were in Wildwood.

"As she lay on the gurney in the emergency room, I just laid my head next to hers and prayed," she said. "This was the end of our journey. I kissed Marianne goodbye and told her that no one would hurt her anymore. She will be with her nanny, her grandfather, and all her aunts, uncles, and friends who had passed away. It was their turn to enjoy her."

Clara's Heart Failure

In August of 2004, her sister, through a friend, got her a part-time job in a warehouse in Newark. "I only worked from 9 am to 1 pm but it was good for me," she said. She also did some work for a company on the second floor of the warehouse. Since there was no elevator, she got winded climbing the stairs. She went in for her regular checkups, got her prescriptions for prednisone, and took what she needed to get through the day.

On Thanksgiving Day of 2004, Clara woke up feeling tightness in her chest and shortness of breath. She took the prednisone and went off to her sister's house for the holiday dinner. But the prednisone didn't work as it usually had. She wasn't getting any relief from the tightness or the trouble breathing. The next day, she called the doctor's office and said she needed to see him right away.

"He examined me, took some X-rays, and thought it best that I see a cardiologist," she recalled. "The cardiologist took me as an emergency and performed an echocardiogram. I was not prepared when the doctor and his assistant walked into the exam room and told me to go straight to the ER. I was in heart failure. I don't remember all of what they did, but I do know that I was placed on amiodarone for the atrial fibrillation and given prednisone."

The amiodarone didn't agree with her. She was nauseous all the time. Her heart wasn't beating right, and she didn't feel well. She stopped taking the amiodarone.

"In February of 2005, it happened again," she said. "I felt that my lungs were collapsing."

She was admitted to the intensive care unit. Physicians inserted an implantable defibrillator and restarted her on amiodarone. The drug caused vomiting and a weird feeling right away, and it was discontinued. She spent weeks in the hospital and it seemed like an eternity.

"They didn't know what was wrong with me because I wasn't responding to anything they gave me," she said. Finally, her doctor decided to transfer her to Mount Sinai Medical Center.

Solving the Puzzle

Clara was admitted to our CCU. After examining her carefully, and reviewing her records, like every other physician who had seen her, we had no idea what was wrong. Because of her unresponsiveness and the lack of a diagnosis, a heart biopsy was performed.

It turned out that Clara had a very unusual condition known as Churg-Strauss syndrome, also known as allergic granulomatosis, first described by Drs. Jacob Churg and Lotte Strauss at our institution in 1951. This inflammatory disease involves the medium to small blood vessels, and it is an autoimmune vasculitis, meaning that the immune system attacks those vessels, restricts them, and leads to tissue death (necrosis). Since it most often damages the vessels of the lungs, it presents as a severe type of asthma late in life, though rhinitis and sinusitis may precede it. It can also affect the heart, gastrointestinal system, peripheral nerves, skin, and kidneys. Fortunately, it is noninheritable and non-transmissible. Undoubtedly, the disease affected Clara's lungs and her heart.

When we established the diagnosis in May of 2005, Clara was relieved to finally find out what was wrong with her after battling the illness for several years.

"Unfortunately, it had run freely for a bit too long and caused other damage to my body," she said. "Now I know what was wrong with me and I have a brilliant team of doctors assigned to my care. Today, I have a special relationship with each of them and have never looked back. God has once again taken care of me."

"It's wonderful that you feel this way," I said. "Your perseverance and fight are exemplary."

We finally stabilized her on medications for heart failure, and the atrial fibrillation came under control after an ablative procedure and on medications. She felt symptomatically much better, and after a lengthy hospital stay, she was discharged. There is no cure for her disease, but we could keep it in check so that she could go on living. Despite her disability, she has regained some quality of life. A few months thereafter, she developed another rapid heart arrhythmia, an atrial flutter, but an ablative procedure readily cured it. Her atrial fibrillation recurred and was ultimately controlled with medications.

As I write, Clara has a strong family that has survived more tragedies than most people will in a lifetime. Her condition has waxed and waned, but with treatment and close follow-up care, she has remained out of the hospital environment. Every time I see her, she always has a broad smile full of optimism. Her family is still carrying many financial burdens, but they are forging ahead. She finally said to me, "I plan on meeting future challenges with the passion I hold in my heart and continue to get out of bed every morning with a positive outlook for whatever lies ahead."

> *Endurance is not just the ability to bear a hard thing, but to turn it into glory.*

—William Barclay

♥

Chapter 28
Old Age: How Long Should We Hope to Live?

Let us never know what old age is. Let us know the happiness time brings, not count the years.

—Decimus Magnus Ausonius

The secret of genius is to carry the spirit of the child into old age, which means never losing your enthusiasm.

—Aldous Huxley

Let's begin by asking: What is old age?

The best answer is probably: old age is when one can no longer function, regardless of chronological age. Consider David Perlman. He was a science writer for the *San Francisco Chronicle*, and on August 4, 2017, he retired—at age 98. He had worked there for 77 years, beginning in 1940, and one of his last pieces was about the 2017 solar eclipse. Such "superagers" retain memory and function as well as much younger people, and scientists know that their brains shrink less and the outer layers, the cerebral cortexes, remain thicker. That thickness matters because the cortex plays a critical role in memory, thought, attention, and consciousness. These lucky people don't age at the same rate. On the other hand, we see individuals below the current average life expectancy of 76 years for men and 81 years for women who have a dismal quality of life and cannot take care of themselves due to a chronic or an acute progressive illness.

Who is really older?

It has always been hard to draw a bright line for old age or even cite a transition zone. And today, when more and more people are living longer, healthier, and more productive lives, it is even harder. In the 1980s, our cutoff for a medical intervention such as major surgery was usually the 70s. Beyond that, we felt the patient might not withstand it. But by 2000, it was extended to the 80s, and today we perform major procedures even in patients over 90, provided they have well-preserved mental faculties. Medically speaking, we have been pushing the boundaries of "old age." And new strategies may push it further.

© The Author(s), under exclusive license to Springer Nature Switzerland AG 2021
J. A. Gomes, *Rhythms of Broken Hearts*,
https://doi.org/10.1007/978-3-030-77382-3_28

The Consequences of Aging

Life is not that bad when you consider the alternative.—Maurice Chevalier

Most people want to live as long as they can, and consequently many in our society embark on exercise programs such as long-distance running, try a host of diets, and consume an assortment of exotic juices, vitamins, and supplements, all for a healthier living and the postponement of the dying process. Is it really a good idea?

According to a 2016 survey of 300,000 adults in Great Britain, the period between 65 and 79 was the happiest of all. The sense of satisfaction and the feeling that life was worthwhile peaked in this period. As we retire, we can enjoy our existence in new ways. We can sit and relax, travel, and do pleasurable things that might have escaped us before—like reading, writing, gardening, cooking, exercising, reminiscing about the past, sharing it with members of our family and friends, partaking of our wisdom, and even rediscovering ourselves.

How will we really be remembered? In fact, as we age into retirement, we can create wonderful memories for those who know us. For instance, people commonly have fond recollections of their grandparents. Indeed, today many seniors are sacrificing for their children, helping them financially and taking care of their grandchildren. It's true that the aging of some parents creates hardships for their children, but those parents have long sacrificed for their children. And children typically have loving memories of their parents regardless of medical problems.

Are older people a burden on society? I don't think so. They have sacrificed for their children and family and contributed to society, their government, and some the world at large. Furthermore, in today's day and age, many seniors are still sacrificing for their children, often helping them financially and care-taking their grandchildren. Their children, our society, and our government have an obligation toward them, for the time and effort spent and for the social infrastructure such as social security and health care to which they contributed in their younger years and continue contributing. However, a growing elderly population is bound to strain federal coffers with rising Social Security and Medicare costs; yet, in old age, they have the right to live with quality and dignity.

Are older people unproductive? Statistics show that 1 in 8 people 65 years and over, and nearly half of those over 80 years, have some disability, and almost half over 85 years have Alzheimer's. That still leaves a large segment of the elderly population relatively intact with decent mental capabilities. To mention some well-known examples, as I write, architect Frank Gehry is still productive at 91 and investor Warren Buffett at 90. Comedian "Professor" Irwin Corey performed often in his 90s, dying in 2017 at the age of 102.

It has been shown that creativity rises rapidly as a career commences, peaks about 20 years into the career, and then slowly diminishes. But the decline, often attributed to age, may not necessarily imply a drop-off in mental function, but rather changing interests or lack of motivation. The fact that Nobel Prize winners in the sciences make their discoveries at a mean age of 48 does not imply that their mental capabilities decline after that. On the contrary, these scientists continue contributing to their fields and mentoring postdocs and other younger scientists. Many doctors, poets, painters, writers, and businessmen keep working and producing far beyond their heydays, often into their 80s and even 90s. A friend of mine, a writer who had coronary bypass surgery more than 20 years ago and who is now over 90, continues to travel between continents and write stories. One can argue that such superagers are outliers, but there are more and more of them around nowadays.

As people age, some feel they need to be productive and go to their place of work as they have all their lives. This habit is quite common in the medical community, as well as among artists and business owners. I have known doctors in their 80s who have continued to go to work until they just couldn't any longer and a couple who were actually found dead in their offices.

Many years ago, I was asked to deliver a lecture in Florida during the winter. The lecture was to start at 7:30 am, and I had flown from New York the night before. I was surprised to see that many attendees were old physicians who were not in my specialty, and probably had no interest in what I had to say. I asked the organizer of the lecture what these folks were doing here, and so early; he said that most were East Coast practitioners who were content to meet friends and colleagues, drink a cup of coffee, and eat a few glazed donuts. I then understood that they were there simply because they had attended lectures all their life in the early morning hours. Often, US doctors in academia dislike retiring because they don't know what to do with their time and have not adjusted to the concept of retirement itself.

But perhaps, the critical issue is how well we'll be as we advance in age.

Is There Compression or Expansion of Morbidity with Age?

In 1977, Dr. Ernest Gruenberg (1915–1991) hypothesized that a decline in mortality would be associated with greater prevalence of disease. Medical research had lengthened our lives, he observed, and thus "at the same time that persons suffering from chronic diseases are getting an extension of life, they are also getting an extension of disease and disability." Paradoxically, medical breakthroughs were increasing suffering, making us worse. Our successes were really failures.

However, in 1980, Dr. James F. Fries introduced the concept of compression of morbidity—that is, ill health—in an article in *The New England Journal of Medicine*. He proposed that along with greater life expectancy would come a *shorter* length of morbidity. With the benefits from good habits like exercise, he posited, we would develop "a radically different view of life span and of society, in which life is physically, emotionally, and intellectually vigorous until shortly before its close." Our successes were successes after all.

This debate has arisen because of a shift in the diseases causing morbidity and mortality. In the early twentieth century, far more people died of infectious ailments, which tended to be short. Today, cardiovascular disease and cancers account for more than half of deaths among the elderly in the United States. The increasing prevalence of obesity and diabetes could further add to morbidity and mortality not just among the aging, but the general population too.

Moreover, unlike patients with heart disease in the 1960s and 1970s, today, many of them will survive because of lifestyle changes and the universal availability of a host of therapies and interventions discussed in previous chapters. However, these patients do not all function to the best of their abilities. In many, the coronary artery disease progresses and requires further intervention, and some will develop heart failure. Yet, with the advent of novel therapies, they will continue to live longer and have a reasonably good quality of life, provided they are mentally competent. In this regard, by postponing death, modern medicine has enabled longer survival with some physical disability. What does it mean? Should we regret it?

In 2010, Drs. Eileen Crimmins and Hiram Beltrán-Sánchez showed that from 1998 to 2006, there was an *increase in life expectancy with disease* and an *increase in expected years with functional loss*. However, the implications of this study can be misleading. "Functional loss" as defined from the National Health Interview Survey meant inability to perform at least one of the following: walk a quarter mile, climb ten flights of stairs, stand or sit for up to 2 hours, and stand, bend, or kneel without using special equipment. Unfortunately, this study did not address quality-of-life issues. In other words, people can enjoy a good quality of life despite having one of the four criteria of "functional loss." They might regularly see movies or plays, go out for dinners and concerts, attend parties and celebrations, listen to music in their homes, have interesting conversations, visit family and friends, travel, and go on vacations.

What is quality of life, really? A friend of mine in his late 80s, a retired physician and a basic scientist, developed heart failure and poor heart function. He already had severe spinal problems and was unable to walk without help and a walker, and he'd had a previous heart attack, coronary angioplasty and stenting, and carotid artery surgery. Although a defibrillator was indicated in his condition according to current guidelines, both his cardiologist and I tried to talk him out of having one, mostly because of his advancing age, physical disability, and the fact that an yearly risk of around 5–7% for sudden cardiac death might not be the worst way for him to make his exit. However, despite his "functional loss" and many problems, he attended concerts and operas, went out for dinner more than once a month and enjoyed a glass of wine and a good conversation, listened to music, and read a lot. He had a wonderful marriage and he had adjusted to his condition. Simply stated, he was happy, adapted, with a good quality of life, and personal choice was paramount. He wholeheartedly expressed a desire to have the implantable defibrillator. He had a strong will to go on living even if he encountered a sudden death situation. He ultimately passed away in his home of terminal heart failure.

It is important to recognize that many patients with heart disease, and even those with heart failure, feel better with drugs, interventions including stenting and heart surgery, and biventricular pacemakers. *Their quality of life improves*, along with their survival.

After heart disease, cancer is the next most important cause of death and disability in the elderly. However, cancer-related morbidity and mortality is more difficult to analyze in view of its complexity. Cancer is really a hundred different diseases. Lung cancer is not the same as prostate cancer, for instance. Each kind has its own screening policies and programs, and each requires its own treatment. Mortality rates differ for each. Cancer also occurs in stages and spreads to other organs. Unlike treatments for heart disease, chemotherapy makes individuals symptomatically worse, with greater disability and a dismal quality of life, and patients can ultimately succumb to the disease as well as the treatment itself. Thus, elderly patients with "advanced cancer" should have palliative care. But in the future, cancer treatment could substantially change to genetically guided immunotherapy, making chemotherapy obsolete, and cancer treatment itself may be more tolerable even in the elderly.

Beyond taking care of ourselves with a sensible lifestyle, there are other approaches which may potentially extend life spans and quality of life. They tend to fall into the categories of hardship (such as caloric restrictions, fasting, and exposure to certain biological agents) and biochemical change. *However, at this time, they remain highly experimental and controversial.* Nonetheless, we cannot indefinitely postpone the aging process, partly because it relates to the environment, our habits, acquired or congenital illnesses, and most importantly our genetic mold. It's likely we never will.

The Scourge of COVID-19

The year 2020 saw the beginnings of a pandemic due to an unusual, highly infectious, and deadly virus, SARS-CO-V2 virus named COVID-19. As of this writing, there are over 186 million COVID cases worldwide with over 4 million deaths. In the United States, there are over 33 million cases with over 600,000 deaths according to Johns Hopkins University database, and the pandemic is not even over. It is noteworthy that age in and of itself carries a greater risk of dying from COVID-19 (Fig. 28.1). As one gets older, the risk of severe illness from COVID-19 increases. People in their 50s are at higher risk for severe illness than people in their 40s, while those in the ages of 60s–70s are at higher risk for severe illness than those in their 50s. Those individuals aged over 85 years are at the greatest risk for severe illness and death (Fig. 28.2). It is noteworthy that 8 out of 10 COVID-19-related deaths in the United States have been among adults aged 65 years and older. Other risk factors include obesity, diabetes, and hypertension that are common in the elderly.

It is of paramount importance for the elderly individuals and those who live with them to reduce the risk of getting COVID-19. The best way of protection and to reduce the spread of the virus that causes COVID-19 is the following:

A: Limit interactions with other people as much as possible.
B: Take precautions such as wearing a mask when going out and social distancing when interacting with others. It is important to keep abreast of the fact that asymptomatic young individuals can potentially infect the elderly.

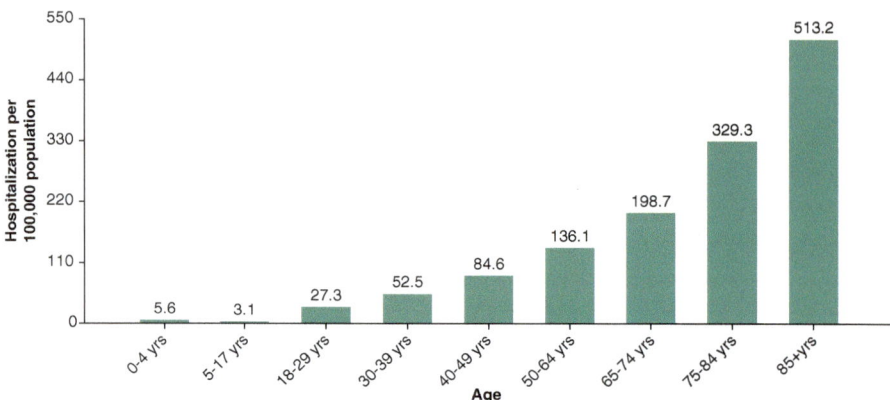

Fig. 28.1 Bar graphs showing coronavirus disease hospitalizations in the United States. Legend: On the X-axis are plotted the age and on the Y-axis hospitalizations per 100,000 population. Note that the number of people hospitalized is age-related with the greatest number 85 years and over. "Materials developed by CDC". "Reference to specific commercial products, manufacturers, companies, or trademarks does not constitute its endorsement or recommendation by the U.S. Government, Department of Health and Human Services, or Centers for Disease Control and Prevention" (https://www.cdc.gov/coronavirus/2019-ncov/need-extra-precautions/older-adults.html)

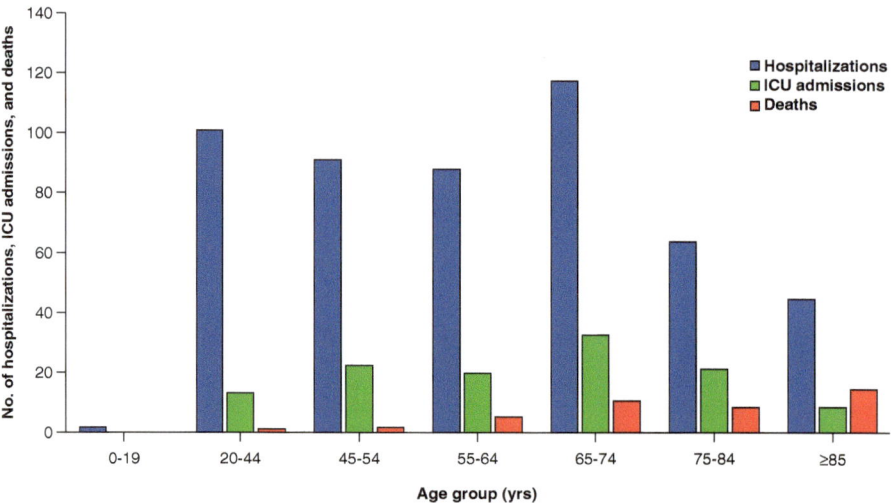

Fig. 28.2 COVID-19 hospitalizations, intensive care unit admissions, and deaths by age group. (Modified from "Materials developed by CDC." "Reference to specific commercial products, manufacturers, companies, or trademarks does not constitute its endorsement or recommendation by the U.S. Government, Department of Health and Human Services, or Centers for Disease Control and Prevention" file:///Users/josephgomes/Desktop/ARTICLES%20FOR%20RBH/Welcome%20to%20CDC%20stacks%20%7C.webarchive)

C: Elderly individuals who feel sick with fever, cough, shortness of breath, loss of smell and taste, weakness and fatigue, and muscle aches should get in touch with the health-care provider within 24 hours. However, it is important to keep into perspective that seniors may respond differently to COVID-19. They may not act like themselves. They might sleep more than usual or stop eating. They may seem unusually apathetic or confused, losing orientation to their surroundings. They may become dizzy and fall or collapse.

D: If the elderly individual lives in a nursing home, assisted living facility, or other types of senior living facility, they need to be concerned about COVID-19. For the protection of the individual and to protect friends and family members in these facilities, CDC has advised that long-term care facilities (1) restrict visitors; (2) require or recommend visitors wear masks over their nose and mouth, if visitors are allowed, (3) regularly check health-care workers and residents for fevers and symptoms; and (4) limit activities within the facility to keep residents distanced from each other and safe.

E: Vaccination: Currently vaccination for COVID-19 is available, and the type of vaccines and availability varies from country to country. At this time in the United States, three vaccines are available: Pfizer-BioNTech and Moderna COVID-19 vaccines based on mRNA technology are given in two dosages weeks apart, while the Johnson & Johnson is a single-dose vaccine. It is likely that more vaccines by other companies should be available in the near future. Elderly subjects, those with comorbidities, and those in nursing homes, assisted living facility, or other types of senior living facility have priority and should be vaccinated. The ultimate goal is to vaccinate all eligible subjects.

Irrespective of precautions, COVID-19 has been a great burden among the aged and elderly leaving them isolated in their homes or apartments or nursing homes without visits from their friends and loved ones. This will have considerable impact on their psyche as well as physical well-being.

End-of-Life Issues

Should we want to live beyond 90? Certainly—especially given the advances that seem to be coming. And if we can still enjoy life. Undoubtedly, the prospect of aging can bring fears of disability; loneliness; desolation; loss of one's home, one's surroundings; and death. But "old age" is not a fall from grace. It can show the way forward into a new grace, a time to contemplate the past and remember moments of joy and sorrow, of love and loss.

As far as I'm concerned, if I'm sane in mind and in decent physical shape, with an acceptable quality of life, I will continue savoring my existence. If I need a pacemaker, a defibrillator, a pacemaker for both chambers, and even a heart surgery, I will consider them with a critical mind by weighing the pros and cons, particularly quality-of-life issues and the risks involved.

Beyond 90, quality of life should assume greater importance than survival alone.

I have encountered several of my elderly patients with terminal heart failure with a dismal quality of life who wanted their defibrillator turned off. I have also come across friends in their 70s and 80s with terminal illness content that their lives should ebb away without heroic measures for survival. In these individuals, I have witnessed a lack of fear and a sense of peace as they faced imminent death.

For my part, if I have terminal heart failure, I will not opt for resuscitation measures including intubation. Moreover, if I already have a defibrillator and years later develop terminal heart failure, I will ask that my defibrillator be turned off. If sudden death comes my way, it will be a blessing rather than a curse.

If I develop advanced cancer, I will choose palliative therapy.

The hospital is the worst place for patients with terminal cancer and terminal heart failure to die. If at all possible, I will seek a compassionate death at home, surrounded by my family. And if I have some appetite left and consciousness, I will celebrate my coming death with champagne in the style of Anton Chekhov. I write this with one caveat: I cannot predict what my attitude, what my feelings will be, until I encounter death face to face!

How we live is our personal choice, and how we approach death can be too, just as much. However, the appearance of the COVID-19 pandemic has had a considerable impact on dying. Almost all elderly and relatively young patients seriously ill with the disease have died in an intensive care unit all alone without their family and friends in attendance. Many of them were intubated and on a respirator comatose on an anesthetic without sensorium. Most of them did not even have a chance to say their goodbyes. Undoubtedly, the lonely deaths due to COVID-19 without the presence of loved ones will leave families grieving and empty for a long time with a strong desire to connect in the afterlife.

A single person is missing for you, and the whole world is empty.—Joan Didion, *The Year of Magical Thinking*

♥

Part X
Heart Care

Chapter 29
Some Heart Care Advice to Live By

Good advice is always certain to be ignored, but that's no reason not to give it.

—Agatha Christie

Medicine offered me a wonderful opportunity to interact with people when they were sick, in pain, when sad and happy, when they returned to health from illness, and when they were close to dying. Today, we often forget that a cheerful disposition, a touch, a few sympathetic words are often more comforting to a sick patient than high-tech medicine we offer. This congruence of humanity and science is what makes the practice of medicine so great, so worthwhile, and its satisfaction cannot be measured on a scale of dollars or sheets of silver and gold. Perhaps, no other profession affords such interaction on a human scale.

It has been a privilege for which I am grateful, a privilege that at times I have not embraced wholeheartedly, limited by my own weaknesses. Nonetheless, I have usually risen above myself when the day was not so good, when I had a physical problem like an illness, when I had a family issue, when I was confounded by institutional politics, or when I wished to be left alone. Doctoring does not afford such privileges. Instead, it elevates us above ourselves. The experience has been vast and sobering and at the same time exciting, one of helping people cope with illness and better still, of steering them back to health with the right treatment.

Illness triggers a crisis within us, a crisis of confidence that makes us question how it could have happened, a crisis that shakes our very foundation, and perhaps for the very first time we face disability and even death. When we have an acute illness such as a heart attack, we suddenly face a new reality. We also enter an unknown landscape: an emergency room, an operating room, an intensive care unit, a hospital bed with its sterile surroundings, a world we may have barely taken in as visitors to other people. But for an active healthy person to suddenly occupy a hospital bed is overwhelming, mind-boggling, and tragic. Whether we like it or not, illness reminds

J. A. Gomes, *Rhythms of Broken Hearts*,
https://doi.org/10.1007/978-3-030-77382-3_29

us of our vulnerability, our transience, our mortality, and the genetic weaknesses that we were born with and were entirely unaware of.

Recently, a 42-year-old woman, a healthy physician who had never been sick before, a wonderful mother, a friend I have known since she was a child, suddenly and unexpectedly suffered a cardiac arrest. Thankfully, she survived. But can we imagine her plight?

The pandemic due to COVID-19 made the world face a new reality—a reality of fear, of acquiring an illness, of possible death, and of economic devastation. Can we imagine the loneliness of the felled individual, alone in the ICU without the loved ones, dying a lonely death, and the predicament, the sadness of the relative, the loved ones of those felled by COVID-19? The awesome insecurity and posttraumatic stress disorder that such an unforeseen and catastrophic event ushered?

In many of my patients, I have encountered loneliness, fear, insecurity, and loss, and the only route remaining is assurance from a carrying doctor and often faith and consolation in a supreme power.

Some medical problems like infections or accidents are random events. But others have a genetic background, like coronary artery disease at a young age, certain heart arrhythmias like the long QT and Brugada syndromes, and many cancers, and they are an ongoing peril.

It is hard to swallow the fact that overall, we have very little control of our lives. Sheer luck has shaped most of it. Our birth parents are a matter of chance, as are the wealth or poverty we are born in, the country of our birth, and more often than not even our marriage partner. Similarly, we have little ultimate control of our future health. All we can do is to live a healthy lifestyle and hope for the best.

When facing illness, we need to adjust, and the faster we do it—entrust ourselves to a good and caring doctor and embrace life all over again—the better off we are. But the collection of scars, the visible ones we see on our body each morning in the bathroom mirror and the invisible ones in the mind, do remain. Over time, perhaps after months or even years, we may seldom think of them. But when we do, we understand that they are marks of life, like tattoos etched into the body, that tell the story of who we are, of what happened to us, and of the hope that carried us onward.

What is life without hope? Physicians often forget to give an inkling of hope, instead immersing patients in discussions of complex statistics and all sorts of complications from the disease, drug, or procedure, information that the person is not even registering. All the patient wants to hear is a kind word! Words illuminated with hope. Remember that hope is the very essence of life. "I am prepared for the worst," said Benjamin Disraeli, "but hope for the best."

The words of a doctor have an awesome impact. Each word he or she utters is measured, repeated in the mind, re-repeated, retold to friends and family, and contemplated by the patient. One wrong word will bring about anxiety, a sense of fear and doom. A physician has an overwhelming responsibility to sound an optimistic note if it is deserved. He needs as well to leave room for elements that are unclear and unknown, and many elements in medicine fall into the latter category. As much as one wrong word can be devastating, a right word can be reassuring and provide a sense of confidence, even euphoria. It can suggest that improvement is down the road, at the corner, around the bend. All my patients want to know the facts, but facts should come in with some optimism if it is deserved. I never hesitate to end my conversations on a positive note, partly because cardiovascular medicine, and particularly electrophysiology, offers complete cures in maladies such as supraventricular tachycardia and protection with an internal defibrillator.

What to Do If Illness Strikes

Here is my advice for anyone who may someday suffer from a cardiovascular illness:

1. *Know yourself physically and mentally, your weaknesses and your strengths.* This knowledge will help you greatly through the process. But acquiring it is easier said than done. Most of us come to understand ourselves only in hindsight when we face a calamity. Calamity is like a reflection in the mirror. It shows us our inner selves.
2. *Learn your family history.* If you find you have a family history of coronary artery disease, with one or more family members who have had a heart attack at an early age, or sudden cardiac death, view this information as a warning sign. Immerse yourself in regular physical activity, watch your weight, and eat healthily.

I recommend a Mediterranean diet consisting mainly of vegetables, fruits, whole grains, nuts, legumes, and fish. Poultry, eggs, milk, and cheese can be enjoyed several times a week. Herbs and spices, rather than excessive salt, can be used for seasoning. Olive oil should replace saturated fats such as butter. Red wine in moderation is encouraged. Red meats and sweets may be enjoyed, but no more than two to four times a month. The Mediterranean diet is minimally processed, is home cooked, and enjoyed with family and friends.

See a physician regularly to check for cholesterol, blood pressure, and diabetes. If you have any of these problems, seek advice from your doctor.

You can calculate your own risk for CAD and a heart attack. Several Internet sites are available, such as http://tools.acc.org/ASCVD-Risk-Estimator-Plus/#!/calculate/estimate. (The "ASCVD" is arteriosclerotic cardiovascular disease.) If you are already on a statin to lower your cholesterol, you can also check your risk over the next 10 years with the Statin Choice Decision Aid from the Mayo Clinic. You will have to know your history of events such as prior heart attack, stroke, acute coronary syndrome, angioplasty, and stents, as well as diabetic status, treated systolic blood pressure, HDL, total cholesterol, and if you are on statins whether you are on a standard or high dose. The website is: https://statindecisionaid.mayoclinic.org

Be aware that the risk calculation will not be 100% accurate. Nothing is, in this area. Moreover, these formulas are based on old studies and may not be sensitive enough in today's day and age. Your risk can also change over time and you may need to recalculate it. Finally, there are many issues about CAD that we don't yet understand. The figure is just a rough guide.

I do not advocate the use of drugs to start with in young, symptomless individuals. I would rather they control the risk factors (high blood pressure, diabetes, smoking, overweight and obesity, and high cholesterol) with a healthy lifestyle, those simple habits such as regular exercise, healthy eating, and relaxation. It is disconcerting that so many people will adopt them only after a catastrophic event in their lives such as a heart attack or survival from a cardiac arrest. If lifestyle improvements do not produce the desired effects, medications may be necessary. Your cardiologist might also consider obtaining a calcium score and/or a high-resolution CT to define your proximal coronary anatomy before committing you to an aggressive LDL- and triglyceride-lowering regimen.

If you have a strong family history of sudden death at a young age or during sports activity, you might want to alert your physician who might consider obtaining an ECG and an echo to exclude certain conditions like the long QT syndrome, Brugada syndrome, right ventricular dysplasia, and hypertrophic cardiomyopathy.

3. *Realize that acute and sudden illness may happen.* The classic example of an acute illness is an unexpected heart attack or a cardiac arrest. Say you are a 60-year-old man who has been doing very well, had regular physical checkups, and received a good bill of health. A few weeks later under a stressful situation, you develop chest discomfort. You call 911. You are taken to a hospital and you are told that you are having a heart attack. This is a startling, extremely upsetting event, and you will then hand your life over to the doctor, in this case a cardiologist/interventionist who will attempt to open your clogged coronary artery. At that moment, the time is so short, that the doctor is your savior. You completely give yourself into his or her hands. You have no choice but to hope that you have an experienced, technically skillful doctor who is doing the right thing for you. If you are in a reputable institution, it is highly likely that you are in good hands.

4. *See a doctor for subacute and chronic illnesses.* Perhaps your condition is not acute. For example, you may notice that you have skipped beats or your heart is beating fast or palpitating. Perhaps you feel faint. You may sense chest discomfort when you walk uphill which goes away immediately when you rest. Even though your condition may not be urgent, you need to see a doctor at once who might refer you to a cardiologist.

5. *Ask questions about the referral.* Learn who the cardiologist is, the quality of his or her reputation, and any other relevant information you can gather. You can do it yourself by Googling the specialist. If you are not satisfied with what you hear and read, seek another physician. One useful guide is "Best Doctors in America," which has names, addresses, and phone numbers of specialist in your area. If you live in New York, *New York* magazine publishes a list of doctors yearly in various specialties in the Tri-State area. Choose a doctor who cares about you and takes time to explain your condition, the treatment options, and the prognosis of your illness.

6. *Ask the cardiologist a lot of questions.* For instance, if your cardiologist wants to take you to the cath. lab, ask what he or she plans to do. Is he going to put in stents? What are the consequences of inserting one? Is it necessary? Similarly, if you are going to have a procedure such as ablation for atrial fibrillation, ask the doctor about his success rate, the complications of the procedure, the long-term outcomes, and, importantly, how many procedures he has done.

7. *Take charge of your illness.* Read about your condition. You can do lots of searches on the Internet. Indeed, there are too many sources, and sometimes they can be confusing. Whenever you are having a procedure, read about it, check the options, and most importantly, ask your doctor whether you need the procedure, that is, whether you can do without it. If you are placed on a drug, read about it and its side effects. Don't forget to ask the doctor whether you need the drug and whether there are other options. Don't believe the surgeon or interventionist who assures you that nothing will go wrong, and all will be well. There are always risks, even if small ones. On the other hand, a doctor who overemphasizes the possibility of complications may be less experienced.

8. *Seek a second opinion. I cannot overstress this.* Especially if your condition doesn't improve, or worsens, or if your doctor seems uncertain, do seek another opinion. "The most important thing to do if you find yourself in a hole is to stop digging," said Warren Buffett. When seeking a second opinion, focus on specialists associated with a reputable institution, in particular a university hospital. Often, they have cutting-edge technologies and novel experimental drugs in their armamentarium that are not available elsewhere.

9. *Favor high-volume institutions for complex procedures.* Some procedures such as a repeat ablation for atrial fibrillation and ventricular tachycardia are best done in these institutions. Find out which institutions and individual doctors in your area perform most of them. These ablations are extremely complicated and can take several hours, and you get the best results at institutions with teams that are well-equipped to handle them. Again, keep in mind that cutting-edge technology is available in only some high-volume centers.

Recently, I was consulted by an 82-year-old patient who had severe three-vessel coronary artery diseases. She also had significant calcification and left main disease and two prior mini-strokes. She was strongly advised coronary bypass surgery, but because of her prior strokes, she was high risk, and she and her family were unwilling to proceed. A friend of the family contacted me regarding the possibility of stenting. I referred her to our superb interventionalists, Dr. Samin Sharma and Dr. Kini, who handle such complex cases that need not only stenting but also removal of coronary calcium by rotor. She had two successful intervention procedures 3 days apart and was discharged home without surgery.

10. *Enjoy life.* Remember that you are as old as you think you are. Age, in and of itself, no longer defines "old age." I have seen people in the 80s and 90s, sharper than some in their 60s and with an excellent quality of life. However, if you have attained "old age," seek quality of life rather than just existence. This decision is probably one of the most difficult one we will face in our lives. And only

you can make it. Blend into old age, not with a heavy heart but with a smile. Remember, old people are more contented and happier than young ones.

In earliest times, the very purpose of the heart was an exotic mystery, much like the universe and beyond today. Eventually, physicians made the heroic discoveries of its mechanical and command systems and devised brilliant strategies that have prolonged and enhanced so many people's lives. And today, we know how to treat heart disease and perhaps in the future prevent most and eradicate certain genetic ailments altogether. Humanity has been on an amazing journey.

Meanwhile, our lives are precious, a marvelous gift, and from my heart to yours, I wish you the best life possible.

♥

About the Author

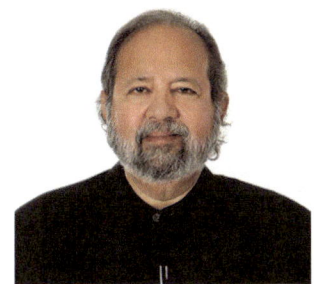

J. Anthony Gomes, MD also known as António Gomes is a professor of medicine at The Icahn School of Medicine, and director of the Cardiac Arrhythmia Consultation Service and senior consultant, The Leona M. and Harry B. Helmsley Charitable Trust Center for Cardiac Electrophysiology, and past director of Cardiac Electrophysiology and Electrocardiography, The Mount Sinai Medical Center, NYC. He has published extensively in medicine, including two textbooks of cardiology, *Signal Averaged Electrocardiography: Basic Concepts Methods and Application* (Kluwer Academic Press, London/Amsterdam, 1993) and *Heart Rhythm Disorders: History, Mechanisms and Treatment Perspectives* (Springer Nature, 2020). He has also published articles in the humanities in anthologies, books, newspapers, and magazines; two books of poetry entitled *Visions from Grymes Hill* (Turn of River Press, Stanford, Connecticut, USA, 1994) and *Mirrored Reflections* (GOA 1556 and Fundacão Oriente, 2013); and novels *The Sting of Peppercorns* (GOA, 1556 & Broadway Books, 2010, second edition, Amaryllis, New Delhi, India, 2017), *Nas Garras Do Destino* (Chiado Editora, Brake Media, Lisbon, Portugal and Brazil, 2019), and *Have A Heart* (Serving House Books, Copenhagen, Denmark and South Orange, NJ, 2020).

Notes

Authors Note

- *The Language of Medicine.* Henrik R. Wulff. *Journal of the Royal Society of Medicine*, v. 97, no. 4, 2004. https://www.ncbi.nlm.nih.gov/pmc/articles/PMC1079361/
- *The aim of science is to discover and illuminate truth. And that, I take it, is the aim of literature, whether biography or history... It seems to me, then, that there can be no separate literature of science.* — From Carson's remarks at her acceptance of the National Book Award for Nonfiction. https://www.fws.gov/refuge/Rachel_Carson/about/rachelcarsonexcerpts2.html
- *Medicine is my lawful wife and literature my mistress; when I get tired of one, I spend the night with the other.* — Anton Chekhov (in a letter written to his friend Alexei Suvorin on 11 September 1888.) https://www.racgp.org.au/afp/2013/september/a-is-for-aphorism/
- *"The physician should not treat the disease but the patient who is suffering from it."* https://www.quotetab.com/quote/by-maimonides/the-physician-should-not-treat-the-disease-but-the-patient-who-is-suffering-from
- *Medicine is the art of engagement with the human condition rather than with disease.* Bernard Lown: The Lost Art of Healing: Practicing Compassion in Medicine. RANDOM HOUSE, Ballentine Books, 1999

J. A. Gomes, *Rhythms of Broken Hearts*, https://doi.org/10.1007/978-3-030-77382-3

Preface

- *For while knowledge defines all we currently know and understand, imagination points to all we might yet discover and create.*—Albert Einstein. What Life Means to Einstein. The Saturday Evening Post, Oct 26,1929, interview by George Sylvester Viereck. http://www.saturdayeveningpost.com/wp- content/uploads/satevepost/what_life_means_to_einstein.pdf
- *Change is the law of life. And those who look only to the past or the present are certain to miss the future.* — John F. Kennedy (*Address in the Assembly Hall at the Paulskirche in Frankfurt, June 26 1963*) https://www.jfklibrary.org/asset-viewer/archives/JFKPOF/045/JFKPOF-045-023.
- *Your work is going to fill a large part of your life, and the only way to be truly satisfied is to do what you believe is great work. And the only way to do great work is to love what you do—Steve Jobs.* Stanford Commencement address on June 12, 2005. https://news.stanford.edu/2005/06/14/jobs-061505/
- *A Look at the 1940 Census.* United States Census Bureau https://www.census.gov/newsroom/cspan/1940census/CSPAN_1940slides.pdf.
- *Heart Disease and Stroke Statistics 2017 at a Glance.* American Heart Association January 25, 2017, p. 1. https://www.heart.org/idc/groups/ahamah-public/@wcm/@sop/@smd/documents/downloadable/ucm_491265.pdf.
- *Heart Disease and Stroke Statistics— 2021 Update.* A Report From the American Heart Association. Circulation: https://www.ahajournals.org/doi/10.1161/CIR.0000000000000950
- *"I Was on That Ground Dead,"* Gabrielle Frank, *Bob Harper Opens Up on 'Widow-maker'* Heart Attack: *Today*, April 4, 2017. http://www.today.com/health/biggest-loser-bob-harper-opens-today-about-recovery-t109956.
- *U.S. Life Expectancy Plummeted in 2020.* Sabrina Tavernise and Abby Goodnough: Covid-19 Live Updates: https://www.nytimes.com/live/2021/02/18/world/covid-19-coronavirus

Part I: The Mythology of the Human Heart

Romanticizing the Heart

- I would rather have eyes that cannot see; ears that cannot hear; lips that cannot speak, than a heart that cannot love. — Robert Tizon. https://www.quotery.com/authors/robert-tizon
- Tears come from the heart and not from the brain. — Leonardo da Vinci. https://thequotesforlife.com/tears-come-from-the-heart-and-not-from-the-brain-leon-ardo-da-Vinci/#.YFD6Ai1h27A
- *Egyptian Mummies: Exploring Ancient Lives.* Uncredited: *Arts Review*, December 21, 2016. http://artsreview.com.au/egyptian-mummies-exploring-ancient-lives/

- *The Meaning and Significance of Heart in Hinduism.* https://www.hinduwebsite. com/hinduism/essays/the-meaning-and-significance-of-heart-in-hinduism.asp *Yoga Philosophy & the Upanishads* https://www.sheffieldyogaschool.co.uk/yoga-philosophy-the-upanishads/
- *Empedocles (c. 492–432 B.C.E.).* Gordon Campbell Internet Encyclopedia of Philosophy. http://www.iep.utm.edu/empedocl/ Stanford Encyclopedia of Philosophy. https://plato.stanford.edu/entries/stoicism/
- *Galen and the Squealing Pig.* Charles G. Gross: *The Neuroscientist,* v. 4, no. 3, 1998. https://www.princeton.edu/~cggross/neuroscientist_4_98_216.pdf
- Pearl S. Buck (American Novelist) http://www.inspiration.rightattitudes.com/authors/pearl-s-buck/
- Ted Hughes. https://www.goodreads.com/quotes/160333-the-only-calibration-that-counts-is-how-much-heart-people
- *The Unbearable Lightness of Being.* Milan Kundera. English translation 1984 by Harper & Row Publishers, Inc.
- *Devotion to the Immaculate Heart of Mary.* Uncredited. heotokos Books. http://theotokos.org.uk/devotion-to-the-immaculate-heart-of-mary/

The Mysteries of the Age-Old Pulse

- *Very often conditions are recorded as observable "under thy fingers"… Among such observations it is important to notice that the pulsations of the human heart are observed.* — James Henry Breasted (1865–1935), archeologist, on the *Edwin Smith Surgical Papyrus,* c. 1600 BCE. https://www.goodreads.com/work/quotes/21574235-the-edwin-smith-surgical-papyrus-vol-1-hieroglyphic-transliteration-t
- *I love yoga… I also see an Ayurvedic doctor, which is an ancient Indian thing. I go and see the doctor to balance my system twice a year; it's preventative. They take my pulse, give me some herbs, and tell me what I should eat and what I should avoid.*— Jerry Hall https://www.brainyquote.com/quotes/jerry_hall_746451
- *The Papyrus Ebers.* Cyril P. Bryan, translated from the German Version, Geoffrey Bles, London, 1930. http://www.ask-force.org/web/India/Bryan-CP-The-Papyrus-Ebers-searchable-1930.pdf
- *History and Development of Traditional Chinese Medicine.* Zhen'guo Wang, Chin Peng, ed., Beijing, Science Press, 1999, p. 99.
- *The Conception of Nadi and Its Examination.* S.K. Ramachandra Rao: *Ancient Science of Life,* v. 4, no. 3, Jan 1985, pp. 148–152, p. 150. https://www.ncbi.nlm.nih.gov/pmc/articles/PMC3331513/pdf/ASL-4-148.pdf
- *Measure of the Heart: Santorio Santorio and the Pulsilogium.* In Richard de Grijs and Daniel Vuillermin. https://arxiv.org/pdf/1702.05211.pdf
- *The First Man/Machine Interaction in Medicine: The Pulsilogium of Sanctorius.* J. Levitt and G. Agarwal: Med Instrumentation, v. 13, no. 1, Jan–Feb 1979, pp. 61–3. https://www.ncbi.nlm.nih.gov/pubmed/370523

- Galileo and the Pendulum Clock. Adrian Johnstone, 2009. http://www.cs.rhul.ac.uk/~adrian/timekeeping/galileo/
- *Sir John Floyer (1649–1734).* Lilian Lindsay: Proceedings of the Royal Society of Medicine, v. 44, 1950, P. 43. http://journals.sagepub.com/doi/pdf/10.1177/003591575104400107
- *The Physician's Pulse Watch.* D.D. Gibbs: *Medical History,* v. 15, no. 2, April 1971, pp. 187–190, p. 189. https://www.ncbi.nlm.nih.gov/pmc/articles/PMC1034144/pdf/medhist00131-0082.pdf

Part II: The Renaissance Period in Heart Rhythm Disorders

Demystifying the Heart

- *Explore, Dream & Discover are three secrets of which the time traveler is unaware. They demystify as the journey advances!* — Vishwanath S. J. https://www.goodreads.com/quotes/tag?id=time+travel&page=16
- *The real voyage of discovery consists not in seeking new landscapes, but in having new eyes*—Marcel Proust. In Search of Lost Time. Modern Library; Slp edition (June 3, 2003). https://www.abebooks.com/readers-books-petworth/3967716/sf
- *"Doth never stop, except it be for eternity."* Quoted in Dario DiFrancesco, *The Role of the Funny Current in Pacemaker Activity.* Circulation Research, v. 106, issue 3, 2010, pp. 434–446, p. 435. http://circres.ahajournals.org/content/106/3/434
- *Walter Gaskell and the Understanding of Atrioventricular Conduction and Block.* Mark E. Silverman and Charles B. Upshaw, Jr., Journal of the American College of Cardiology, v. 39, no. 10, 2002, pp. 1574–1580, p. 1577. https://www.ncbi.nlm.nih.gov/pubmed/12020482
- *Discovery of the Sinus Node by Keith and Flack: On the Centennial of Their 1907 Publication.* Mark E. Silverman and Arthur Hollman *Heart,* v. 93, October 2007, pp. 1184–1187, p. 1185. https://www.ncbi.nlm.nih.gov/pmc/articles/PMC2000948/
- *"He had discovered in the right auricle [atrium] of the mole, just where the superior vena cava enters that chamber."* In Mark E. Silverman and Arthur Hollman, "Discovery of the Sinus Node by Keith and Flack: On the Centennial of Their 1907 Publication," *Heart,* vol. 93, no. 10, October 2007, pp.1184–1187, p. 1184. https://www.ncbi.nlm.nih.gov/pmc/articles/PMC2000948/
- *"Resembles a tree, having a beginning, or root, and branches."* In Mark E. Silverman et al: *Why Does the Heart Beat?* Circulation, vol. 113, issue 23, June 12, 2006, pp. 2775–2781, p. 2778. http://circ.ahajournals.org/content/113/23/2775
- YouTube: *Sodium – Potassium Pump Animated Lecture*: Prakash B. *https://www.youtube.com/watch?v=xweYA-IJTqs).2015*

Understanding Heart Rhythm Disorders: The Birth of Clinical Cardiac Electrophysiology

- *I am one of those who think like Nobel, that humanity will draw more good than evil from new discoveries.* — Marie Curie. https://www.mariecurie.org.uk/who/our-history/marie-curie-the-scientist
- *There is not a discovery in science, however revolutionary, however sparkling with insight, that does not arise out of what went before. 'If I have seen further than other men,' said Isaac Newton, 'it is because I have stood on the shoulders of giants.''* — Isaac Asimov, Adding a Dimension: Seventeen Essays on the History of Science, Lancer Books, 1969
- *Einthoven's String Galvanometer.* Moises Rivera-Ruiz, Christian Cajavilca, and Joseph Varon *Texas Heart Institute Journal*, v. 35, no. 2, 2008, pp. 174–78. P. 175. https://www.ncbi.nlm.nih.gov/pmc/articles/PMC2435435/
- Willem Einthoven—Biographical. Unknown, in *Nobel Lectures, Physiology or Medicine 1922–1941*, Amsterdam, Elsevier, 1965. https://www.nobelprize.org/nobel_prizes/medicine/laureates/1924/einthoven-bio.html
- *Historic Timeline.* Mount Sinai Heart History. Mountsinai.org
- *Oct. 30, 1958: Medical Oops Leads to First Coronary Angiogram.* Hadley Leggett, *Wired*, October 30, 2009. https://www.wired.com/2009/10/1030first-coronary-angiogram/
- Benjamin J. Scherlag, PhD. Unknown. https://www.oumedicine.com/heartrhythm-institute/our-staff/benjamin-j-scherlag-phd
- *The Development of the His Bundle Recording Technique.* Benjamin J. Scherlag: *Pacing and Electrophysiology*, v. 2, issue 2, March 1979, pp. 230–233, p. 230. http://onlinelibrary.wiley.com/doi/10.1111/j.1540-8159.1979.tb05206.x/full
- *"We were able to initiate and terminate tachycardia by appropriately timed stimuli. This was the birth of programmed stimulation of the heart, over 50 years ago, and we danced in the catheterization lab!"* Personal communication, the late, Dr. Hein J.J. Wellens

Part III: Galloping Away in the Atrium

Living With a Galloping Heart

- Among my stillness was a pounding heart.—Shannon A. Thomson, *Seconds before Sunrise* Clean Teen Publishing (August 25, 2015)
- Having this thing totally wrecked my life. I felt so scared and helpless because I never knew when I'd have another episode, how bad that episode would be, if this new drug would work … because many of them didn't… or if it never stopped racing… would I die?—Kathryn A. Wood, RN, PhD, Carolyn L. Wiener, PhD, and Jeanie Kayser-Jones, RN, PhD, FAAN

- Supraventricular Tachycardia and the Struggle to be Believed. Eur J Cardiovasc Nurs. 2007 Dec; 6(4): 293–302.
- *Paroxysmal Tachycardia.* Thomas Lewis, *Heart*, v. 1, July 1 1909, pp. 43–72.
- *Obituary: Sir John Parkinson.* William Evans, *British Heart Journal*, v. 38, 1976, pp. 1105–1107, p. 1107. http://heart.bmj.com/content/heartjnl/38/10/1105.full.pdf

Radical Ideas: The Road to Conquering Supraventricular Tachycardia

- *Over every mountain there is a path, although it may not be seen from the valley.* Theodore Roethke. https://www.brainyquote.com/quotes/theodore_roethke_120661
- *First comes thought; then organization of that thought, into ideas and plans; then transformation of those plans into reality. The beginning, as you will observe, is in your imagination.* Napoleon Hill. https://www.brainyquote.com/quotes/napoleon_hill_393412

- *In the early 1980s electrical shocks via a catheter were used to ablate the AV Junction.* Dr. Melvin N. Sheinman and the late Dr. John J. Gallagher: Personal Communication.

Atrial Fibrillation: The Heart's Tap Dance

- *Don't let anyone, especially your doctor, tell you that A-Fib isn't that serious, or you should just learn to live with it.* —Steve S. Ryan, *Beat Your A-Fib: The Essential Guide to Finding Your Cure.* https://a-fib.com/graphic-quote-dont-let-anyone-tell-you-a-fib-isnt-that-serious/
- *The Yellow Emperors Classic of Medicine.* Maoshing Ni, Ph.D: Shambala, Boston and London 1995.
- From rebellious palpitations to the discovery of auricular fibrillation. Mark E. Silverman: Contributions of Mackenzie, Lewis and Einthoven. The Am. J. Cardiol 1994; 73: 384–389
- *Afflicts between 2.7 and 6.1 million people in the United States.* Unknown, *Atrial Fibrillation Fact Sheet.* Centers for Disease Control and Prevention, August 2015. https://www.cdc.gov/dhdsp/data_statistics/fact_sheets/fs_atrial_fibrillation.htm
- *"Their results were magic to me,"* he said. Unknown, "Michel Haïssaguerre," *Cardiac Rhythm News*, February 6, 2009. https://cardiacrhythmnews.com/michel-haissaguerre/
- *"Variants in chromosomes 16q22, 1q21, and a few others are associated with it too".* Moritz F. Sinner at al., Genome-Wide Association Studies of Atrial Fibrillation:

Past, Present, and Future," *Cardiovascular Research*, v. 89, no. 4, March 1, 2011, pp. 701–709. https://www.ncbi.nlm.nih.gov/pmc/articles/PMC3039249/
- *"30% of people with AF may also have a relative with it."* Rekha Mankad, *Does Atrial Fibrillation Run in Families?* Mayo Clinic, October 22, 2014. http://www.mayoclinic.org/diseases-conditions/atrial-fibrillation/expert-answers/atrial-fibrillation-genetics/faq-20111614
- *A-Fib and cardioversion.* David H. Neuman: A Brief History. Epmonthly.com
- *Atrial Fibrillation & the Cox Maze Procedure*—Dr. James Cox, StopAfib.org Interviews, February 20, 2013. https://www.youtube.com/watch?v=GuMsUaqmAQc

The Sawtooth Rhythm: Atrial Flutter

- *The gloom encroaches upon my mind, and my heart flutters like a bird held fast in a fist* —Hannah Kent. Burial Rites (ed. Pan Macmillan, 2013)
- *The foxglove, with its stately bells Of purple, shall adorn thy dells.*—David Macbeth Moir
  https://www.quotemaster.org/qa90c7ba276bf4c58349fcadf0ecf5584
- *Solitude! if I must with thee dwell, Let it not be among the jumbled heap Of murky buildings: climb with me the steep, Nature's observatory whence the dell, In flowery slopes, its river's crystal swell, May seem a span; let me thy vigils keep 'Mongst boughs pavilion'd, where the deer's swift leap Startles the wild bee from the foxglove bell...* —John Keats (Sonnet VII [O Solitude! if I must with thee dwell])
- *An Account of the Foxglove and Some of Its Medical Uses.* Withering W: M. Swinney, Birmingham (1785) (The Classics of Medicine Library, Special Edition, 1979)
- *William Withering and An Account of the Foxglove.* Silverman ME, Clin. Cariol. 1989, 12: 416–418.
- *Sir Thomas Lewis (1881–1945).* Cygankiewicz I: Cardiology Journal. 2007, Vol. 14, No. 6, pp. 605–606.

Part IV: Abnormal Rhythms Arising from the Ventricles

The Elusive Extrabeat

- *lab/dab ------ lab/dab --- dab ------------- lab/dab*

  My heart skips: the ventricular premature beat¬ the heart tumbles, the chest heaves

  pain, dizziness, delirium. What is it white knight? An impending infarction, or death?

Out of my lungs, the last breath? lab/dab ------ lab/dab --- dab ------------- lab/dab

António Gomes — Modified from *Mirrored Reflections* (GOA 1556 and Fundacão Oriente, 2013)

- *Karel Frederick Wenckebach (1864–1940).* Pérez-Riera, Andrés Ricardo; Femenía, Francisco et al: A giant of medicine, Cardiology Journal 2011, Vol. 18, No. 3, pp. 337–339
- *"Or, 'You're a very unhealthy man. No smoking, please."* In Rick Newby, *From Norman Jefferis 'Jeff' Holter: A Serendipitous Life: An Essay in Biography. Drumlummon Views*, Fall 2008. http://www.drumlummon.org/images/DV_vol2-no1-PDFs/DV_vol2-no1_Newby1.pdf

A Catastrophic Event: Sudden Cardiac Death

- *Sudden cardiac death has left no age untouched; sparing neither saint nor sinner, it has Burdened man with a sense of insecurity and fragility.* — Bernard Lown. Sudden cardiac death: The major challenge confronting contemporary cardiology. The American Journal of Cardiology, 1979; 43 (2):313–328
- *A death from a long illness is very different from a sudden death. It gives you time to say goodbye and time to adjust to the idea that the beloved will not be with you anymore.* — Meghan O'Rourke: "Normal" vs. "Complicated" Grief. SLATE, MARCH 05, 2009
  https://slate.com/human-interest/2009/03/the-long-goodbye-normal-vs-complicated-grief.html
- *Facts Every Second Counts.* Rural and Community Access to Emergency Devices. https://www.heart.org/idc/groups/heart-public/@wcm/@adv/documents/downloadable/ucm_301646.pdf
- *Denkmiler Agyptischer Sculptur.* Bissing Von, FW: (Explanatory Text and Plates I, 1–57), Mfinehen, F. Bruckmann, 1914, Plate 18B.
- *Eccguidelines.heart.org*
- *Cardioversion: Past, Present, and Future. Circulation*, vol. 120, no. 16, October 20, 2009, pp. 1623–1632. https://www.ncbi.nlm.nih.gov/pmc/articles/PMC2782563/

Strange Occurrences in Life's Channels

- *Death is a distant rumor to the young.* — Andy A. Rooney. 60 Years of Wisdom and Wit (Public Affairs; Reprint edition, 2010)

  https://www.goodreads.com/quotes/926408-death-is-a-distant-rumor-to-the-young

- *Your life was a hypothesis. Those who die old are made of the past. Thinking of them, one thinks of what they have done. Thinking of you, one thinks of what you could have become. You were, and you will remain, made up of possibilities.*— Édouard Levé: SUICIDE, Gallimard Education; 0 edition, 2009. https://www.goodreads.com/quotes/427474-your-life-was-a-hypothesis-those-who
- *"It is the ingenuity of our genome that is the secret to our complexity."* Siddhartha Mukherjee, *The Gene*, New York, Scribner, 2016, pp. 322–23.
- *"Her story was told to me by Professor Dr. Peter Schwartz of the University of Milan."* Personal communication from Dr. Peter Schwartz.
- *"What I learned from that case, and since then always tell my students, is that children and adolescents suffering from a life-threatening arrhythmia should be told to come back to the out-patient clinic often, again and again, telling them, but also the parents and eventual partners, that taking their medication is crucial."* The late Hein J.J. Wellens, personal communication.
- *"But all this angst that everybody else had was making me a bit nervous."* Regina Nuzzo, "Biography of Mark T. Keating," *Proceedings of the National Academy of Sciences (PNAS)*, vol. 102, no. 23, pp. 8086–8088, p. 8087. http://www.pnas.org/content/102/23/8086.full
- *"I was getting anxious about the whole process."* Regina Nuzzo, "Biography of Mark T. Keating," *Proceedings of the National Academy of Sciences (PNAS)*, vol. 102, no. 23, pp. 8086–8088, p. 8087. http://www.pnas.org/content/102/23/8086.full
- *"Unfortunately for me, the revolutions weren't happening in San Francisco."* Regina Nuzzo. Biography of Mark T. Keating. In Proceedings of the National Academy of Sciences of the United States of America, 2005; 102, no 23: 8086–8088
- *"I was doing it all with my own hands. At the time, it wasn't clear we would ever succeed. I was getting anxious about the whole process."* Regina Nuzzo. Biography of Mark T. Keating. In Proceedings of the National Academy of Sciences of the United States of America, 2005; 102, no 23: 8086–8088
- *"There is nothing new,"* he said. *"Everything has already been done."* The defibrillator was not yet invented, and decoding the human genome was a dream. *"Just imagine what a bad prediction that was,"* said Dr. Brugada much later. Pioneers in cardiology: Pedro Brugada, MD, PhD. Ingrid Torjesen, Circulation, 2008: f38–f39 (http://circ.ahajournals.org/content/circulationaha/117/7/f37.full.pdf)
- *"The major contribution of that boy was to put the whole genetics of cardiac arrhythmias another context."* Ingrid Torjesen, "Pioneers in Cardiology: Pedro Brugada, MD, PhD," *Circulation*, February 19, 2008, pp. f38–f39.

A Heart Braking Calamity: Sudden Death in the Athlete

- *Today, the road all runners come, Shoulder-high we bring you home, And set you at your threshold down, Townsman of a stiller town.* — A.E. Houseman, To an Athlete Dying Young.

  https://www.poetryfoundation.org/poems/46452/to-an-athlete-dying-young
- *Sudden death in young competitive athletes usually is precipitated by physical activity and may be due to a heterogeneous spectrum of cardiovascular disease, most commonly hypertrophic cardiomyopathy.* — Dr. Barry J. Maron: Sudden Death in Young Competitive Athletes. Clinical, Demographic, and Pathological Profiles. *JAMA*. 1996;276(3):199–204.
  https://jamanetwork.com/journals/jama/article-abstract/405465
- "*Soon after, he died. He was 23.*" Bill Dwyre, "25 Years After It Happened, Hank Gathers' Death Still Brings a Shudder," *Los Angeles Times*, March 4, 2015. http://www.latimes.com/sports/la-sp-hank-gathers-dwyre-20150304-column.html
- "*He can return to professional basketball without limitations.*" Christine Gorman, "Did Reggie Lewis Have to Die?" *Time*, Sunday, June 24, 2001. http://content.time.com/time/magazine/article/0,9171,162165,00.html
- "*He didn't put his arms out to break his fall, or anything, he just dropped.*" Euan Ferguson, "78 Minutes in the Life (and Near Death) of Fabrice Muamba," *The Guardian*, March 24, 2012. https://www.theguardian.com/football/2012/mar/25/muamba-collapse-minute-by-minute

Conquering the Arrhythmia Substrate: The Scalpel and the Source

- *In order to conquer, what we need is to dare, still to dare, and always to dare.* — Georges Jacques Danton. https://welikequotes.com/author/georges-jacques-danton-1759/in-order-to-conquer-what-we-need-is-to-dare-still-to-dare
- "*These patients had a well-tolerated VT, due to a previous heart attack or unknown causes,*" he said. "*None of them developed VF during stimulation in the laboratory...*" Personal communication, the late, Dr. Hein J.J. Wellens
- *Heart Rhythms—Rhythms in History*: Interview with Mark E. Josephson
- "*The Josephson School of electrophysiology.*" Hein J.J. Wellens, Alfred E. Buxton, Frank F. Marchlinski, Peter Zimelbaum: Josephson School: A Legacy of Important Contributions to Electrophysiology 1st Edition, 2015. Cardiology Publishing LLC, Minneapolis, Mn. 55410s

A Revolutionary Idea: The Implantable Defibrillator—A Lifesaver

- *Political revolutions, the writer Amitav Ghosh writes, often occur in the court-yards of palaces, in spaces on the cusp of power, located neither outside nor inside. Scientific revolutions, in contrast, typically occur in basements, in buried-away places removed from mainstream corridors of thought.*— Siddhartha Mukherjee, *The Emperor of All Maladies,* Scribner; 1st edition (August 1, 2011)
- *"But that's not me. Nobody nursed me along."* John A. Kastor, "Michel Mirowski and the Automatic Implantable Defibrillator," *The American Journal of Cardiology*, vol. 63, issue 15, May 1, 1989, pp. 1121–1126, p. 1121. http://www.ajconline.org/article/0002-9149(89)90090-8/pdf

To Freeze and Not to Fry

- *The same water that will kill you, drown you, give you hypothermia is the same water that will help you survive.* — Joe Teti

  https://www.wisefamousquotes.com/quotes-about-hypothermia/
- *The Edwin Smith Papyrus*: Joost J. van Middendorp, Gonzalo M. Sanchez, and Alwyn L. Burridge. The Edwin Smith papyrus: a clinical reappraisal of the oldest known document on spinal injuries. Eur Spine J. 2010 Nov; 19(11): 1815–1823.
- *"By 1803, the Russians were covering people with snow as they tried to resuscitate them."* Lioudmila V. Karnatovskaia, Katja E. Wartenberg, and William D. Freeman, "Therapeutic Hypothermia for Neuroprotection: History, Mechanisms, Risks, and Clinical Applications," *The Neurohospitalist*, vol. 4, no. 3, 2014, pp. 153–163, p. 153. https://www.ncbi.nlm.nih.gov/pmc/articles/PMC4056415/
- *Memoirs of Military Surgery, and Campaigns of the French Armies*. Baltimore, MD: Dominique Jean Larrey (1766–1842). Published by Joseph Cushing, 6, North Howard street, 1814.
- *"Similar patients treated without hypothermia have rarely survived."* G. Rainey Williams, Jr., and Frank C. Spencer, "The Clinical Use of Hypothermia Following Cardiac Arrest," *Annals of Surgery*, vol. 148, no. 3, September 1958, pp. 462–466, p. 465. https://www.ncbi.nlm.nih.gov/pmc/articles/PMC1450838/pdf/ann-surg01227-0170.pdf
- *"She woke up without any brain damage and recovered completely after a few months."* Lecia Bushak, "Induced Hypothermia: How Freezing People After heart Attacks Could Save Lives," *Newsweek*, December 20, 2014. http://www.newsweek.com/2015/01/02/induced-hypothermia-how-freezing-people-after-heart-attacks-could-save-lives-293598.html

- *"This Is How a Norwegian Woman Survived The Lowest Body Temperature Ever Recorded."* Fiona MacDonald: Science Alert, October 14, 2016, https://www.sciencealert.com/this-woman-survived-the-lowest-body-temperature-ever-recorded.
- *"She took a job at the hospital that saved her life."* Fiona MacDonald, *"This Is How a Norwegian Woman Survived The Lowest Body Temperature Ever Recorded,"* Science Alert, October 14, 2016, https://www.sciencealert.com/this-woman-survived-the-lowest-body-temperature-ever-recorded.
- *BACK TO LIFE: THE SCIENCE OF REVIVING THE DEAD.* NEWSWEEK STAFF: 7/22/07 AT 8:00 PM EDT
- *"Induced Hypothermia: How Freezing People After Heart Attacks Could Save Lives."* Lecia Bushak: Newsweek, December 20, 2014. http://www.newsweek.com/2015/01/02/induced-hypothermia-how-freezing-people-after-heart-attacks-could-save-lives-293598.html

Of Scintillating Lights, Tunnels, and Astral Encounters

- *I am incapable of conceiving infinity, and yet I do not accept finity. I want this adventure that is the context of my life to go on without end.* — Simone de Beauvoir. The Coming of Age (1970), Pt. 2, Ch. 2: Time, activity, history, pg. 412
- *I depart as air—I shake my white locks at the runaway sun, I effuse my flesh in eddies, and drift it in lacy jags. I bequeath myself to the dirt to grow from the grass I love.* — Walt Whitman: Section 52, *Song of Myself.* http://www.yourdailypoem.com/listpoem.jsp?poem_id=856
- *Life After Life.* Raymond A. Moody Jr, MD: HarperCollins, 2015
- *Plato's Republic: The Myth of ER.* George A Charalampidis: *An unconventional interpretation of the Universe in the first description of an out-of-body experience in Plato's Republic.* Akakía Publications, 2016, London, UK.
- *Assent of the Blessed.* Hieronymus Bosch https://en.wikipedia.org/wiki/Ascent_of_the_Blessed.
- *What Happens When We Die.* Sam Parnea, M.D: Ph.D: Hay House Inc. Carlsbad CA 92018-5100. https://books.google.com/books?id=-vBTm4CuDkYC&pg=PA10&lpg=PA10&dq=the+19th+Century,+the+accounts+of+the+survivors+of+a+Swiss+mountaineering+accident&source=bl&ots=tsb14MDkjL&sig=ACfU3U3EOU5_oeB668tCywmt1oCHQJxN8w&hl=en&sa=X&ved=2ahUKEwi45snioPvuAhUdRTABHRcwB2IQ6AEwA3oECAYQAw#v=onepage&q=the%2019th%20Century%2C%20the%20accounts%20of%20the%20survivors%20of%20a%20Swiss%20mountaineering%20accident&f=false
- *Tangshan Earthquake Survivors Recount Their History*: story. http://english.cctv.com/2016/07/28/VIDEoA5i32lMOQ6k65MM3LAX160728.shtml
- *Is there Finality in Death?* Anthony Gomes, In the Wrath-Bearing Tree, May 2020.

Part V: The Break Down

The Broken Heart

- *For my part, I prefer my heart to be broken. It is so lovely, dawn-kaleidoscopic within the crack.* — D. H. Lawrence "Pomegranate" in *Birds, Beasts, and Flowers: Poems By D. H. Lawrence,* (David R. Godine, 2007) pages 13–14
- *If I can stop one heart from breaking, I shall not live in vain.* — Emily Dickinson from the poem "If I can stop one heart from breaking." The Complete Poems. Boston: Little, Brown, 1924, New York: BARTLEBY.COM, 2000
- *"Hearts have been broken thousands of times more often in these past months either directly or indirectly due to COVID-19. Loss of loved ones, loss of potential lovers or existing lovers, loss of touch, of being held, loss of taste and smell, loss of work, of motivation, of freedoms and even of a raison d'etre. The idea that one heart must bear so much and yet maintain a rhythm sufficient to keep one alive is almost heart stopping in itself. Such a great demand on a thing the size of a fist."* Linda Thorson, personal communication.
- *"Voodoo" death.* Walter B. Cannon: *American Anthropologist.* 1942; 44:169–181.

Part VI: The Slow Down

The Ubiquitous Faint

- *He felt the whole vision turn to darkness and his very feet give way. His head went round; he was going; he had gone.* — Henry James, "The Jolly Corner"—Gutenberg eBook The Jolly Corner.
- *I tended to faint when I saw accident victims in the emergency ward, during surgery, or while drawing blood.* — Michael Crichton. On why he gave up medicine. https://quotably.io/michael-crichton-quotes/i-tended-3/
- *"Ubi pulsus sit rarus semper expectanda est syncope."* O Aquilina. A brief history of cardiac pacing. Images Paediatr Cardiol. 2006 Apr-Jun; 8(2): 17–81.
- *"Epilepsy with a slow pulse."* Berndt Luderitz: Historical Perspectives of Cardiac Electrophysiology. Hellenic J Cardiol 2009; 50: 3–16; J. Anthony Gomes, MD: Heart Rhythm Disorders: History, Mechanisms and Management Perspectives, pg. 412 (Springer, 2020)
- *"A person awakes and then either faints in bed or on standing up."* David L. Jardine et al., "Sympatho-vagal Responses in Patients with Sleep and Typical Vasovagal Syncope," *Clinical Science*, vol. 117, pp. 345–353, p. 346. http://www.clinsci.org/content/117/10/345
- *"Many will swoon when they do look on blood."* William Shakespeare, *As You Like It*, act IV, scene 3, line 2165.

- *"But about a quarter of its victims are unable to work."* Postural Orthostatic Tachycardia Syndrome, Dysautonomia International, 2012. http://www.dysautonomiainternational.org/page.php?ID=30
- *"They can presumably reduce the counter response that slows the heart down and causes fainting."* Blair P. Grubb, *The Fainting Phenomenon*, Wiley-Blackwell, 2007, p. 101. https://books.google.com/books?id=YuUdjCGHCV4C&pg=PA101&lpg=PA101&dq=serotonin+fainting&source=bl&ots=edvD34Of eX&sig=QJZMkTiizveahiGhif4Y7y_WdT0&hl=en&sa=X&ved=0ahUKEwio vu3v7ZDVAhVHj1QKHaeIAYY4ChDoAQg4MAM#v=onepage&q=seroto nin%20fainting&f=false

The Stuttering Maestro: The Sick Sinus

- *And the maestro surely wielded the chairman's baton with extraordinary skill.* — Alan Blinder

  https://www.azquotes.com/quote/1200726
- *You can't teach the old maestro a new tune.* — Jack Kerouac. On the Road (Penguin Classics, 1999). https://www.goodreads.com/work/quotes/1701188-on-the-road
- *"Slow heart rates due to a reduction in their open funny channels...."* Alicia D'Souza et al., "Exercise Training Reduces Resting Heart Rate via Downregulation of the Funny Channel HCN4," *Nature Communications*, published online May 13, 2014, pp. 1–12, p. 1. https://www.nature.com/articles/ncomms4775
- *"Total failure of the sinus node took 7 to 29 years, with an average of 13 years."* Wen-Pin Lien et al., "The Sick Sinus Syndrome. Natural History of Dysfunction of the Sinoatrial Node," *Chest*, vol. 72, issue 5, November 1977, pp. 628–634, p. 628. http://journal.chestnet.org/article/S0012-3692(16)38008-4/fulltext, https://www.researchgate.net/publication/22242099_The_sick_sinus_syndrome_Natural_history_of_dysfunction_of_the_sinoatrial_node

Of Disconnected Highways: AV Blocks

- *If the R is far from the P. Then you have a first degree. Longer, longer, longer, drop! Then you have a Wenckebach block. If some P's just don't go through, Then you have a Mobitz II. And if P's and Q's just don't agree, Then you have a third degree.* The Heart Block Poem The Princeton Surgical Group and Nurses Labs) https://nurseslabs.tumblr.com/post/91133209935/the-heart-block-poem-if-you-liked-this-check-out

- *"The term 'block' to refer to any artificial obstacle in the passage of current to the muscle of a jellyfish."* Gerald L. Geison, *Michael Foster and the Cambridge School of Physiology*, Princeton NJ, Princeton University Press, 1978, p. 294. https://books.google.com/books?id=E3V9BgAAQBAJ&pg=PA293&lpg=PA29 3&dq=romanes+jellyfish+block&source=bl&ots=beJ1NFed2X&sig=6RGrQDi miqsKshHpQacVplorgrE&hl=en&sa=X&ved=0ahUKEwiQpN3nvqfVAhUmq VQKHSg4B0QQ6AEIKDAA#v=onepage&q=romanes%20jellyfish%20 block&f=false
- *Walter Gaskell and the Understanding of Atrioventricular Conduction and Block.* Mark E. Silverman and Charles B. Upshaw, Jr., Journal of the American College of Cardiology, v. 39, no. 10, 2002, pp. 1574–1580, p. 1577. https://www. ncbi.nlm.nih.gov/pubmed/12020482
- *"In a 1904 book entitled Die Unregelmassige Hertztatigkeit (Arhythmia of the Heart)."* K.F. Wenckebach, *Arythmia of the Heart*, trans. Thomas Snowball, Edinburgh and London, William Green & Sons, 1904. https://books.google.com/ books?id=ckBAAAAAIAAJ&pg=PA70&lpg=PA70&dq=luciani+periods&sour ce=bl&ots=73iwuEyZhh&sig=kiekCKt2TgX3t96rg9zscv2ir8o&hl=en&sa=X& ved=0ahUKEwiE__KN-qHVAhUK72MKHdJGAkU4ChDoAQg6MAU#v= onepage&q=luciani%20periods&f=false
- *"The heart sounds were weak, but pure."* K.F. Wenckebach, *Arythmia of the Heart*, trans. Thomas Snowball, Edinburgh and London, William Green & Sons, 1904, p. 69. https://books.google.com/books?id=ckBAAAAAIAAJ& pg=PA70&lpg=PA70&dq=luciani+periods&source=bl&ots=73iwuEyZhh &sig=kiekCKt2TgX3t96rg9zscv2ir8o&hl=en&sa=X&ved=0ahUKEwiE__ KN-qHVAhUK72MKHdJGAkU4ChDoAQg6MAU#v=onepage&q=luciani%20 periods&f=false
- *"He stated that the cause of it lay in the heart itself, not the brain, as contemporaries believed."* Eoin T. O'Brien, "Dublin Masters of Clinical Expression II: Robert Adams (1791–1875)," *Journal of the Irish Colleges of Physicians and Surgeons*, vol. 3, no. 4, April 1974, pp. 127–129, p. 128. http://www.eoinobrien. org/wp-content/uploads/2008/08/dublin-masters-of-clinical-expression-ii-rob-ert-adams.pdf
- *"The pulsation of veins is of a kind which we have never before witnessed."* J.D. Cantwell, Profiles in Cardiology: William Stokes (1804–1878)," *Clinical Cardiology*, vol. 11, no. 12, 1988, pp. 856–858, p. 857. http://onlinelibrary.wiley. com/store/10.1002/clc.4960111213/asset/4960111213_ftp.pdf;jsessioni d=48785889CC7DECEC3F29093853152662.f03t04?v=1&t=j5lhmcsj&s=983c abe04af886c9f400dec0c77ab9da6cd392f2
- *"The power of independent rhythmical contraction decreases regularly as we pass from the sinus to the ventricle."* In Mark E. Silverman and Charles B. Upshaw, Jr., *Walter Gaskell and the Understanding of Atrioventricular Conduction and Block. Journal of the American College of Cardiology*, vol. 39, no. 10, May 15, 2002, pp. 1574–1580, p. 1576. http://www.sciencedirect.com/ science/article/pii/S0735109702018399

Part VII: A Brand-New Rhythm: A Brand-New Heart

The Artificial Pacemaker: A Life Giver

- *That's one small step for man, one giant leap for mankind.* — Neil Armstrong; July 20, 1969

  https://www.nasa.gov/mission_pages/apollo/apollo11.html
- *At some point in every person's life, you will need an assisted medical device - whether it's your glasses, your contacts, or as you age and you have a hip replacement or a knee replacement or a pacemaker. The prosthetic generation is all around us.* — Aimee Mullins: Life, You, Age, Glasses. https://www.quote-pub.com/quote/aimee-mullins-at-some-point-in-every-persons-life-you-will-need-an-assisted-medical-device
- *Paul M. Zoll and Electrical Stimulation of the Human Heart.* W. H. Abelmann *Clinical Cardiology*, vol. 9, 1986, pp. 131–135, p. 132. http://onlinelibrary.wiley.com/store/10.1002/clc.4960090311/asset/4960090311_ftp.pdf;jsessionid=AFA 1A54D167E65CF20E078EC9CFCF8A5.f01t03?v=1&t=j3x96ixp&s=2973bbd fe9b497f7e29e0f5ea032cb80936f55a0
- *Faculty of Medicine Online Museum and Archive.* Lidwill, Mark C. https://sydney.edu.au/medicine/museum/mwmuseum/index.php/Lidwill,_Mark_C
- *History of Pacemakers* – Biotele
  https://www.biotele.com/pacemakers.htm
- *Five Giants in Electrophysiology.* Kevin O'Sullivan: *EP Lab Digest*, vol. 8, issue 7, July 2008. http://www.eplabdigest.com/article/8941
- *Oral History: Wilson Greatbatch.* In Rik Nebeker, interviewer: Engineering and Technology History Wiki, undated. http://ethw.org/Oral-History:Wilson_Greatbatch
- *The Effect of Cardiac Resynchronization on Morbidity and Mortality in Heart Failure.* John G. F. Cleland et al., *New England Journal of Medicine*, vol. 352, no. 15, April 14, 2005, pp. 1539–1549, p. 1546. http://www.nejm.org/doi/pdf/10.1056/NEJMoa050496

When All Is Said and Done: Waiting for a Heart Transplant

- *For a dying man it is not a difficult decision to agree to become the world's first heart transplant ... because he knows he is at the end. If a lion chases you to the bank of a river filled with crocodiles, you will leap into the water convinced you have a chance to swim to the other side. But you would not accept such odds if there were no lion.*— Christiaan Barnard. Kathirvel Subramaniam, Tesuro Sakai,

Editors. Anesthesia and Perioperative Care for Organ Transplantation, Springer, 233 Spring Street, NY, 2017

https://www.pbs.org/wgbh/aso/databank/entries/bmbarn.html
- *If a man will begin with certainties, he shall end in doubts; but if he will be content to begin with doubts, he shall end in certainties.* — Francis Bacon. The Oxford Francis Bacon IV: The Advancement of Learning. https://www.goodreads.com/quotes/51-if-a-man-will-begin-with-certainties-he-shall-end
- *"I do not bring any special talent to solving those problems."* Patricia Sullivan, "Adrian Kantrowitz; Performed First U.S. Heart Transplant," *Washington Post*, November 20, 2008. http://www.washingtonpost.com/wp-dyn/content/article/2008/11/19/AR2008111903948.html
- *"Look, the leaves are so green. The sky is so blue—isn't it beautiful?"* Eileen Blaiberg, "Philip Blaiberg Was Dying—This Time for Certain," *Chicago Tribune*, October 12, 1969. http://archives.chicagotribune.com/1969/10/12/page/254/article/philip-blaiberg-was-dying-this-time-for-certain
- *"But he died of hepatitis and organ rejection after 592 days."* Margaret M. Lock, *Twice Dead: Organ Transplants and the Reinvention of Death*, Berkeley, University of California Press, 2001, p. 97. https://books.google.com/books?id=VQF-onQX3m8C&pg=PA97&lpg=PA97&dq=philip+blaiberg+cause+of+death&source=bl&ots=lrg_pqTCYH&sig=CcXZyXsXgbgvdLWFBb-VJdEAEGs&hl=en&sa=X&ved=0ahUKEwiM9ZPwh__UAhVV3WMKHXYbB0Y4ChDoAQhJMAw#v=onepage&q=philip%20blaiberg%20cause%20of%20death&f=false
- *"The company decided to continue with it, mainly as a prestige project."* David Hamilton, *A History of Organ Transplantation: Ancient Legends to Modern Practice*, Pittsburgh, University of Pittsburgh Press, 2012, p. 382. https://books.google.com/books?id=4uS1eem2SbMC&pg=PA381&lpg=PA381&dq=cyclosporine+April+1976+meeting+of+the+British+Society+for+Immunology&source=bl&ots=FPPphzpyYp&sig=Y8R2TjLR_BxgAF3tugWQkuJEWZY&hl=en&sa=X&ved=0ahUKEwjgkbG0iv_UAhVH6mMKHZp8CUIQ6AEIJzAA#v=onepage&q=cyclosporine%20April%201976%20meeting%20of%20the%20British%20Society%20for%20Immunology&f=false
- *"Adding prednisone made an effective and much safer anti-immune cocktail."* Clyde F. Barker and James F. Markmann, "Historical Overview of Transplantation," *Cold Spring Harbor Perspectives in Medicine*, vol. 3, no. 4, April 2013. https://www.ncbi.nlm.nih.gov/pubmed/23545575
- *"She lived five more years and did not die from rejection of the tissue."* Sara Wykes, "5 Questions: Bruce Weitz Recalls First Successful heart-Lung Transplant," Stanford Medicine News Center, undated. https://med.stanford.edu/news/all-news/2016/03/bruce-reitz-recalls-the-worlds-first-heart-lung-transplant.html
- *"There were almost 9,000 kidney transplants in the United States alone."* Author unknown, "History of Kidney Transplants," National Kidney Center, undated.

http://www.nationalkidneycenter.org/treatment-options/transplant/history-of-transplants/

- *"Over 20% of the company's pharmaceutical sales and 40% of the profits."* David K. C. Cooper and Robert P. Lanza, *Xeno: The Promise of Transplanting Animal Organs into Humans*, Oxford, UK, Oxford University Press, 2000, pp. 237–38.
- *The mind bending effects of feeling two hearts.* https://www.bbc.com/future/article/20141205-the-man-with-two-hearts
- *"I long to give her something—a new life?—yet I'm afraid to temper with such dignity,"* he writes. *"And so I smile as best I can, and say: Namaste!"* *"Good morning!"* How absurd. And her voice follows as we go away, a small clear smiling voice,—"Namaste!"—a Sanskrit word for greeting and parting, which means, "I salute you!"* Peter Matthiessen: The Snow Leopard. Penguin, 1978

Part VIII: The Quest to Overcome Heart Attacks

Of Bypasses and Clot Busters

- *What is wanted is not the will to believe, but the will to find out, which is the exact opposite.* — Bertrand Russell. Conway memorial Lecture. Free Thought and Official Propaganda. (public library). https://www.brainpickings.org/2016/05/18/bertrand-russell-free-thought-propaganda-doubt/
- *Scientists have become the bearers of the torch of discovery in our quest for knowledge.* Stephen Hawking and Leonard Mlodinow. *The Grand Design*, Bantam, 2012. https://www.age-of-the-sage.org/stephen_hawking/philosophy_is_dead.html
- *WILLIAM HEBERDEN ON ANGINA PECTORIS, 1772*: http://www.epi.umn.edu/cvdepi/essay/william-heberden-on-angina-pectoris-1772/
- "The Vineberg Legacy," J. L. Thomas: *Texas Heart Institute Journal*, 1999. https://www.ncbi.nlm.nih.gov/pmc/articles/PMC325613/pdf/thij00017-0018.pdf
- *The Heart Healers*, In James Forrester, New York, Macmillan, 2015, p. 145.
- *Vasilii I. Koselov: A Surgeon to Remember.* Igor E. Konstantinov, *Texas Heart Institute Journal*, 2004, 31:4, 349–358, p. 353. https://www.ncbi.nlm.nih.gov/pmc/articles/PMC548233/
- *A Cardiac Conundrum.* Alice Park, *Harvard Magazine*, March-April 2013. http://harvardmagazine.com/2013/03/a-cardiac-conundrum.
- *Coronary Artery Bypass Graft Surgery: The Past, Present, and Future of Myocardial Revascularization.* Michael Diodato and Edgar G. Chedrawy: *Surgery Research and Practice*, v. 2014, January 2, 2014. https://www.hindawi.com/journals/srp/2014/726158/.

A Riveting New Era: The Birth of Interventional Cardiology

- *Discovery is seeing what everybody else has seen and thinking what nobody else has thought.*— Albert Szent-Gyorgyi. https://www.goodreads.com/quotes/1187791-discovery-consists-of-seeing-what-everybody-has-seen-and-thinking
- *Imagination is more important than knowledge. Knowledge is limited. Imagination encircles the world.* — Albert Einstein. The Saturday Evening Post, 1929 https://www.saturdayeveningpost.com/2010/03/imagination-important-knowledge/
- *"May make it not improperly be called angina pectoris."* In "Description of Angina Pectoris by William Heberden." http://rwjms1.umdnj.edu/shindler/heberden.html
- *In Search of Andreas Roland Gruntzig, MD (1939–1985).* Robert Short, Circulation, 2007; 116 (9):f49–53.
- *"Herr Grüntzig, Sie werden mir die Patienten wegnehmen, aber legen sie los!"* Matthias Barton Johannes Grüntzig, Marc Husmann, and Josef Rösch et al., "Balloon Angioplasty—The Legacy of Andreas Grüntzig, M.D.," *Frontiers in Cardiovascular Medicine*, vol. 1, article 15, December 2014, pp. 1–25, p. 13. https://www.ncbi.nlm.nih.gov/pmc/articles/PMC4671350/
- *"But the idea was consuming him all the time."* Matthias Barton et al., *Balloon Angioplasty—The Legacy of Andreas Grüntzig, M.D. Frontiers in Cardiovascular Medicine*, vol. 1, article 15, December 2014, pp. 1–25, p. 13. https://www.ncbi.nlm.nih.gov/pmc/articles/PMC4671350/
- *Journey into the Heart.* David Monagan with David O. Williams. Gotham Books, Published by Penguin Books, 375 Hudson Street, New York, NY 10014, 2007
- Charles Theodore Dodder: The Father of Intervention. Misty M. Payne, *Texas Heart Institute Journal*, vol. 28, no. 1, pp. 28–38, p. 29. https://www.ncbi.nlm.nih.gov/pmc/articles/PMC101126/
- *"If a plumber can do it to pipes, we can do it to blood vessels."* Misty M. Payne, "Charles Theodore Dodder: The Father of Intervention," *Texas Heart Institute Journal*, vol. 28, no. 1, pp. 28–38, p. 29. https://www.ncbi.nlm.nih.gov/pmc/articles/PMC101126/
- *"There were a lot of bad vibes in the room by now."* David Monagan, *Journey into the Heart*, New York, Penguin, 2007, p. 200. https://books.google.com/books?id=m04e-NHGFUcC&pg=PA199&lpg=PA199&dq=geoffrey+hartzler&source=bl&ots=EpWxJpdtmO&sig=RiSL5usrAIU19sZyDEFxbmdfnHQ&hl=en&sa=X&ved=0ahUKEwi52Zff-NHVAhVeVWMKHfBgAWs4FBDoAQhFMAY#v=onepage&q=geoffrey%20hartzler&f=falseCHAPTER XXIII
- *In Memoriam Geoffrey O. Hartzler (1946–2012).* James T. Willerson, MD Tex Heart Inst J. 2012; 39(3): 317–318.
- *Geoffrey O. Hartzler, MD A Tribute.* Barry D. Rutherford, MD; Joel K. Kahn, MD; David Strelow, David R. Holmes, Jr, MD, *Circulation.* 2012;125:2958–2960

- *"A man who in 2001 would purchase a Las Vegas strip club for funds to further his research."* Eric Malnic, *Surgeon Uses Strip Club to Bankroll His Research. Los Angeles Times*, November 9, 2001. http://articles.latimes.com/2001/nov/09/local/me-2049
- *Medscape Radiology*: An Expert Interview With Dr. Julio Palmaz: Part I -- Serendipity and the Stent, May 06, 2004
- *Medscape Radiology:* An Expert Interview With Dr. Julio Palmaz: Part II -- Drug-Eluting and "Interactive" Stents May 13, 2004
- *National Inventors Hall of Fame.* "Hall of Fame Induction Info: Julio Palmaz." https://web.archive.org/web/20090207151259/http://invent.org/hall_of_fame/1_3_0_induction_palmaz.asp

Part IX: Stories of Survival

A Family Affair

- *When everything goes to hell, the people who stand by you without flinching—they are your family.* — Jim Butcher

  https://www.goodreads.com/quotes/66608-when-everything-goes-to-hell-the-people-who-stand-by
- *Death leaves a heartache no one can heal, love leaves a memory no one can steal.*—From a Headstone in Ireland. https://quotefancy.com/quote/29627/Richard-Puz-Death-leaves-a-heartache-no-one-can-heal-love-leaves-a-memory-no-one-can
- *Standby automatic defibrillator.* Mirowski M, Mower MM, Staewen WS, et al. An approach to prevention of sudden coronary death. Arch Intern Med 1970;126:158–161.

Cruising Through Complications of a Heart Attack

- *Nothing can dim the light which shines from within*—Maya Angelou

  https://www.goodreads.com/quotes/67751-nothing-can-dim-the-light-which-shines-from-within
- *The weak overcome its menace, the strong overcomes itself. What is there like fortitude! What sap went through that little thread to make the cherry red!* — Marianne Moore from the poem *Nevertheless.* https://allpoetry.com/Nevertheless
- *Complications of Acute Myocardial Infarction.* Dr Laurence Knott. https://patient.info/doctor/complications-of-acute-myocardial-infarction

- *Left ventricular assist device (LVAD).* (https://www.mayoclinic.org/tests-proce-dures/ventricular-assist-device/multimedia/left-ventricular-assist-device/img-20006714)
- *Repairing the heart with stem cells.* (https://www.health.harvard.edu/heart-health/repairing-the-heart-with-stem-cells)

A Missed Diagnosis: A Lifetime of Endurance

- *As any doctor can tell you, the most crucial step toward healing is having the right diagnosis. If the disease is precisely identified, a good resolution is far more likely. Conversely, a bad diagnosis usually means a bad outcome, no matter how skilled the physician.* — Andrew Weil: The Wrong Diagnosis

  https://www.huffpost.com/entry/the-wrong-diagnosis_b_254227
- *Every calamity is to be overcome by endurance.* — Virgil
  https://www.brainyquote.com/quotes/virgil_145417
- 10 Commonly Misdiagnosed Conditions. Ariana Marini. (https://www.every-dayhealth.com/pictures/commonly-misdiagnosed-conditions/)
- *Allergic granulomatosis, allergic angiitis, and periarteritis nodosa.* CHURG J, STRAUSS L. Am J Pathol. 1951; 27(2):277–301.

Old Age: How Long Should We Hope to Live?

- *Let us never know what old age is. Let us know the happiness time brings, not count the years.* — Decimus Magnus Ausonius

  https://quotesgram.com/ausonius-quotes/
- *The secret of genius is to carry the spirit of the child into old age, which means never losing your enthusiasm.* — Aldous Huxley
  https://www.goodreads.com/quotes/130291-the-secret-of-genius-is-to-carry-the-spirit-of
- *"He was a science writer for the San Francisco Chronicle, and on August 4, 2017 he retired—at age 98."* Interview, "A Newspaperman Looks Back On A 77-Year Career," NPR, July 28, 2017. http://www.npr.org/2017/07/28/539945623/a-newspaperman-looks-back-on-a-77-year-career
- *"Their brains shrink less and their cortexes remain thicker."* Knvul Sheikh, *"'Super Agers' Have Brains That Look Young,"* Scientific American Mind, March 1, 2017. https://www.scientificamerican.com/article/ldquo-super-agers-rdquo-have-brains-that-look-young/
- *Life is not that bad when you consider the alternative.* — Maurice Chevalier. https://quoteinvestigator.com/2014/07/10/old-age/

- *"The sense of satisfaction and the feeling the life was worthwhile peaked in this period."* Unknown, *Measuring National Well-Being: At What Age Is Personal Well-Being the Highest?* UK Office for National Statistics, February 2, 2016. https://www.ons.gov.uk/peoplepopulationandcommunity/wellbeing/articles/measuringnationalwellbeing/atwhatageispersonalwellbeingthehighest
- *"They are also getting an extension of disease and disability."* Ernest M. Gruenberg, "The Failures of Success," reprinted in *The Milbank Quarterly*, vol. 83, no. 4, December 2005, pp. 779–800, p. 779. https://www.ncbi.nlm.nih.gov/pmc/articles/PMC2690285/
- *"Life is physically, emotionally, and intellectually vigorous until shortly before its close."* James F. Fries, "Aging, Natural Death, and the Compression of Mortality," *New England Journal of Medicine*, vol. 303, no. 3, July 17, 1980, pp. 130–135, p. 135. https://www.ncbi.nlm.nih.gov/pmc/articles/PMC2567746/pdf/11984612.pdf
- *"There was an increase in life expectancy with disease and an increase in expected years with functional loss."* Eileen Crimmins and Hiram Beltrán-Sánchez, *The Journals of Gerontology. Series B, Psychological Sciences and Social Sciences*, vol. 66B, no. 1, January 2011, pp. 75–86. https://www.ncbi.nlm.nih.gov/pmc/articles/PMC3001754/
- *The most studied and reproducible non-genetic intervention known to extend healthspan and/or lifespan in organisms.* Changhan Lee and Valter Longo, "Dietary Restriction With and Without Caloric Restriction for Healthy Aging," *F1000Research*, 5(F1000 Faculty Rev): 117, pp. 1–7, p. 3. https://www.ncbi.nlm.nih.gov/pmc/articles/PMC4755412/pdf/f1000research-5-7686.pdf
- *Fasting may provide effective strategies to reduce weight, delay aging, and optimize health.* Valter Longo and Mark Mattson, *Cell Metabolism*, vol. 19, no. 2, February 4, 2014, pp. 181–192, p. 181. http://ac.els-cdn.com/S1550413113005032/1-s2.0-S1550413113005032-main.pdf?_tid=9d7a1f40-8c3b-11e7-9439-00000aab0f27&acdnat=1503957513_53d8ed60b460ac5e5f938416c59825b8
- *"A single person is missing for you, and the whole world is empty."*— Joan Didion, *The Year of Magical Thinking*. https://www.goodreads.com/work/quotes/1659905-the-year-of-magical-thinking

Part X: Heart Care

Some Heart Care Advice to Live By

- *Good advice is always certain to be ignored, but that's no reason not to give it.* — Agatha Christie. https://www.goodreads.com/quotes/296358-good-advice-is-always-certain-to-be-ignored-but-that-s
- *ASCVD RISK ESTIMATOR PLUS*: http://tools.acc.org/ASCVD-Risk-Estimator-Plus/#!/calculate/estimate/
- *The New Statin Choice Decision Aid*: https://shareddecisions.mayoclinic.org/2014/11/19/the-new-statin-choice-decision-aid/

Selected Bibliography

Romanticizing the Heart

A history of the heart. https://web.stanford.edu/class/history13/earlysciencelab/body/heartpages/heart.html.

Aird WC. Discovery of the cardiovascular system: from Galen to William Harvey. J Thromb Haemost. 2011;9(1):118–29. https://www.ncbi.1lm.nih.gov/pubmed/21781247.

Avicenna's canon of medicine – Internet archive. https://archive.org/stream/.../9670940-Canon-of-Medicine_djvu.txt.

Boon B. Leonardo da Vinci on atherosclerosis and the function of the sinuses of Valsalva. Neth Heart J. 2009;17(12):496–9.

el Tatawi MD. Der Lungenkreislauf nach el Koraschi. Wortlich Iibersetzt nach seinem Kommentar zum Teschrih Avicenna (Medical dissertation). Freiburg: University of Freiburg; 1924.

Gomes JA. Discovery of the circulatory system. In: Heart rhythm disorders: history, mechanisms, and management perspectives. Cham: Springer; 2020.

Harvey W. Exercitatio anatomica de motu cordis et sanguinis in animalibus. With an english translation and annotations by Chauncey D. Leake. Tercentennial edition. Published by Charles C. Thomas, Springfield, 1928.

Lubitz SA. Early reactions to harvey's circulation theory: the impact on medicine. Mt Sinai J Med. 2004;71(4):274–80.

Mahdi M, Gutas D, Abed SB, et al. Avicenna. Encyclopedia Iranica, vol. 3. London: Routledge and Kegan Paul; 1987. [Google Scholar].

Mark JJ. Ancient Egyptian medical text. https://www.ancient.eu/article/1015/ancient-egyptian-medical-texts/.

Merlo L. The anatomic location of the soul from the heart, through the brain, to the whole body, and beyond: a journey through Western history, science and philosophy. Neurosurgery. 2009;65(4):633–43.

Petrescu L. Descartes on the heartbeat: the Leuven affair. Perspect Sci. 2013;21(4):400. http://www.mitpressjournals.org/doi/pdf/10.1162/POSC_a_00110A ml.

Saba MM, Ventura HO, Saleh M, Mehra MR. Ancient Egyptian medicine and the concept of heart failure. J Card Fail. 2006;12(6):416–21.

© The Editor(s) (if applicable) and The Author(s), under exclusive license to Springer Nature Switzerland AG 2021
J. A. Gomes, *Rhythms of Broken Hearts*,
https://doi.org/10.1007/978-3-030-77382-3

Stefanadis C, Karamanou M, Androutsos G. Michael Servetus (1511-1553) and the discovery of pulmonary circulation. Hell J Cardiol. 2009;50:373–8. http://www.hellenicjcardiol.org/archive/full_text/2009/5/2009_5_373.pdf.

West JB. Ibn al-Nafis, the pulmonary circulation, and the Islamic Golden Age. J Appl Physiol. 1985;105(6):1877–80. https://www.ncbi.nlm.nih.gov/pmc/articles/PMC2612469/7.

The Mysteries of the Age-Old Pulse

Floyer JS. The physician's pulse-watch; or, An essay to explain the old art of feeling the pulse, and to improve it by the help of a pulse-watch ... to which is added, an extract out of Andrew Cleyer, concerning the Chinese art of feeling the pulse, S. Smith and B. Walford, London, 1707.

Kanada M. The natural movement or beating of the pulse. (KRL Gupta, Trans.),. Sage Kanad on Pulse; 1987.

Nima G, Maziar Zafari A. A brief journey into the history of the arterial pulse. Cardiology Research and Practice; 2011. https://www.hindawi.com/journals/crp/2011/164832/.

Upadhyay VGP. The science of pulse examination in Ayurveda. New Delhi: Sri Satguru Publication; 1997.

Demystifying the Heart

Akiyama T, Tawara S. Discoverer of the atrioventricular conduction system of the heart. Cardiol J. 2010;17(4):428–33.

Augustus O. Grant. Cardiac ion channels. Circ Arrhythmia Electrophysiol. 2009;2:185–94.

Bellis M. Biography of Luigi Galvani. Developed theory of animal electricity. In: Humanities history and culturte. 24 Jan 2018.

Das TS. Reizleitungssystem des Säugetierherzens. Gustav Fischer. Jena; 1906. Google Scholar.

DiFrancesco D. Pacemaker mechanisms in cardiac tissue. Annu Rev Physiol. 1993;55(1):455–72, (IF: 11.12).

Fye WB. Disorders of the heartbeat: a historical overview from antiquity to the mid-20th century. Am J Cardiol. 1993;72:1055–70.

Gomes JA. The road to unearthing the conducting system of the heart, Chapter 2. In Heart rhythm disorders: history, mechanisms, and management perspectives. Cham: Springer; 2020.

Gomes JA, Winters SL. The origins of the sinus pacemaker complex in man: demonstration of dominant and subsidiary foci. J Am Coll Cardiol. 1987;9:45–52.

Hodgkin AL, Huxley AF. A quantitative description of membrane current and its application to conduction and excitation in nerve. J Physiol. 1952;117:500–44.

Mazurak M, Kusa J. Jan Evangelista Purkinje: a passion for discovery. Tex Heart Inst J. 2018;45(1):23–6.

Roguin A. Wilhelm His Jr. (1863-1934)--the man behind the bundle. Heart Rhythm. 2006;3(4):480–3.

Siegel RE. Galen's system of physiology and medicine, vol. 45. New York: S. Karger; 1968.

Silverman ME, Hollman A. Discovery of the sinus node by Keith and Flack: on the centennial of their 1907 publication. Heart. 2007;93:1184–7.

Silverman ME, Grove D, Upshaw CB Jr. Why does the heartbeat? The discovery of the electrical system of the heart. Circulation. 2006;113(23):2775–81.

Understanding Heart Rhythm Disorders: The Birth of the ECG and Clinical Cardiac Electrophysiology

Amagishi T. A short biography of Takemi Taro, the president of the Japan Medical Association. J Nanzan Acad Soc Soc Sci. 2011;1:49–56.

Burchell HE. A centennial note on Waller and the first human electrocardiogram. Am J Cardiol. 1987;59:979–83.

Coumel P, Cabrol C, Fabiato A, et al. Tachycardie permanente par rythme reciproque. Arch Mal Coeur Vaiss. 1967;60:1830–64.

Cranefield PF, Hoffman BF. The electrical activity of the heart and the electrocardiogram. J Electrocardiol. 1968;1(1):2–4.

Damato AN, Lau SH, Berkowitz WD et al. Recording of specialized conducting fibers (AV nodal, His bundle and right bundle branch) in man using an electrode catheter technique. Circulation. 1969;39:435–47.

Durrer D, Schoo L, Schuilenburg RM, Wellens HJJ. The role of premature beats in the initiation and the termination of supraventricular tachycardia in the Wolff-Parkinson-White syndrome. Circulation. 1967;36:644–62.

Gomes JA. Birth of clinical cardiac electrophysiology, Chapter 3. In: Heart rhythm disorders: history, mechanisms, and management perspectives. Cham: Springer; 2020.

Gomes JA, Damato AN, Bobb GA, Lau SH. The effect of digitalis on refractoriness of the intact canine His-Purkinje system. Circulation. 1978;58(2):284–94.

Hurst JW. Naming of the waves in the ECG, with a brief account of their genesis. Circulation. 1998;98:1937–42.

Moe GK, Abildskov JA. Atrial fibrillation as a self-sustaining arrhythmia independent of focal discharge. Am Heart J. 1959;58(1): 59–70.

Rivera-Ruiz M, Cajavilca C, Varon J. Einthoven's string galvanometer the first electrocardiograph. Tex Heart J. 2008;35(2):174–8.

Scherlag BJ, Lau SH, Helfant RH, et al. Catheter techniques for recording His bundle activity in man. Circulation. 1969;39:13.

Sones FM Jr, Shirey EK. Cine coronary arteriography. Mod Concepts Cardiovasc Dis. 1962;31:735–8.

Wellens HJ, Schuilenberg RM, Durrer D. Electrical stimulation of the heart in patients with Wolff-Parkinson-White syndrome, type A. Circulation. 1971;43(1):99–114.

Wellens HJ, Schuilenburg RM, Durrer D. Electrical stimulation of the heart in patients with ventricular tachycardia. Circulation. 1972;46(2):216–26.

Living with a Galloping Heart

Becker AE, Anderson RH, Path MRC, Durrer D, Wellems HJJ. The anatomic substrates of Wolff-Parkinson-White syndrome. A clinicopathologic correlation in seven patients. Circulation. 1978;57:870–9.

Blomström-Lundqvist C, Scheinman MM, Aliot EM, et al. ACC/AHA/ESC guidelines for the management of patients with supraventricular arrhythmias—executive summary. A report of the American College of Cardiology/American Heart Association Task Force on Practice Guidelines and the European Society of Cardiology Committee for Practice Guidelines (writing committee to develop guidelines for the management of patients with supraventricular arrhythmias) developed in collaboration with NASPE-Heart Rhythm Society. JACC. 2003;42(8):1494–531.

Brechenmacher C. Atrio-His bundle tracts. Br Heart J. 1975;37:853–5.

Coumel P, Attuel P. Reciprocating tachycardia in overt and latent pre-excitation: influence of functional bundle branch block on the rate of the tachycardia. Eur J Cardiol. 1974;1:423–36.

Durrer D, Roos JP. Epicardial excitation of ventricles in patient with Wolff-Parkinson-White syndrome (type B). Circulation. 1967;35:15–21.

Gallagher JJ, Oritchett ELC, Sealey WC, et al. The preexcitaion syndromes. Prog Cardiovasc Dis. 1978;20:285–327.

Goldreyer BN, Damato AN. The essential role of A-V conduction delay in the initiation of paroxysmal supraventricular tachycardia in man. Circulation. 1971;43:679–87.

Gollob MH, Tang A, Karibe A, et al. Identification of a gene responsible for familial Wolff–Parkinson–White syndrome. N Engl J Med. 2001;344:1823–31. http://www.nejm.org/doi/full/10.1056/nejm200106143442403#t=article.

Gomes JA. Atrioventricular nodal reentry, Chapter 6. In: Heart rhythm disorders: history, mechanisms, and management perspectives. Cham: Springer; 2020.

Gomes JA. Wolff-Parkinson-White syndrome, Chapter 7. In: Heart rhythm disorders: history, mechanisms, and management perspectives. Cham: Springer; 2020.

Gomes JAC, Damato AN, Dhatt MS, Rubenson D. Electrophysiologic evidence for selective retrograde utilization of specialized conduction system in atrioventricular nodal reentrant tachycardia. Am J Cardiol. 1979;43:687–98.

Hariman RA, Gomes JAC, El-Sherif N. Catecholamine-dependent atrioventricular nodal reentrant tachycardia. Circulation. 1983;67:681–6.

Jackman WM. Participation of atrial myocardium (posterior septum) in AV nodal reentrant tachycardia: evidence from resetting by atrial extrastimuli. Pacing Clin Electrophysiol. 1991;14:646.

Kent AFS. A conducting path between the right auricle and the external wall of the right ventricle in the heart of the mammal. J Physiol. 1914;48:57.

Klein GJ, Yee R, Sharma AD. Longitudinal electrophysiologic assessment of asymptomatic patients with the Wolff–Parkinson–White electrocardiographs. Pattern N Engl J Med. 1989;320:1229–33.

Lockwood DJ, Nakagawa H, Jackman WM. Electrophysiological characteristics of atrioventricular nodal reentrant tachycardia implications for the reentrant circuits. In: Zipes DP, Jalif J, editors. Cardiac electrophysiology: from cell to bedside. Philadelphia: Elsevier Health Sciences; 2017.

Mahaim I, Benatt A. Nouvelles recherches sur les connexions superieures de la branche gauche du faisceau de His-Tawara avec la cloison inter-ventriculaire. Cardiologia. 1937;1:61–73.

Mines GR. On dynamic equilibrium in the heart. J Physiol. 1913;46(4–5):349–81. http://onlinelibrary.wiley.com/doi/10.1113/jphysiol.1913.sp001596/epdf

Moe GK, Preston JB, Burlington H. Physiologic evidence for a dual A-V transmission system. Circ Res. 1956;4:357–75.

Otomo K, Suyama K, Okamura H, et al. Participation of a concealed atriohisian tract in the reentrant circuit of the slow–fast type of atrioventricular nodal reentrant tachycardia. Heart Rhythm. 2007;4:703–10.

Pappone C, Santinelli V, Rosanio S, et al. Usefulness of invasive electrophysiologic testing to stratify the risk of arrhythmic events in asymptomatic patients with Wolff-Parkinson-White pattern: results from a large prospective long-term follow-up study. J Am Coll Cardiol. 2003;41:239–44.

Spurrell RAJ, Krikler D, Sowton E. Two or more intra AV nodal pathways in association with either a James or Kent extranodal bypass in 3 patients with paroxysmal supraventricular tachycardia. Br Heart J. 1973;35:113–22.

Wolff L, Parkinson J, White PD. Bundle-branch block with short P-R interval in healthy young people prone to paroxysmal tachycardia. Am Heart J. 1930;5:685–704.

Wood FC, Wolferth C, Geckeler G. Histological demonstration of accessory muscular connections between auricle and ventricle in a case of short P-R interval and prolonged QRS complex. Am Heart J. 1943;25(4):454–62. http://www.ahjonline.com/article/S0002-8703(43)90484-3/pdf

Wu P, Denes C, Wyndham F, Amat-y-Leon RC, Dhingra KM. Rosen demonstration of dual atrio-ventricular nodal pathways utilizing a ventricular extrastimulus in patients with atrioventricular nodal reentrant paroxysmal supraventricular tachycardia. Circulation. 1975;52:789–98.

Zipes DP, Drjoseph RL, Rothbaum DS. Unusual properties of accessory pathways. Circulation. 1974;49:1200–11.

Radical Ideas: The Road to Conquering Supraventricular Tachycardia

Borggrefe M, Budde T, Podczeck A, Breithardt G. High frequency alternating current ablation of an accessory pathway in humans. J Am Coll Cardiol. 1987;10(3):576–82. http://www.online-jacc.org/content/accj/10/3/576.full.pdf.

Calkins H, Sousa J, el Atassi R, et al. Diagnosis and cure of the Wolff-Parkinson-White syndrome or paroxysmal supraventricular tachycardias during a single electrophysiologic test. N Engl J Med. 1991;324:1612–8.

Cobb FR, Blumenschein S, Sealy WC, Boineau JP, Wagner GS, Wallace AG. Successful surgical interruption of the bundle of Kent in a patient with Wolff-Parkinson-White syndrome. Circulation. 1968;38:1018–29. http://circ.ahajournals.org/content/38/6/1018

Gallagher JJ, Svenson RH, Kasell JH. Catheter technique for closed-chest ablation of the atrioventricular conduction system – a therapeutic alternative for the treatment of refractory supraventricular tachycardia. N Engl J Med. 1982;306:194–200.

Gomes JA. Ablative therapy of bypass tracts, AV junction, and AV nodal reentrant tachycardia, Chapter 8. In: Heart rhythm disorders: history, mechanisms, and management perspectives. Cham: Springer; 2020.

Guiraudon GM, Klein GJ, Sharma AD, Yee R, McLennan DG. Surgery for the Wolff-Parkinson-White syndrome: the epicardial approach. Semin Thorac Cardiovasc Surg. 1989;1:21–33.

Huang SK, Jordan N, Graham A, et al. Closed-chest catheter desiccation of atrio-ventricular junction using radiofrequency energy - a new method for catheter ablation [abstract]. Circulation. 1985;72:111–389.

Jackman WM, Wang X, Friday KJ, Roman CA, et al. Catheter ablation of accessory atrioventricular pathways (Wolff-Parkinson-White syndrome) by radiofrequency current. N Engl J Med. 1991;324(23):1605–11. https://doi.org/10.1056/NEJM199106063242301.

Jackman WM, Beckman KJ, McClelland JH, et al. Treatment of supraventricular tachycardia due to atrioventricular nodal reentry, by radiofrequency catheter ablation of slow-pathway conduction. N Engl J Med. 1992;327:313–8.

Kuck KH, Schlüter M, Geiger M, Siebels J, Duckeck W. Radiofrequency current catheter ablation of accessory atrioventricular pathways. Lancet. 1991;337:1557–61.

Mehta D, Gomes JA. Long term results of fast pathway ablation in AV nodal reentry tachycardia using a modified technique. Br Heart J. 1995;74:671–5.

Page RL, Joglar JA, Caldwell MA, et al. 2015 ACC/AHA/HRS guideline for the management of adult patients with supraventricular tachycardia. A report of the American College of Cardiology/American Heart Association Task Force on Clinical Practice Guidelines and the Heart Rhythm Society. Circulation. 2016;133:e506–74.

Scheinman MM, Morady F, Hess DS, Gonzalez R. Catheter-induced ablation of the atrioventricular junction to control refractory supraventricular arrhythmias. JAMA. 1982;248:851–5.

Winters SL, Gomes JAC. Electrode catheter recordings of atrioventricular bypass tracts in Wolff-Parkinson-White syndrome: technique, electrophysiologic characteristics and demonstration of concealed and decremental propagation. J Am Coll Cardiol. 1986;7:1392–403.

Atrial Fibrillation: The Heart's Tap Dance

Allessie MA, Lammers WEJEP, Bonke FIM, Hollen J. Experimentalevaluation of Moe's multiple wavelet hypothesis of atrial fibrillation. In: Zipes DP, Jalife J, editors. Cardiac electrophysiology and arrhythmias. Orlando: Grune & Stratton; 1985. p. 265–75.

Benjamin EJ, Levy D, Vaziri SM, et al. Independent risk factors for atrial fibrillation in a population-based cohort. The Framingham Heart Study. JAMA. 1994;271:840–4.

Boersma LV, Schmidt B, Betts TR, et al. Implant success and safety of left atrial appendage closure with the WATCHMAN device: peri-procedural outcomes from the EWOLUTION registry. Eur Heart J. 2016;37:2465–74.

Cappato R, Calkins H, Chen SA, et al. Updated worldwide survey on the methods, efficacy, and safety of catheter ablation for human atrial fibrillation. Circ Arrhythm Electrophysiol. 2010;3:32–8.

Chugh SS, Blackshear JL, Shen WK, et al. Epidemiology and natural history of atrial fibrillation: clinical implications. J Am Coll Cardiol. 2001;37:371–8.

Clark DM, Plumb VJ, Epstein AB, Kay GN. Hemodynamic effects of an irregular sequence of ventricular cycle lengths during atrial fibrillation. J Am Coll Cardiol. 1997;30:1039–45.

Coumel P, Attuel P, Lavallee J, Flammang D, Leclercq JF, Slama R. The atrial arrhythmia syndrome of vagal origin. Arch Mal Coeur Vaiss. 1978;71:645–56.

Cox JL. A perspective of postoperative atrial fibrillation in cardiac operations. Ann Thorac Surg. 1993;56:405–9.

Cox JL, Schuessler RB, Boineau JP. The development of the maze procedure for the treatment of atrial fibrillation. Semin Thorac Cardiovasc Surg. 2000;12:2–14.

Coyne KS, Paramore C, Grandy S, et al. Assessing the direct costs of treating nonvalvular atrial fibrillation in the United States. Value Health. 2006;9:348–56.

Frustaci A, Cameli S, Zeppilli P. Biopsy evidence of atrial myocarditis in an athlete developing transient sinoatrial disease. Chest. 1995;108:1460–2.

Furberg CD, Psaty BM, Manolio TA, et al. Prevalence of atrial fibrillation in elderly subjects (the Cardiovascular Health Study). Am J Cardiol. 1994;74:236–41.

Go AS, Hylek EM, Phillips KA, et al. Prevalence of diagnosed atrial fibrillation in adults: national implications for rhythm management and stroke prevention: the anticoagulation and risk factors in atrial fibrillation (ATRIA) study. JAMA. 2001;285:2370–5.

Gomes JA. Atrial fibrillation, Chapter 11. In: Heart rhythm disorders: history, mechanisms, and management perspectives. Cham: Springer; 2020.

Gómez-Outes A, Terleira-Fernández AI, Calvo-Rojas G, et al. Dabigatran, rivaroxaban, or apixaban versus warfarin in patients with nonvalvular atrial fibrillation: a systematic review and meta-analysis of subgroups. Thrombosis. 2013;2013, Article ID 640723, 18 pages

Haissaguerre M, Jais P, Shah DC, et al. Spontaneous initiation of atrial fibrillation by ectopic beats originating in the pulmonary veins. N Engl J Med. 1998;339:659–66.

Hart G, Benavente O, Mc Bride R, Pierce LA. Antithrombotic therapy to prevent strokes in atrial fibrillation. Ann Inter Med. 1999;131(7):492–50.

Hollowell J, Ruigómez A, Johansson S, et al. The incidence of bleeding complications associated with warfarin treatment in general practice in the United Kingdom. Br J Gen Pract. 2003;53:312–4.

Holmes DR Jr, Kar S, Price MJ, et al. Prospective randomized evaluation of the Watchman Left Atrial Appendage Closure device in patients with atrial fibrillation versus long-term warfarin therapy: the PREVAIL trial. J Am Coll Cardiol. 2014;64:1–12.

Holmes DR Jr, Doshi SK, Kar S, et al. Left atrial appendage closure as an alternative to warfarin for stroke prevention in atrial fibrillation: a patient-level meta-analysis. J Am Coll Cardiol. 2015;65:2614–23.

Holmes DR, Reddy VY, Turi ZG, et al. PROTECT AF Investigators. Percutaneous closure of the left atrial appendage versus warfarin therapy for prevention of stroke in patients with atrial fibrillation: a randomised non-inferiority trial. Lancet. 2009;374:534–42.

Jaïs P, Weerasooriya R, Shah DC, et al. Ablation therapy for atrial fibrillation (AF): past, present and future. Cardiovasc Res. 2002;54:337–46.

January CT, Wann LS, Alpert JS, et al. 2014 AHA/ACC/HRS guideline for the management of patients with atrial fibrillation: a report of the American College of Cardiology/American Heart Association Task Force on Practice Guidelines and the Heart Rhythm Society. J Am Coll Cardiol. 2014;64:e1–e76.

January CT, Wann LS, Calkins H, et al. 2019 AHA/ACC/HRS focused update of the 2014 guideline for management of patients with atrial fibrillation. A report of the American College of Cardiology/American Heart Association Task Force on Clinical Practice Guidelines, and the Heart Rhythm Society. J Am Coll Cardiol. 2019;74(1):104–32. https://doi.org/10.1016/j.jacc.2019.01.011.

Lafuente-Lafuente C, Mouly S, Longas-Tejero MA. Antiarrhythmic drugs for maintaining sinus rhythm after cardioversion of atrial fibrillation: a systematic review of randomized controlled trials. Arch Intern Med. 2006;166:719–28.

Lee JW, Park NH, Choo SJ, et al. Surgical outcome of the maze procedure for atrial fibrillation in mitral valve disease: rheumatic versus degenerative. Ann Thorac Surg. 2003;75:57–61.

Lip GY, Nieuwlaat R, Pisters R, et al. Refining clinical risk stratification for predicting stroke and thromboembolism in atrial fibrillation using a novel risk factor-based approach: the euro heart survey on atrial fibrillation. Chest. 2010;137:263–72.

Loardi C, Alamanni F, Veglia F, et al. Modified maze procedure for atrial fibrillation as an adjunct to elective cardiac surgery: predictors of mid-term recurrence and echocardiographic follow-up. Tex Heart Inst J. 2015;42(4):341–7.

Lown B, Perlroth MG, Kaidbey S, Abe T, Harken DE. "Cardioversion" of atrial fibrillation: a report on the treatment of 65 episodes in 50 patients. N Engl J Med. 1963;269:325–31. [PubMed: 13931297].

Lubitz SA, Yin X, Fontes JD, et al. Association between familial atrial fibrillation and risk of new-onset atrial fibrillation. JAMA. 2010;304:2263–9.

Moe GK, Abildskov JA. Atrial fibrillation as a self-sustaining arrhythmia independent of focal discharge. Am Heart J. 1959;58:59–70.

Nathan H, Eliakim M. The junction between the left atrium and the pulmonary veins. An anatomic study of human hearts. Circulation. 1966;34:412–22.

Niemerovsky D, Hutter R, Gomes JA. The electrical substrate of vagal atrial fibrillation as assessed by the signal-averaged electrocardiogram. PACE. 2008;31:308–13.

Ott A, Breteler MM, de Brune MC, et al. Atrial fibrillation in a population based study. The Rotterdam Study. Stroke. 1997;28(2):316–21.

Packer DL, Mark DB, Robb RA, et al. Effect of catheter ablation vs antiarrhythmic drug therapy on mortality, stroke, bleeding, and cardiac arrest among patients with atrial fibrillation. The CABANA randomized clinical trial. JAMA. 2019;321(13):1261–74. https://doi.org/10.1001/jama.2019.0693.

Pappone C, Rosanio S, Oreto G, et al. Circumferential radiofrequency ablation of pulmonary vein ostia: a new anatomic approach for curing atrial fibrillation. Circulation. 2000;102:2619–28.

Reddy VY, Holmes D, Doshi SK, Neuzil P, Kar S. Safety of percutaneous left atrial appendage closure: results from the Watchman Left Atrial Appendage System for Embolic Protection in Patients with AF (PROTECT AF) clinical trial and the Continued Access Registry. Circulation. 2011;123:417–24.

Reddy VY, Neuzil P, Koruth JS, et al. Pulsed field ablation for pulmonary vein isolation in atrial fibrillation. J Am Coll Cardiol. 2019;74:315–26.

Reddy VY, Sievert H, Halperin J, et al. Percutaneous left atrial appendage closure vs warfarin for atrial fibrillation. A randomized clinical trial. JAMA. 2014;312(19):1988–98.

Reddy VY, Gibson DN, Kar S, et al. Post-approval U.S. experience with left atrial appendage closure for stroke prevention in atrial fibrillation. J Am Coll Cardiol. 2017;69:253–61.

Saint LL, Bailey MS, Sunil Prasad M, et al. Cox-maze IV results for patients with lone atrial fibrillation versus concomitant mitral disease. Ann Thorac Surg. 2012;93(3):789–95.

Santoro G, Meucci F, Stolcova M, et al. Percutaneous left atrial appendage occlusion in patients with non-valvular atrial fibrillation: implantation and up to four years follow-up of the AMPLATZER Cardiac Plug. EuroIntervention. 2016;11:1188–94.

Shinbane JS, Wood MA, Jensen DN, et al. Tachycardia-induced cardiomyopathy: a review of animal models and clinical studies. J Am Coll Cardiol. 1997;29:709–15.

Wardrop D, Keeling D. The story of the discovery of heparin and warfarin. Br J Haematol. 2008;141:757–63.

Wolf PA, Abbott RD, Kannel WB. Atrial' fibrillation as an independent risk factor for stroke: the Framingham Study. Stroke. 1991;22:983–8.

Wolff L. Familial auricular fibrillation. N Engl J Med. 1943;229:396–8.

Wyse DG, Waldo AL, DiMarco JP, et al. A comparison of rate control and rhythm control in patients with atrial fibrillation. N Engl J Med. 2002;347:1825–33.

The Sawtooth Rhythm: Atrial Flutter

Cosio FG, Lopez-Gil M, Goicolea A, Arribas F, Barroso JL. Radiofrequency ablation of the inferior vena cava-tricuspid valve isthmus in common atrial flutter. Am J Cardiol. 1993;71:705–9.

Cosio FG, Martin-Penato A, Pastor A, Nunez A, Goicolea A. Atypical flutter: a review. Pacing Clin Electrophysiol. 2003;26:2157–69.

Feld GK, Fleck RP, Chen PS, et al. Radiofrequency catheter ablation for the treatment of human type 1 atrial flutter. Identification of a critical zone in the reentrant circuit by endocardial mapping techniques. Circulation. 1992;86:1233–40.

Gomes JA. Atrial flutter, Chapter 10. In: Heart rhythm disorders: history, mechanisms, and management perspectives. Cham: Springer; 2020.

Haft JI, Kosowsky BD, Lau SH, Stein E, Damato AN. Termination of atrial flutter by rapid electrical pacing of the atrium. Am J Cardiol. 1967;20(2):239–44.

Jais P, Shah DC, Haissaguerre M, et al. Mapping and ablation of left atrial flutters. Circulation. 2000;101:2928–34.

Klein GJ, Guiraudon GM, Sharma AD, Milstein S. Demonstration of macroreentry and feasibility of operative therapy in the common type of atrial flutter. Am J Cardiol. 1986;57:587–91.

Lee KW, Yang Y, Scheinman MM. Atrial Flutter: a review of its history, mechanisms, clinical features, and current therapy. Curr Probl Cardiol. 2005;30:121–68.

Mangat I, Tschopp DR Jr, Yang Y, Cheng J, Keung EC, Scheinman MM. Optimizing the detection of bidirectional block across the flutter isthmus for patients with typical isthmus-dependent atrial flutter. Am J Cardiol. 2003;91:559–64.

Waldo AL, MacLean WA, Karp RB, Kouchoukos NT, James TN. Entrainment and interruption of atrial flutter with atrial pacing: studies in man following open heart surgery. Circulation. 1977;56:737–45.

Willems S, Weiss C, Ventura R, et al. Catheter ablation of atrial flutter guided by electroanatomic mapping (CARTO): a randomized comparison to the conventional approach. J Cardiovasc Electrophysiol. 2000;11:1223–30.

The Elusive Extrabeat

Baman TS, Lange DC, Ilg KJ, et al. Relationship between burden of premature ventricular complexes and left ventricular function. Heart Rhythm. 2010;7:865–9.

Blaye-Felice MS, Hamon D, Sacher F, Lellouche N, et al. Premature ventricular contraction-induced cardiomyopathy: related clinical and electrophysiologic parameters. Heart Rhythm. 2016;13(1):103–10. http://www.heartrhythmjournal.com/article/S1547-5271(15)01076-0/abstract.

Bogun F, Latchamsetty R. Premature ventricular complexes. In: Zipes DP, editor. Cardiac electrophysiology: from cell to bedside. Philadelphia: Elsevier Health Sciences; 2018.

Bogun F, Crawford T, Reich S, et al. Radiofrequency ablation of frequent, idiopathic premature ventricular complexes: comparison with a control group without intervention. Heart Rhythm. 2007;4:863–7.

Buxton AE, Lee KL, DiCarlo L, et al. Electrophysiologic testing to identify patients with coronary artery disease who are at risk for sudden death. N Engl J Med. 2000;342:1937–45.

Duffee DF, Shen WK, Smith HC. Suppression of frequent premature ventricular contractions and improvement of left ventricular function in patients with presumed idiopathic dilated cardiomyopathy. Mayo Clin Proc. 1998;73:430–3.

Echt DS, Lierson PR, Mitchell LB, et al. Mortality and morbidity in patients receiving encainide, flecainide, or placebo: the cardiac arrhythmia suppression trial. N Engl J Med. 1991;324(12):781–8.

Gomes JA. The ventricular premature complex, Chapter 12. In: Heart rhythm disorders: history, mechanisms, and management perspectives. Cham: Springer; 2020.

Gomes JAC, Carambas C, Moran H, Matthews L, et al.. Inotropic effect of post stimulation potentiation in man: an echocardiographic study. Am J Cardiol. 1979;43:745–52.

Gomes JAC, Hariman RI, et al.. Programmed electrical stimulation in patients with high-grade ventricular ectopy: Electrophysiologic findings and prognosis for survival. Circulation. 1984;70:43–51.

Haissaguerre M, Shah DC, Jais P, et al. Role of Purkinje conducting system in triggering of idiopathic ventricular fibrillation. Lancet. 2002;359:677–8.

Jose C Pachon M, Lobo TJ, Enrique I Pachon M. Idiopathic VPC: distribution of FOCI and tips of ablation. JAFIB. 2016;8(6):92–5.

Kennedy HL, Whitlock JA, Sprague MK. Long-term follow-up of asymptomatic healthy subjects with frequent and complex ventricular ectopy. N Engl J Med. 1985;312:193–7.

Kotler MN, Tabatznik B, Mower MM, Tominaga S. Prognostic significance of ventricular ectopic beats with respect to sudden death in the late post-infarction period. Circulation. 1973;47:959–66.

Latchamsetty R, Yokokawa M, Morady F, et al. Multicenter outcomes for catheter ablation of idiopathic premature ventricular complexes. J Am Coll Cardiol EP. 2015;1:116–23.

Lie KI, Wellens HJ, Durrer D. Characteristics and predictability of primary ventricular fibrillation. Eur J Cardiol. 1974;1(4):379–84.

Lown B, Wolf M. Approaches to sudden death from coronary artery disease. Circulation. 1971;44:130–42.

Maggioni AP, Zuanetti G, Franzosi MG, et al. Prevalence and prognostic significance of ventricular arrhythmias after acute myocardial infarction in the fibrinolytic era GISSI-2 results. Circulation. 1993;87(2):312–22.

Miller MA, Dukkipati SR, Turagam M, et al. Arrhythmic mitral valve prolapse. J Am Coll Cardiol. 2018;72:2904–14.

Moss AJ, Davis HT, DeCamilla J, Bayer LW. Ventricular ectopic beats and their relation to sudden death and non-sudden cardiac death after myocardial infarction. Circulation. 1979;60:998–1003.

Schulze RA, Strauss HW, Pit B. Sudden death in the year following myocardial infarction: relation to ventricular premature contractions in the late hospital phase and left ventricular ejection fraction. Am J Med. 1977;62:192–9.

Stamler J, Horowitz S, Gomes JA, et al. The effect of stress and fatigue on cardiac arrhythmias in medical interns. J Electrocardiol. 1992;25:333–8.

The Multicenter Postinfarction Research Group. Risk stratification and survival after myocardial infarction. N Engl J Med. 1983;309:331–6.

Yokokawa M, Kim HM, Good E, et al. Impact of QRS duration of frequent premature ventricular complexes on the development of cardiomyopathy. Heart Rhythm. 2012;9:1460–4.

A Catastrophic Event: Sudden Cardiac Death

Albert CM, Chae CU, Grodstein F, Rose LM, Rexrode KM, Ruskin JN, Stampfer MJ, Manson JE. Prospective study of sudden cardiac death among women in the United States. Circulation. 2003;107:2096–101. [PubMed].

Benjamin EJ, Virani SS, Callaway CW, et al. AHA statistical update heart disease and stroke statistics— 2018 update. A report from the American Heart Association. Circulation. 2018;137:e67–e492.

Bezzina CR, Pazoki R, Bardai A, et al. Genome-wide association study identifies a susceptibility locus at 21q21 for ventricular fibrillation in acute myocardial infarction. Nat Genet. 2010;42:688–91. [PMC free article] [PubMed].

Chan PS, McNally B, et al. Recent trends in survival from out-of-hospital cardiac arrest in the United States. Circulation. 2014;130:1876–82.

Davies MJ, Thomas AC. Plaque fissuring—the cause of acute myocardial infarction, sudden ischaemic death, and crescendo angina. Br Heart J. 1985;53:365–73.

de Luna B, Coumel P, Leclercq JF, et al. Ambulatory sudden cardiac death: mechanisms of production of fatal arrhythmias on the basis of data from 157 cases. Am Heart J. 1989;117:151–9.

Deo R, Albert CM. Epidemiology and genetics of sudden cardiac death. Circulation. 2012;125(4): 620–37.

Farb A, Tang AL, Burke AP, et al. Sudden coronary death frequency of active coronary lesions, inactive coronary lesions, and myocardial infarction. Circulation. 1995;92:1701–9.

Gomes JA. Sudden cardiac death, Chapter 17. In Heart rhythm disorders: history, mechanisms, and management perspectives. Cham: Springer; 2020.

Gomes JAC, Alexopoulos D, Winters SL, et al. The role of silent ischemia, the arrhythmic substrate and the short-long sequence in the genesis of sudden death. J Am Coll Cardiol. 1989;14:1618–25.

Gomes JA, Mehta D, Ip J, Winters S, Camunas J, Ergin A, Newhouse T, Pe E. Predictors of long -term survival in patients with malignant ventricular arrhythmias. Am J Cardiol. 1997;79:1054–60.

Leclercq JF, Maisonblanche F, Canchemez B, et al. Respective role of cardiac pauses in the genesis of 62 cases of ventricular fibrillation recorded during monitoring. Eur J Cardio. 1988;9:1276–83.

Mehta D, Curwin J, Gomes JA and Fuster V. Sudden death in coronary artery disease. Acute ischemia versus myocardial substrate. Circulation. 1997;96:3215–23.

Myerburg RJ, Castellanos A. Cardiac arrest and d sudden cardiac death. In: Braunwald E, editor. Heart disease: a textbook of cardiovascular medicine. Philadelphia: WB Saunders; 1992. p. 756–89.

Myerburg RJ, Goldberger JJ. Sudden death in adults. In: Zipes DP, Jalife J, Stevenson WG, editors. Cardiac electrophysiology: from cell to bedside. 7th ed. Philadelphia: Elsevier Health Sciences; 2018. p. 19103–22899.

Vaillancourt C, Everson-Stewart S, Christenson J, et al. the Resuscitation Outcomes Consortium Investigators. The impact of increased chest compression fraction on return of spontaneous circulation for out-of-hospital cardiac arrest patients not in ventricular fibrillation. Resuscitation. 2011;82:1501–7.

Walter L. Bruetsch. The earliest record of sudden death possibly due to atherosclerotic coronary occlusion. Circulation. 1959;20:438–41.

Weisfeldt ML, Everson-Stewart S, Sitlani C, et al. Resuscitation Outcomes Consortium Investigators. Ventricular tachyarrhythmias after cardiac arrest in public versus at home. N Engl J Med. 2011;364:313–21.

Winters SL, Cohen M, Greenberg S, Stein B, Camunas J, Elena P, Gomes JA. Sustained ventricular tachycardia associated with sarcoidosis: assessment of the underlying cardiac anatomy and the prospective utility of programmed ventricular stimulation, drug therapy and an implantable antitachycardia device. J Am Coll Cardiol. 1991;18:937–43.

Wissenberg M, Lippert FK, Folke F, et al. Association of National Initiatives to improve cardiac arrest management with rates of bystander intervention and patient survival after out-of-hospital cardiac arrest. JAMA. 2013;310(13):1377–84.

Strange Occurences in Life's Channels

Ackerman MJ, Priori SG, Willems S, et al. HRS/EHRA expert consensus statement on the state of genetic testing for the channelopathies and cardiomyopathies: this document was developed as a partnership between the Heart Rhythm Society (HRS) and the European Heart Rhythm Association (EHRA). Heart Rhythm. 2011;8:1308–39.

Bagnall RD, Weintraub RG, Ingles J et al. A prospective study of sudden cardiac death among children and young adults. N Engl J Med. 2016;374:2441–52.

Brugada P, Brugada J. Right bundle branch block, persistent ST segment elevation and sudden cardiac death: a distinct clinical and electrocardiographic syndrome. A multicenter report. J Am Coll Cardiol. 1992;20:1992–391.

Brugada J, Brugada R, Brugada P. Determinants of sudden cardiac death in individuals with the electrocardiographic pattern of Brugada syndrome and no previous cardiac arrest. Circulation. 2003;108:3092–6.

Chen Q, Kirsch GE, Zhang D, et al. Genetic basis and molecular mechanism for idiopathic ventricular fibrillation. Nature. 1998;392:293–6.

Conte G, Sieira J, Ciconte G, et al. Implantable cardioverter-defibrillator therapy in Brugada syndrome: a 20-year single-center experience. J Am Coll Cardiol. 2015;65:879–88.

Curran ME, Splawski I, Timothy KW, et al. A molecular basis for cardiac arrhythmia: HERG mutations cause long QT syndrome. Cell. 1995;80:795–803.

Dessertenne F. Ventricular tachycardia with 2 variable opposing foci [in French]. Arch Mal Coeur Vaiss. 1966;59:263–72.

Gehi AK, Duong TD, Metz LD, et al. Risk stratification of individuals with the Brugada electrocardiogram: a meta-analysis. J Cardiovasc Electrophysiol. 2006;17:577–83.

Giustetto C, Schimpf R, Mazzanti A, et al. Long-term follow-up of patients with short QT syndrome. J Am Coll Cardiol. 2011;58:587–95.

Gomes JA. The channelopathies and sudden daeth. In: Heart rhythm disorders: history, mechanisms, and management perspectives. Cham: Springer; 2020.

Jervell A, Lange-Nielsen F. Congenital deaf-mutism, functional heart disease with prolongation of the Q-T interval and sudden death. Am Heart J. 1957;54:59–68.

Keating M, Atkinson D, Dunn C, et al. Linkage of a cardiac arrhythmia, the long QT syndrome, and the Harvey ras-1 gene. Science. 1991;252:704–6.

Lahat H, Pras E, Olender T, et al. A missense mutation in a highly conserved region of CASQ2 is associated with autosomal recessive catecholamine-induced polymorphic ventricular ventricular tachycardia in Bedouin families from Israel. Am J Hum Genet. 2001;69:1378–84.

Leenhardt A, Lucet V, Denjoy I, et al. Catecholaminergic polymorphic ventricular tachycardia in children. A 7-year follow-up of 21 patients. Circulation. 1995;91:1512–9.

Levine SA, Woodworth CR. Congenital deaf-mutism, prolonged QT interval, syncopal attacks and sudden death. N Engl J Med. 1958;259:412–7.

Moss AJ, McDonald J. Unilateral cervicothoracic sympathetic ganglionectomy for the treatment of long QT interval syndrome. N Engl J Med. 1971;285:903–4.

Moss AJ, Schwartz PJ. Delayed repolarization (QT or QTU prolongation) and malignant ventricular arrhythmias. Modern Concepts Cardiovasc Dis. 1982;51:85–90.

Moss AJ, Schwartz PJ. 25th Anniversary of the International Long-QTSyndrome Registry. An ongoing quest to uncover the secrets of long-QT syndrome. Circulation. 2005;111:1199–201.

Nademanee K, Veerakul G, Chandanamattha P, et al. Prevention of ventricular fibrillation episodes in Brugada syndrome by catheter ablation over the anterior right ventricular outflow tract epicardium. Circulation. 2011;123:1270–9.

Outcome of apparently unexplained cardiac arrest: results from investigation and follow-up of the prospective cardiac arrest survivors with preserved ejection fraction registry. Circ Arrhythm Electrophysiol. 2016; 9:e004012. https://doi.org/10.1161/CIRCEP.116.004012.

Priori SG, Napolitano C, Tiso N, et al. Mutations in the cardiac ryanodine receptor gene (hRyR2) underlie catecholaminergic polymorphic ventricular tachycardia. Circulation. 2001;103:196–200.

Priori SG, Napolitano C, Gasparini M, et al. Natural history of Brugada syndrome: insights for risk stratification and management. Circulation. 2002;105:1342–7.

Priori SG, Wilde AA, Horie M, et al. HRS/EHRA/APHRS expert consensus statement on the diagnosis and management of patients with inherited primary arrhythmia syndromes. Heart Rhythm. 2013;10(12):1932–63. https://doi.org/10.1016/j.hrthm.2013.05.014.

Remme CA, Wever EF, Wilde AA, et al. Diagnosis and long-term follow-up of the Brugada syndrome in patients with idiopathic ventricular fibrillation. Eur Heart J. 2001;22:400–9.

Romano C, Gemme G, Pongiglione R. Rare cardiac arrhythmias of the pediatric age. II. Syncopal attacks due to paroxysmal ventricular fibrillation. (Presentation of 1st case in Italian pediatric literature) [in Italian]. Clin Pediatr (Bologna). 1963;45:656–83.

Schwartz PJ. The idiopathic long QT syndrome: the need for a prospective registry. Eur Heart J. 1983;4:529–31.

Schwartz PJ, Periti M, Malliani A. The long Q-T syndrome. Am Heart J. 1975;89:378–90.

Schwartz PJ, Priori SG, Spazzolini C, et al. Genotype-phenotype correlation in the long-QT syndrome gene-specific triggers for life-threatening arrhythmias. Circulation. 2001;103:89–95.

Schwartz PJ, Ackerman MJ, George AL Jr, Wilde AM. Impact of genetics on the clinical management of channelopathies. J Am Coll Cardiol. 2013;62:169–80.

Schwartz PJ, Priori SG, Cerrone M, et al.. Left cardiac sympathetic denervation in the management of high-risk patients affected by the long-QT syndrome. Circulation. 2004;109:1826–33.

Survivors of out-of-hospital cardiac arrest with apparently normal heart. Need for definition and standardized clinical evaluation. Consensus Statement of the Joint Steering Committees of the Unexplained Cardiac Arrest Registry of Europe and of the Idiopathic Ventricular Fibrillation Registry of the United States. Circulation. 1997; 95:265.

Wang Q, Shen J, Splawski I, et al. SCN5A mutations associated with an inherited cardiac arrhythmia, long QT syndrome. Cell. 1995;80:805–11.

Wellens HJ, Vermeulen A, Durrer D. Ventricular fibrillation occurring on arousal from sleep by auditory stimuli. Circulation. 1972;46:661–5.

Yanowitz F, Preston JB, Abildskov JA. Functional distribution of right and left stellate innervation to the ventricles. Production of neurogenic electrocardiographic changes by alteration of sympathetic tone. Circ Res. 1966;18:416–28.

A Heartbraking Calamity: Sudden Death in the Athlete

Abernethy WB, Choo JK, Hutter AM Jr. Echocardiographic characteristics of professional football players. J Am Coll Cardiol. 2003;41:280–4.

Balady GJ, Cadigan JB, Ryan TJ. Electrocardiogram of the athlete: an analysis of 289 professional football players. Am J Cardiol. 1984;53:1339–43.

Billea K, Figueirasb D, Schamaschc P, et al. Sudden cardiac death in athletes: the Lausanne recommendations. Eur J Cardiovasc Prev Rehabil. 2006;13:859–87.

Coonar AS, Protonotarios N, Tsatsopoulou A, Needham EW, Houlston RS, Cliff S, et al. Gene for arrhythmogenic right ventricular cardiomyopathy with diffuse nonepidermolytic palmoplantar keratoderma and woolly hair (Naxos disease) maps to 17q21. Circulation. 1998;97:2049–58. https://doi.org/10.1161/01.CIR.97.20.2049. [PubMed] [CrossRef].

Corrado D, Basso C, Pavei A, Michieli P, Schiavon M, Thiene G. Trends in sudden cardiovascular death in young competitive athletes after implementation of a preparticipation screening program. JAMA. 2006;296:1593–601.

Eckart RE, Scoville SL, Campbell CL, et al.. Sudden death in young adults: a 25-year review of autopsies in military recruits. Ann Intern Med. 2004;141:829–34.

Finocchiaro G, Papadakis M, Robertus J-L, et al. Etiology of sudden death in sports insights from a United Kingdom Regional Registry. J Am Coll Cardiol. 2016;67:2108–15.

Finocchiaro G, Behr ER, Tanzarella G, et al. Anomalous coronary artery origin and sudden cardiac death: clinical and pathological insights from a National Pathology Registry. JACC: Clin Electrophysiol. 2019; https://doi.org/10.1016/j.jacep.2018.11.015.

Fontaine G, Guiraudon G, Frank R, Vedel J, Grosgogeat Y, Cabrol C, et al. In: Kulbertus H, et al., editors. Stimulation studies and epicardial mapping in ventricular tachycardia: study of mechanisms and selection for surgery. MTP Pub: Lancaster; 1977. p. 334–50.

Fontaine G, Fontaliran F, Frank R. Arrhythmogenic right ventricular cardiomyopathies: clinical forms and main differential diagnoses. Circulation. 1998;97:1532–5. https://doi.org/10.1161/01.CIR.97.16.1532. [PubMed] [CrossRef].

Gersh BJ, Maron BJ, Bonow RO, et al. 2011 ACCF/AHA guideline for the diagnosis and treatment of hypertrophic cardiomyopathy. A report of the American College of Cardiology Foundation/American Heart Association Task Force on Practice Guidelines. J Am Coll Cardiol. 2011;58:e212–60. https://doi.org/10.1016/j.jacc.2011.06.011. [PubMed].

Gomes JA. Sudden cardiac death in athletes, Chapter 18. In: Heart rhythm disorders: history, mechanisms, and management perspectives. Cham: Springer; 2020.

Harmon KG, Asif IM, Klossner D, Drezner JA. Incidence of sudden cardiac death in National Collegiate Athletic Association athletes. Circulation. 2011;123:1594–600.

Israel Sport Law 5748-1988 and The Sport (Medical Tests) Regulations 5757-1997. http://www.nevo.co.il/Law_word/law06/TAK-5828.pdf.

Link MS. Commotio cordis ventricular fibrillation triggered by chest impact–induced abnormalities in repolarization. Circ Arrhythm Electrophysiol. 2012;5:425–32.

Marcus FI, Fontaine GH, Guiraudon G, et al. Right ventricular dysplasia: a report of 24 adult cases. Circulation. 1982;65(20):384–98.

Marcus FI, McKenna WJ, Sherrill D, Basso C. Diagnosis of arrhythmogenic right ventricular cardiomyopathy/dysplasia. Proposed modification of the task force criteria. Circulation. 2010;121:1533–41.

Maron B. American College of Cardiology/European Society of Cardiology Clinical Expert Consensus Document on Hypertrophic Cardiomyopathy. A report of the American College of Cardiology Foundation Task Force on Clinical Expert Consensus Documents and the European Society of Cardiology Committee for Practice Guidelines. Eur Heart J. 2003;24:1965–91. https://doi.org/10.1016/s0195-668x(03)00479-2. [PubMed].

Maron BJ. Distinguishing hypertrophic cardiomyopathy from athlete's heart: a clinical problem of increasing magnitude and significance. Heart. 2005;91:1380–2.

Maron BJ.. Sudden death in young athletes. N Engl J Med. 2003;349:1064–75.

Maron BJ, Estes NA 3rd. Commotio cordis. N Engl J Med. 2010;362:917–27.

Maron BJ, Maron MS. Hypertrophic cardiomyopathy. Lancet. 2013;381:242–55.

Maron BJ, Poliac LC, Kaplan JA, Mueller FO. Blunt impact to the chest leading to sudden death from cardiac arrest during sports activities. N Engl J Med. 1995;333:337–42.

Maron BJ, Douglas PS, Graham TP, Nishimura RA, Thompson PD. Task force 1: preparticipation screening and diagnosis of cardiovascular disease in athletes. J Am Coll Cardiol. 2005;45:1322–6.

Maron BJ, Thompson PD, Ackerman MJ, et al. Recommendations and considerations related to preparticipation screening for cardiovascular abnormalities in competitive athletes: 2007 update a scientific statement from the American Heart Association Council on Nutrition, Physical Activity, and Metabolism. Circulation. 2007;115:1643–55.

Maron BJ, Doerer JJ, Hass TS, et al. Sudden death in young competitive athletes. Analysis of 1866 deaths in the United States, 1980-2006. Circulation. 2009;119:1085–92.

Barry J. Maron; Douglas P. Zipes; Richard J. Kovacs; on behalf of the American Heart Association Electrocardiography and Arrhythmias Committee of the Council on Clinical Cardiology, Council on Cardiovascular Disease in the Young, Council on Cardiovascular and Stroke Nursing, Council on Functional Genomics and Translational Biology, and the American College of Cardiology Eligibility and Disqualification Recommendations for Competitive Athletes With Cardiovascular Abnormalities: Preamble, Principles, and General Considerations. A Scientific Statement From the American Heart Association and American College of Cardiology. Circulation. 2015;132:e256–61.

Maron BJ, Haas TS, Ahluwalia A, et al. Demographics and epidemiology of sudden deaths in young competitive athletes: from the United States National Registry. Am J Med. 2016;129:1170–7.

Nesbitt AD, Cooper PJ, Kohl P. Rediscovering commotio cordis. Lancet. 2001;357:1195–7.

Protonotarios N, Tsatsopoulou A, Patsourakos D, Alexopoulos D, Gezerlis P, Simitsis S. Cardiac abnormalities in familial palmoplantar keratosis. Br Heart J. 1986;56:321–6. https://doi.org/10.1136/hrt.56.4.321. [PMC free article] [PubMed] [CrossRef].

Roma-Rodrigues C, Fernandes AR. Genetics of hypertrophic cardiomyopathy: advances and pitfalls in molecular diagnosis and therapy. Appl Clin Genet. 2014;7:195–208.

Steinvil A, Chundadze T, Zeltser D, et al. Mandatory electrocardiographic screening of athletes to reduce their risk for sudden death proven fact or wishful thinking. J Am Coll Cardiol. 2011;57:1291–6.

Conquering the Arrhythmia Substrate: The Scalpel and the Source

Calkins H, Epstein A, Packer D, et al. Catheter ablation of ventricular tachycardia in patients with structural heart disease using cooled radiofrequency energy: results of a prospective multicenter study. J Am Coll Cardiol. 2000;35:1905–14.

Di Biase L, Burkhardt JD, Lakkireddy D, et al. Ablation of stable VTs versus substrate ablation in ischemic cardiomyopathy: the VISTA randomized multicenter trial. J Am Coll Cardiol. 2015;66:2872–82.

Dukkipati SR, Koruth JS, Choudry S, et al. Catheter ablation of ventricular tachycardia in structural heart disease: indications, strategies, and outcomes—part II. J Am Coll Cardiol. 2017;70(23):2924–41.

El-Sherif N, Gough WB, Zeiler RH, Hariman R. Reentrant ventricular arrhythmias in the late myocardial infraction period. 12. Spontaneous versus induced reentry and intramural versus epicardial circuits. J Am Coll Cardiol. 1985;6:124–32.

Ghanbari H, Baser K, Yokokawa M, et al. Noninducibility in postinfarction ventricular tachycardia as an end point for ventricular tachycardia ablation and its effects on outcomes: a meta-analysis. Circ Arrhythm Electrophysiol. 2014;7:677–83.

Gomes JA, Winters SL, Ergin A, et al. Clinical and electrophysiologic determinants, treatment and survival of patients with sustained malignant ventricular tachyarrhythmias occurring late after myocardial infarction. J Am Coll Cardiol. 1991;17(2):320–6.

Gomes J, Winters SL, Ergin A, et al. Clinical and electrophysiologic determinants, treatment and survival of patients with sustained malignant ventricular tachyarrhythmias occurring late after myocardial infarction. J Am Coil Cardiol. 1991;17:320–6.

Guiraudon G, Fontaine G, Frank R, et al. Encircling endocardial ventriculotomy: a new surgical treatment for life-threatening ventricular tachvcardias resistant to medical treatment following myocardial infarction. Ann Thorac Surg. 1978;26:438–44.

Horowitz LN, Harken AH, Kastor JA, Josephson ME. Ventricular resection guided by epicardial and endocardial mapping for treatment of recurrent ventricular tachycardia. N Engl J Med. 1980;302:589–93.

Josephson ME, Horowitz LN, Farshidi A. Continuous local electrical activity. A mechanism of recurrent ventricular tachycardia. Circulation. 1978;57:659–65.

Josephson ME, Harken AH, Horowitz LN. Endocardial excision: a new surgical technique for the treatment of recurrent ventricular tachycardia. Circulation. 1979;60:1430–9.

Khatib SM, Stevenson WG, Ackerman MJ, et al. 2017 AHA/ACC/HRS guidelines for management of patients with ventricular arrhythmias and the prevention of sudden cardiac death. Heart Rhythm. 2018;15(10):e73–e189.

Kuck KH, Schaumann A, Eckardt L, et al. Catheter ablation of stable ventricular tachycardia before defibrillator implantation in patients with coronary heart disease (VTACH): a multicentre randomised controlled trial. Lancet. 2010;375(9708):31–40.

Littmann L, Svenson RH, Gallagher JJ, et al. Functional role of the epicardium in postinfarction ventricular tachycardia. Observations derived from computerized epicardial activation mapping, entrainment, and epicardial laser photoablation. Circulation. 1991;83:1577–91.

Marchlinski FE, Callans DJ, Gottlieb CD, Zado E. Linear ablation lesions for control of unmappable ventricular tachycardia in patients with ischemic and nonischemic cardiomyopathy. Circulation. 2000;101:1288–96.

Marchlinski FE, Haffajee CI, Beshai JF, et al. Long-term success of irrigated radiofrequency catheter ablation of sustained ventricular tachycardia: post-approval THERMOCOOL VT trial. J Am Coll Cardiol. 2016;67:674–83.

Maskoun W, Saad M, Abualsuod A. Outcome of catheter ablation for ventricular tachycardia in patients with ischemic cardiomyopathy: a systematic review and meta-analysis of randomized clinical trials. Int J Cardiol. 2018;267:107–13.

Mason JW, Stinson EB, Winkle RA, et al. Relative efficacy of blind left ventricular aneurysm resection for the treatment of recurrent ventricular tachycardia. AJC. 1982;40:241–8.

Mehra R, Zeiler RH, Gough WB, El-Sherif A. Reentrant ventricular arrhythmias in the late myocardial infarction period 9. Electrophysiologic-anatomic correlation of reentrant circuits. Circulation. 1983;67:11–24.

Miller MA, Dukkipati SR, Mittnacht AJ, et al. Activation and entrainment mapping of hemodynamically unstable ventricular tachycardia using a percutaneous left ventricular assist device. J Am Coll Cardiol. 2011;58:1363–71.

Reddy VY, Reynolds MR, Neuzil P, et al. Prophylactic catheter ablation for the prevention of defibrillator therapy. N Engl J Med. 2007;357:2657–65.

Santangeli P, Frankel DS, Tung R, et al. Early mortality after catheter ablation of ventricular tachycardia in patients with structural heart disease. J Am Coll Cardiol. 2017;69:2105–15.

Sapp JL, Wells GA, Parkash R, et al. Ventricular tachycardia ablation versus escalation of antiarrhythmic drugs. NEJM. 2016;375:111–21.

Stevenson WG, Soejima K. Catheter ablation for ventricular tachycardia. Circulation. 2007;115:2750–60.

Stevenson WG, Weiss J, Weiner I, et al. Localization of slow conduction in a ventricular tachycardia circuit: implications for catheter ablation. Am Heart J. 1987;114:1253–6.

Stevenson WG, Khan H, Sager P, et al. Identification of reentry circuit sites during catheter mapping and radiofrequency ablation of ventricular tachycardia late after myocardial infarction. Circulation. 1993;88(4 Pt 1):1647–70.

Tanner H, Hindricks G, Volkmer M, et al. Catheter ablation of recurrent scar-related ventricular tachycardia using electroanatomical mapping and irrigated ablation technology: results of the prospective multicenter Euro-VT-study. J Cardiovasc Electrophysiol. 2010;21:47–53.

Tung R, Vaseghi M, Frankel DS, et al.. Freedom from recurrent ventricular tachycardia after catheter ablation is associated with improved survival in patients with structural heart disease: an International VT Ablation Center Collaborative Group study. Heart Rhythm. 2015:12: 1997–2007.

Wit AL, Allessie MA, Bonke FIM, et al. Electrophysiological mapping to determine the mechanism of experimental ventricular tachycardia initiated by premature impulses. Experimental approach and initial results demonstrating reentrant excitation. Am J Cardiol. 1982;49:166–85.

A Revolutionary Idea: The Implantable Defibrillator—A Lifesaver

Adduci C, Palano F, Francia P. Safety, efficacy and evidence base for use of the subcutaneous implantable cardioverter defibrillator. J Clin Med. 2018;7:53.

Al-Khatib SM, Stevenson WG, Ackerman MJ, et al. 2017 AHA/ACC/HRS guideline for management of patients with ventricular arrhythmias and the prevention of sudden cardiac death. Heart Rhythm. 2018;15(10):e73–e189. https://doi.org/10.1016/j.hrthm.2017.10.036.

AVID Investigators. Causes of death in the antiarrhythmics versus implantable defibrillators (AVID) trial. J Am Coll Cardiol. 1999;34:1552–9.

Bardy GH, Lee KL, et al. Amiodarone or an implantable cardioverter–defibrillator for congestive heart failure. N Engl J Med. 2005;352:225–37.

Bardy GH, Smith WM, Hood MA, et al. An entirely subcutaneous implantable cardioverter-defibrillator. N Engl J Med. 2010;363:36–44.

Bristow MR, Saxon LA, Boehmer J, et al. Cardiac resynchronization therapy with or without an implantable defibrillator in advanced chronic heart failure. N Engl J Med. 2004;350:2140–50.

Buxton AE, Lee KL, Fisher JD, Josephson ME, Prystowsky EN, Hafley G. A randomized study of the prevention of sudden death in patients with coronary artery disease. Multicenter Unsustained Tachycardia Trial Investigators. N Engl J Med. 1999;341:1882–90.

Connolly SJ, Hallstrom AP, Cappato R, et al. Meta-analysis of the implantable cardioverter defibrillator secondary prevention trials. AVID, CASH, and CIDS studies. Eur Heart J. 2000;21:2071.

Connolly SJ, Gent M, Roberts RS, et al.. Canadian Implantable Defibrillator Study (CIDS): a randomized trial of the implantable defibrillator against amiodarone. Circulation. 2000;101:1297–1302.

Dixon EG, Tang AS, Wolf PD, et al. Improved defibrillation thresholds with large contoured epicardial electrodes and biphasic waveforms. Circulation. 1987;76:1176–84.

Ezzat VA, Lee V, Ahsan S, et al. A systematic review of ICD complications in randomised controlled trials versus registries: is our 'real-world' data an underestimation? Open Heart. 2015;2:e000198.

Gomes JA. The implantable defibrillator: a historical overview and its use in secondary and primary prevention, Chapter 24. In: Heart rhythm disorders: history, mechanisms, and management perspectives. Cham: Springer; 2020.

Gomes JA, Cain ME, Buxton AE, Josephson ME, Lee KL, Hafley GE. Prediction of long-term outcomes by signal-averaged electrocardiography in patients with nonsustained ventricular tachycardia, coronary artery disease, and left ventricular dysfunction. Circulation. 2001;104:306–441.

Kadish A, Dyer A, Daubert JP, et al. Prophylactic defibrillator implantation in patients with non-ischemic dilated cardiomyopathy. N Engl J Med. 2004;350:2151–8.

Kastor JA. Michel Mirowski and the automatic implantable defibrillator. Am J Cardiol. 1989;63:1121–6.

Kuck KH, Cappato R, Siebels J, Ruppel R. Randomized comparison of antiarrhythmic drug therapy with implantable defibrillators in patients resuscitated from cardiac arrest: the Cardiac Arrest Study Hamburg (CASH). Circulation. 2000;102:748–54.

Lown B, Axelrod P. Implanted standby defibrillators. Circulation. 1972;46:637–9. [PubMed:5072764].

Mirowski M, Mower MM, Staewen WS, et al. Standby automatic defibrillator. An approach to prevention of sudden coronary death. Arch Intern Med. 1970;126:158–61.

Mirowski M, Reid PR, Mower MM, et al. Termination of malignant ventricular arrhythmias with an implanted automatic defibrillator in human beings. N Engl J Med. 1980;303:322–4.

Moss AJ, Hall WJ, Cannom DS, et al. Improved survival with an implanted defibrillator in patients with coronary disease at high risk for ventricular arrhythmia. Multicenter Automatic Defibrillator Implantation Trial Investigators. N Engl J Med. 1996;335:1933–40. [PMID: 8960472].

Moss AJ, Zareba W, Hall WJ, Klein H, Wilber DJ, Cannom DS, et al. Multicenter Automatic Defibrillator Implantation Trial II Investigators. Prophylactic implantation of a defibrillator in patients with myocardial infarction and reduced ejection fraction. N Engl J Med. 2002;346:877–83.

Moss, A.J.; Zareba, W.; Hall, W.J.; et al.. Prophylactic implantation of a defibrillator in patients with myocardial infarction and reduced ejection fraction. N Engl J Med. 2002:346:877–83.

Schuder JC. Completely implanted defibrillator. JAMA. 1970;214:1123. [PubMed: 5536262].

Schuder JC, Stoeckle H, Gold JH, et al. Experimental ventricular defibrillation with an automatic and completely implanted system. Trans Amer Soc Artif Intern Organs. 1970;16:207–12.

Strickburger SA, Hummel JD, Bartlett TG, et al. Amiodarone versus implantable cardioverter-defibrillator: randomized trial in patients with nonischemic dilated cardiomyopathy and asymptomatic nonsustained ventricular tachycardia--AMIOVIRT. J Am Coll Cardiol. 2003;42(10):1707–12.

The Antiarrhythmics Versus Implantable Defibrillators (AVID) Investigators. A comparison of antiarrhythmic drug therapy with implantable defibrillators in patients resuscitated from near-fatal ventricular arrhythmias. N Engl J Med. 1997;337:1576–83.

Weiss R, Knight BP, Gold MR, et al. Safety and efficacy of a totally subcutaneous implantable-cardioverter defibrillator. Circulation. 2013;128:944–53.

Westman SB, El-Chami M. The subcutaneous implantable defibrillator—review of recent data. J Gerriatr Cardiol. 2018;15:222–8.

Wever EF, Hauer RN, vanCapelle FL, et al. Randomized study of implantable defibrillator as first-choice therapy versus conventional strategy in postinfarct sudden death survivors. Circulation. 1995;91:2195–203.

To Freeze and Not to Fry

Bradley SM, Liu W, McNally B, et al. Temporal trends in the use of therapeutic hypothermia for out-of-hospital cardiac arrest. JAMA Netw Open. 2018;1(7):e184511.

Chan PS, Berg RA, Tang Y, et al. Association between therapeutic hypothermia and survival after in-hospital cardiac arrest. JAMA. 2016;316(13):1375–82.

Ewy GA. Cardiocerebral resuscitation the new cardiopulmonary resuscitation. Circulation. 2005;111:2134–42.

Hazinski MF, Nadkarni VM, Hickey RW, et al. Major changes in the 2005 AHA guidelines for CPR and ECC. Reaching the tipping point for change. Circulation. 2005;112:IV-206–11.

Jalali R, Rezaei M. A comparison of the Glasgow Coma Scale score with full outline of unresponsiveness scale to predict patients' traumatic brain injury outcomes in intensive care units. Crit Care Res Pract. 2014;2014:289803. Published online 2014 Jun 10. https://doi.org/10.1155/2014/289803.

Karnatovskaia LV, Wartenberg KE, Freeman WD. Therapeutic hypothermia for neuroprotection: history, mechanisms, risks, and clinical applications. Neurohospitalist. 2014;4(3):153–63. https://www.ncbi.nlm.nih.gov/pmc/articles/PMC4056415/.

Kochanek PM, Drabeck T, Tishweman SA. Therapeutic hypothermia: the Safar vision. J Neurotrauma. 2009;26(3):417–20.

Nielsen N, Wetterslev J, Cronberg T, et al. Targeted temperature management at 33°C versus 36°C after cardiac arrest. N Engl J Med. 2013;369:2197–206.

Nolan JP, Morley PT, Vanden Hock TL, Hickey RW. ILCOR advisory statement. Therapeutic hypothermia after cardiac arrest. An advisory statement by the advanced life support task force of the International Liaison Committee on Resuscitation. Circulation. 2003;108:118–21.

Rainey Williams G Jr, Spencer FC. The clinical use of hypothermia following cardiac arrest. Ann Surg. 1958;148(3):462–6. https://www.ncbi.nlm.nih.gov/pmc/articles/PMC1450838/pdf/annsurg01227-0170.pdf.

Safar PJ, Kochanek PM. Therapeutic hypothermia after cardiac arrest. N Engl J Med. 2002;346:612–3.

The Hypothermia after Cardiac Arrest Study Group. Mild therapeutic hypothermia to improve the neurologic outcome after cardiac arrest. N Engl J Med. 2002;346:549–56.

Varon J, Acosta P. Therapeutic hypothermia: past, present, and future. Chest. 2008;133(5):1267–74. [PubMed].

Yenari MA, Han HS. Neuroprotective mechanisms of hypothermia in brain ischaemia. Nat Rev Neurosci. 2012;13(4):267–78. [PubMed].

Of Scintillating Lights, Tunnels, and Astral Encounters

Ammirati F, Colivicchi F, Di Battista G, et al. Electroencephalographic correlates of vasovagal syncope induced by head-up tilt testing. Stroke. 1998;29:2347–51.

Greyson B, Holden JM, Paul Mounsey J. Failure to elicit near-death experiences in induced cardiac arrest. J Near-Death Stud. 2006;25(2):85–98.

Long J. Near-death experiences evidence for their reality. Mo Med. 2014;111(5):372–80.

Milne CT. Cardiac electrophysiology studies and the near-death experience. Can Assoc Crit Care Nurs. 1995;6:6–19.

Moss J, Rockoff M. EEG monitoring during cardiac arrest and resuscitation. J Am Med Assoc. 1980;244:2750–1.

Parnia S, Spearpoint K, de Vos G, Farber M, et al. AWARE-AWAreness during resuscitation – a propective study. Resuscitation. 2012;85:1799–805.

Scherlag B. Stentor coeruleus: do these tiny cells have out-of-body experiences? https://researchoutreach.org/articles/stentor-coeruleus-out-body-experiences/.

Sun G, Montell DJ. Q&A: cellular near death experiences-what is anastasis? BMC Biol. 2017;15:92–7.

van Lommel P, van Wees R, Myers V, Meyers V, Elfferich I. Near-death expirience in survivors of cardiac arrest: a prospective study in the Netherlands. Lancet. 2001;358:2045.

The Broken Heart

Cannon WB. "VOODOO" death. Am J Public Health. 2002;92(10):1593–6.

Eitel I, von Knobelsdorff-Brenkenhoff F, Bernhardt P, Carbone I, et al. Clinical characteristics and cardiovascular magnetic resonance findings in stress (takotsubo) cardiomyopathy. JAMA. 2011;306(3):277–86.

Ghadri JR, Wittstein IS, Prasad A, et al. International expert consensus document on takotsubo syndrome (part I): clinical characteristics, diagnostic criteria, and pathophysiology. Eur Heart J. 2018;39(22):2032–46.

Kurisu S, Sato H, Kawagoe T, Ishihara M, et al. Tako-tsubo-like left ventricular dysfunction with ST-segment elevation: a novel cardiac syndrome mimicking acute myocardial infarction. Am Heart J. 2002;143(3):448–55.

Kurisu S, Sato H, Kawagoe T, Ishihara M, et al.. Tako-tsubo-like left ventricular dysfunction with ST-segment elevation: a novel cardiac syndrome mimicking acute myocardial infarction. Am Heart J. 2002;143(3):448–55.

Sato H. Tako-tsubo like ventricular dysfunction due to multivessle coronary spasm. In: Kodama K, Haze K, editors. Clinical aspects of myocardial injury from ischemia to heart failure. Toykio: Kagakuhyoronsha Publishin Co; 1990. p. P56–64; (article in Japanese).

Sharkey SW, Windenburg DC, Lesser JR, Maron MS, et al. Natural history and expansive clinical profile of stress (Tako-Tsubo) cardiomyopathy. J Am Coll Cardiol. 2010;55(4):333–41.

Steinberg JS, Arshad A, Kowalski M, Kukar A, et al. Increased incidence of life-threatening ventricular arrhythmias in implantable defibrillator patients after the World Trade Center attack. JACC. 2004;44(6):1261–4.

Syed FF, Asirvatham SJ, Francis J. Arrhythmia occurrence with takotsubo cardiomyopathy: a literature review. Europace. 2011;13:780–8.

Taggart P, Boyett MR, Logantha SJRJ, Lambiase PD. Anger, emotion, and arrhythmias: from brain to heart. Front Physiol. 2011;2:67.

Templin C, Ghadri JR, Diekmann J, Napp LC, et al. Clinical features and outcomes of takotsubo (stress) cardiomyopathy. N Engl J Med. 2015;373(10):929–38. http://www.nejm.org/doi/pdf/10.1056/NEJMoa1406761.

Wittstein IS, Thiemann DR, Lima JA, Baughman KL, et al. Neurohumoral features of myocardial stunning due to sudden emotional stress. N Engl J Med. 2005;352:539–48.

The Ubiquitous Faint

Brignole M, Menozzi C, Moya A, et al. Pacemaker therapy in patients with neurally mediated syncope and documented asystole: Third International Study on Syncope of Uncertain Etiology (ISSUE-3): a randomized trial. Circulation. 2012;125:2566–71.

Brignole M, Donateo P, Tomaino M, et al. Benefit of pacemaker therapy in patients with presumed neurally mediated syncope and documented asystole is greater when tilt test is negative: an analysis from the Third International Study on Syncope of Uncertain Etiology (ISSUE-3). Circ Arrhythm Electrophysiol. 2014;7:10–6.

Chopra HK, Nanda NC (editors) History of syncope. In: Textbook of cardiology: a clinical and historical perspective. 1st ed. Jaypee Brothers Medical Publishers Ltd, New Delhi, Panama City, London, Dhaka, Kathmar, 2013.

Connolly SJ, Sheldon R, Roberts RS, Gent M. The North American Vasovagal Pacemaker Study (VPS): a randomized trial of permanent cardiac pacing for the prevention of vasovagal syncope. J Am Coll Cardiol. 1999;33:16–20.

Connolly SJ, Sheldon R, Thorpe KE, et al. Pacemaker therapy for prevention of syncope in patients with recurrent severe vasovagal syncope: second Vasovagal Pacemaker Study (VPS II): a randomized trial. JAMA. 2003;289:2224–9.

Di Girolamo E, Di Iorio C, Sabatini P, et al. Effects of paroxetine hydrochloride, a selective serotonin reuptake inhibitor, on refractory vasovagal syncope: a randomized, double-blind, placebo-controlled study. J Am Coll Cardiol. 1999;33:1227–30.

Ditting T, Hilgers KF, Scrogin KE, et al. Mechanosensitive cardiac C-fiber response to changes in
left ventricular filling, coronary perfusion pressure, hemorrhage, and volume expansion in rats.
Am J Physiol Heart Circ Physiol. 2005;288:H541–52.

Freeman R, Wieling W, Axelrod FB, et al. Consensus statement on the definition of orthostatic
hypotension, neutrally mediated syncope and the postural tachycardia syndrome. Auton
Neurosci. 2011;161:46–8.

Girolamo Mercuriale – Wikipedia. https://en.wikipedia.org/wiki/Girolamo_Mercuriale.

Goldstein DS, Holmes C, Frank SM, et al. Sympathoadrenal imbalance before neurocardiogenic
syncope. Am J Cardiol. 2003;91:53–8.

Gomes JA. Neurocardiogenic syncope. In: Heart rhythm disorders: history, mechanisms, and management perspectives. Cham: Springer; 2020.

Gordon VM, Opfer-Gehrking TL, Novak V, Low PA. Hemodynamic and symptomatic effects of
acute interventions on tilt in patients with postural tachycardia syndrome. Clin Auton Res.
2000;10:29–33.

Grubb BP, Karas BJ. The potential role of serotonin in the pathogenesis of neurocardiogenic syncope and related autonomic disturbances. J Interv Card Electrophysiol. 1998;2:325–32.

Kapoor WN, Smith MA, Miller NL. Upright tilt testing in evaluating syncope: a comprehensive
literature review. Am J Med. 1994;97:78–88.

Kenny RA, Ingram A, Bayliss J, Sutton R. Head-up tilt: a useful test for investigating unexplained
syncope. Lancet. 1986;1:1352–5.

Low PA, Opfer-Gehrking TL, Textor SC, et al. Postural tachycardia syndrome (POTS). Neurology.
1995;45:S19–25.

Morillo CA, Eckberg DL, Ellenbogen KA, et al. Vagal and sympathetic mechanisms in patients
with orthostatic vasovagal syncope. Circulation. 1997;96:2509–13.

Palmisano P, Zaccaria M, Luzzi G, et al. Closed-loop cardiac pacing versus conventional dual-
chamber pacing with specialized sensing and pacing algorithms for syncope prevention
in patients with refractory vasovagal syncope: results of a long-term follow-up. Europace.
2012;14:1038–43.

Perez-Luogones A, Schweikert R, Pavia S, et al. Usefulness of midodrine in patients with
severely symptomatic neurocardiogenic syncope: a randomized control study. J Cardiovasc
Electrophysiol. 2001;12:935–8.

Porzionato A, Macchi V, Stecco C, et al. The Anatomical School of Padua. Anat Rec.
2012;295(6):902–16.

Probst MA, Kanzaria HK, Gbedemah M, et al. National trends in resource utilization associated
with ED visits for syncope. Am J Emerg Med. 2015;33:998–1001.

Raviele A, Giada F, Menozzi C, et al. A randomized, double-blind, placebo-controlled study of
permanent cardiac pacing for the treatment of recurrent tilt-induced vasovagal syncope: the
vasovagal syncope and pacing trial (SYNPACE). Eur Heart J. 2004;25:1741–8. 46.

Salim MA, Di Sessa TG. Effectiveness of fludrocortisone and salt in preventing syncope recurrence in children: a double-blind, placebo-controlled, randomized trial. J Am Coll Cardiol.
2005;45:484–8.

Schondorf R, Low PA. Idiopathic postural orthostatic tachycardia syndrome: an attenuated form of
acute pandysautonomia? Neurology. 1993;43:132–7.

Sebastian A. Dictionary of the history of medicine. Rutledge; 2018.

Sheldon RS, Grubb BP, Olshansky B, et al. 2015 Heart Rhythm Society expert consensus statement on the diagnosis and treatment of postural tachycardia syndrome, inappropriate sinus
tachycardia, and vasovagal syncope. Heart Rhythm. 2015;12:e41–63.

Sun BJ, Emond JA, Camargo CA. Direct medical costs of syncope-related hospitalizations in the
United States. Am J Cardiol. 2005;95:668–71.

Sutton R, Brignole M, Menozzi C, et al. Dual-chamber pacing in the treatment of neurally mediated tilt-positive cardioinhibitory syncope: pacemaker versus no therapy: a multicenter randomized study. Circulation. 2000;102:294–9.
Van Dijk N, Quartieri F, Blanc JJ, et al. Effectiveness of physical counterpressure maneuvers in
preventing vasovagal syncope: the Physical Counterpressure Manoeuvres Trial (PC-Trial). J
Am Coll Cardiol. 2006;48:1652–7.
Winker R, Barth A, Bidmon D, et al. Endurance exercise training in orthostatic intolerance: a randomized, controlled trial. Hypertension. 2005;45:391–8.

The Stuttering Maestro: The Sick Sinus

2018 ACC/AHA/HRS guideline on the evaluation and management of patients with bradycardia
and cardiac conduction delay. https://doi.org/10.1016/j.hrthm.2018.10.037.
Asseman P, Bergin B, Desry D, et al. Persistent sinus nodal electrograms during abnormally prolonged post-pacing atrial pauses in sick sinus syndrome in humans: sinoatrial block vs. over-
drive, suppression. Circulation. 1983;68:33–41.
Benditt DG, Benson DW Jr, Kreitt J, et al. Electrophysiologic effects of theophylline in young
patients with recurrent symptomatic bradyarrhythmias. Am J Cardiol. 1983;52:1223–9.
Desai J, Scheinman MM, Strauss HC, et al. Electrophysiologic effects of combined autonomic
blockade in patients with sick sinus syndrome. Circulation. 1981;63:953–9.
Gilette PC, Wampler DG, Shannon C, et al. Use of atrial pacing in a young population.
PACE. 1985;8:94.
Gomes JA. The sick sinus syndrome, Chapter 28. In: Heart rhythm disorders: history, mechanisms,
and management perspectives. Cham: Springer; 2020.
Gomes JA. The sick sinus syndrome and evaluation of the patient with sinus node disorders. In:
Parmley C, et al., editors. Cardiology. Philadelphia: JP Lipincort; 1987.
Gomes JA, Winters SL. The origins of the sinus node pacemaker complex in man: demonstration
of dominant and subsidiary foci. J Am Coll Cardiol. 1987;9:45–52.
Gomes JAC, Kang PS, El-Sherif N. The sinus node electrogram in patients with and without
sick sinus syndrome: techniques and correlation between directly measured and indirectly esti-
mated sinoatrial conduction time. Circulation. 1982;66:864–73.
Gomes JAC, Hariman RI, Chowdry IA. New application of direct sinus node recordings in man:
assessment of sinus node recovery time. Circulation. 1983;70:663–71.
Hudson REB. The human pacemaker and its pathology. Br Heart J. 1960;22:153–67.
Irene Ferrer M. The sick sinus syndrome. Circulation. 1973;47:635–41.
Jordan JL, Yamaguchi I, Mandel WJ. Studies on the mechanism of sinus node dysfunction in the
sick sinus syndrome. Circulation. 1977;57:217–23.
Kang PS, Gomes JAC, et al. Role of autonomic regulatory mechanism on sinoatrial conduction and
sinus node automaticity in sick sinus syndrome. Circulation. 1981;64:832–8.
Kang PS, Gomes JAC, et al. Differential effects of functional autonomic blockade on the variables
of sinus node automaticity in sick sinus syndrome. Am J Cardiol. 1982;49:273–82.
Lown B. Electrical reversion of cardiac arrhythmias. Br Heart J. 1967;29:469–89.

Of Disconnected Highways: Heart Blocks

Aste M, Brinole M. Syncope and paroxysmal atrioventricular block. J Arrhythm. 2017;33:562–7.
Cantwell JD. Profiles in cardiology: William stokes (1804-1878). Clin Cardiol. 1988;11(2):856–8.

Damato AN, et al. A study of heart block in man using His bundle recordings. Circulation. 1969;39:297–305.

Demoulin JC, Kulbertus HE. Left hemiblocks revisited from the histopathological view point. Am Heart J. 1973;86:712–3.

European Society of Cardiology (ESC), European Heart Rhythm Association (EHRA), Brignole M, et al. 2013 ESC guidelines on cardiac pacing and cardiac resynchronization therapy: the task force on cardiac pacing and resynchronization therapy of the European Society of Cardiology (ESC). Developed in collaboration with the European Heart Rhythm Association (EHRA). Europace. 2013;15:1070–118.

Gomes JAC, Damato AN. His bundle electrocardiograph and intracardiac stimulation in the evaluation of patients with atrioventricular conduction defects and sick sinus syndrome. In: Varialle P, editor. Cardiac pacing. Lea and Febiger; 1979. p. 97–122.

Gomes JAC, El-Sherif N. His bundle recordings: contributions to clinical electrophysiology. In: Samet P, El-Sherif N, editors. Cardiac pacing. Grune and Stratton; 1979. p. 375–407.

Gomes JAC, El-Sherif N. Atrioventricular block: mechanism, clinical presentation and therapy. Medical Clinics of North America Cardiac Arrhythmias I. 1984;68:955–67.

Haft JI, Weinstock M, De Guia R. Electrophysiologic studies in Mobitz type II second degree heart block. Am J Cardiol. 1971;27:682–8.

Hindman MC, Wagner GS, JaRo M, et al. The clinical significance of bundle branch block complicating acute myocardial infarction 1: clinical characteristics; hospital mortality and one year follow-up. Circulation. 1978;58:679–88.

Kelly DT, Brodsky SJ, Mirowski M, Krovetz LJ, Rowe RD. Bundle of His recordings in congenital complete heart block. Circulation. 1972;46:277–81.

Kusumoto FM, Schoenfeld MH, Barrett C, et al. 2018 ACC/AHA/HRS guideline on the evaluation and management of patients with bradycardia and cardiac conduction delay. Circulation. 2019;140:e382–482. https://doi.org/10.1016/j.hrthm.2018.10.037.

Lasser RP, Haft JI, Friedberg CK. Relationship of right bundle branch block and and marked left axis duration (with left parietal peri-infarction block) to complete heart block and syncope. Circulation. 1968;37:429–37.

Lau SH, Damato AN. Mechanism of AV Blocks. Cardiovasc Clin. 1970;2:50.

Mobitz W. Über die unvollständige Störung der Erregungsüberleitung zwischen Vorhof und Kammer des menschlichen Herzens [on the partial block of impulse conduction between atrium and ventricle of human hearts]. Z Gesamte Exp Med. 1924;41:180–237.

Narula OS, Samet P. Wenckebach and Mobitz II A-V Block due to block within the His bundle and bundle branches. Circulation. 1970;41:947–65.

O'Brien ET. Dublin masters of clinical expression II: Robert Adams (1791-1875). Journal of the Irish Colleges of Physicians and Surgeons. 1974;3(4):127–9.

Pérez-Riera AR, Femenía F, McIntyre WF, Baranchuk A. Karel Frederick Wenckebach (1864–1940): a giant of medicine. Cardiol J. 2011;18(3):337–9.

Rosen KM, et al. Site of block in acute myocardial infarction. Circulation. 1970;42:925–33.

Rosenbaum MB, Elizari MV, Lazzari JO. The Hemiblocks. Tampa: Tracings; 1970.

Scheinman MM, Peters RW, Modin G, et al. Prognostic value of infranodal conduction time in patients with chronic bundle branch block. Circulation. 1977;56:240–4.

Silverman ME, Upshaw CB Jr, Lange HW. Woldemar Mobitz and His 1924 classification of second-degree atrioventricular block. Circulation. 2004;110:1162–7.

Tawara S. Die topographie und histologie der bruckenfaser: ein beitrag zur lehre vonder bedeutung der Purkinjeschen faden. Zantralbl Physiol. 1906;19:70–9.

Tawara S. Das Reizleitungssystem des Saeugetierherzens Eine anatomisch-histologische Studie uber das Atrioventrikularbundel und die Purkinjeschen Faden. Jena: Verslag Gustav Fischer; 1906. pp. 35–201.

The Artificial Pacemaker: A Life-Giver

Abbasi AS, Eber LM, MacAlpin RN, et al. Paradoxical motion of the interventricular septum in left bundle branch block. Circulation. 1974;49:423–7.

Abraham WT, Fisher WG, Smith AL, et al. Cardiac resynchronization in chronic heart failure. N Engl J Med. 2002;346(24):1845–53.

Aquilina O. A brief history of cardiac pacing. Images Pediatr Cardiol. 2006;8(2):1–29.

Arnold AD, Shun-Shin MJ, Keene D, et al. His resynchronization versus biventricular pacing in patients with heart failure and left bundle branch block. J Am Coll Cardiol. 2018;72:3112–22.

Auricchio A, Prinzen FW. Non-responders to cardiac resynchronization therapy:the magnitude of the problem and the issues. Circ J. 2011;75:521–7.

Auricchio A, Klein H, Tockman B, et al. Transvenous biventricular pacing for heart failure: can the obstacles be overcome? Am J Cardiol. 1999;83:136D–42D.

Auricchio A, Ding J, Spinelli JC, et al. Cardiac resynchronization therapy restores optimal atrio-ventricular mechanical timing in heart failure patients with ventricular conduction delay. J Am Coll Cardiol. 2002;39:1163–9.

Auricchio A, Delnoy PP, Regoli F, et al., for the Collaborative Study Group. First-in-man implantation of leadless ultrasound-based cardiac stimulation pacing system: novel endocardial left ventricular resynchronization therapy in heart failure patients. Europace 2013;15:1191–7.

Bakker PFA. Cardiac stimulation as nonpharmalogical treatment for heart failure. In: Van Hemel NM, Wittkampf FHM, Ector H, editors. The pacemaker clinic of the 90's. Dordrecht: Kluwer Academic Publishers; 1995. p. 185–97.

Bowers DL. New pacemaker devices from a technical point of view. In: HJT T, Harthorne JW, editors. To pace or not to pace: controversial subjects in cardiac pacing. The Hague: M. Nijhoff; 1978. p. 126–30.

Bracke FA, van Gelder BM, Dekker LRC, et al. Left ventricular endocardial pacing in cardiac resynchronisation therapy: moving from bench to bedside. Neth Heart J. 2012;20:118–24.

Bui AL, Horwich TB, Fonarow GC. Epidemiology and risk profile of heart failure Nat rev Cardiol. Jan. 2011;8(1):30–41.

Cazeau S, Ritter P, Bakdach S, et al. Four chamber pacing in dilated cardiomyopathy. Pacing Clin Electrophysiol. 1994;17:1974–9.

Cazeau S, Leclercq C, Lavergne T, et al. Effects of multisite biventricular pacing in patients with heart failure and intraventricular conduction delay. N Engl J Med. 2001;344(12):873–80.

Chardack WM. Recollections 1958–1961. PACE. 1981;4:592–6.

Chardack WM, Gage AA, Greatbatch W. A transistorized, self-contained, implantable pacemaker for the long-term correction of complete heart block. Surgery. 1960;48:643–54.

Clark AL, Godde K, Cleland JGE. The prevalence and incidence of left bundle branch block in ambulant patients with chronic heart failure. Eur J Heart Fail. 2008;10:696–702.

Daubert JC, Ritter P, Le Breton H, et al. Permanent left ventricular pacing with transvenous leads inserted into the coronary veins. Pacing Clin Electrophysiol. 1998;21:239–45.

Daubert C, Behar N, Martins RP, Mabo P, Leclercq C. Avoiding non-responders to cardiac resynchronization therapy: a practical guide. Eur Heart J. 2017;38:1463–72.

Deshmukh P, Casavant DA, Romanyshyn M, Anderson K. Permanent, direct His-Bundle pacing. Circulation. 2000;101:869–77.

Doll N, Opfermann UT, Rastan AJ, et al. Facilitated minimally invasive left ventricular epicardial lead placement. Ann Thorac Surg. 2005;79:1023–5.

Ellenbogen KA, Wilkoff BL, Kay GN. Clinical cardiac pacing, defibrillation and resynchronization therapy. Philadelphia: WB Saunders Company; 2000.

Ellenbogen KA, Hellkamp AS, Wilkoff BL, et al. Complications arising after implantation of DDD pacemakers: the MOST experience. Am J Cardiol. 2003;92:740–1.

El-Sherif N, Amat-Y-Leon P, Schoenfield C, et al. Normalization of bundle branch block patterns by distal His bundle pacing. Clinical and experimental evidence of longitudinal dissociation in the pathologic His bundle. Circulation. 1978;57:473.

Epstein AE, DiMarco JP, Ellenbogen KA, et al. ACC/AHA/HRS 2008 guidelines for device-based therapy of cardiac rhythm abnormalities: a report of the American College of Cardiology/American Heart Association Task Force on Practice Guidelines (writing committee to revise the ACC/AHA/ NASPE 2002 guideline update for implantation of cardiac pacemakers and antiarrhythmia devices). Circulation. 2008;117:e350–408.

Epstein AE, DiMarco JP, Ellenbogen KA, et al. 2012 ACCF/AHA/HRS focused update incorporated into the ACCF/AHA/HRS 2008 guidelines for device-based therapy of cardiac rhythm abnormalities. J Am Coll Cardiol. 2013;61(3):e6–e75.

Furman S. Recollections of the beginning of transvenous cardiac pacing. PACE. 1994;17:1697–705.

Gabor S, Prenner G, Wasler A, et al. A simplified technique for implantation of left ventricular epicardial leads for biventricular resynchronisation using video-assisted thoracoscopy (VATS). Eur J Cardio Thorac Surg. 2005;28:797–800.

Gomes JA. The artificial pacemaker: a historical overview, Chapter 31. In: Heart rhythm disorders: history, mechanisms, and management perspectives. Cham: Springer; 2020.

Gomes JAC, Damato AN, Akhtar M, et al. Ventricular septal motion and LV dimensions during abnormal ventricular activation. Am J Cardiol. 1977;30:641–7.

Gott VL. C. Walton Lillehei (1918-1999). J Thorac Cardiovasc Surg. 1999;118(4):774–5.

Greatbatch W. Achieving reliable pacemakers. In: Watanabe Y, editor. Proceedings of the Vth international symposium, Tokyo, March 14–18, 1976. Amsterdam: Excerpta Medica; 1977. p. 364–8.

Greatbatch W. Interview. In: Brown KA, editor. Inventors at work. Redmond: Tempus Books; 1988. p. 19–44.

Jaïs P, Douard H, Shah DC, et al. Endocardial biventricular pacing. Pacing Clin Electrophysiol. 1998;21:2128–31.

Kirkfeldt RE, Johansen JB, Nohr EA, et al. Pneumothorax in cardiac pacing: a population-based cohort study of 28,860 Danish patients. Europace. 2012;14:1132–8.

Kirkfeldt RE, Johansen JB, Nohr EA, et al. Complications after cardiac implantable electronic device implantations: an analysis of a complete, nationwide cohort in Denmark. Eur Heart J. 2014;35:1186–94. https://doi.org/10.1093/eurheartj/eht511.

Knops RE, Tjong FV, Neuzil P, et al. Chronic performance of a leadless cardiac pacemaker: 1-year follow-up of the LEADLESS trial. J Am Coll Cardiol. 2015;65:1497–504.

Leclercq C, Gras D, Le Helloco A, et al. Hemodynamic importance of preserving the normal sequence of ventricular activation in permanent cardiac pacing. Am Heart J. 1995;129:1133–41.

Leclercq F, Hager FX, Macia JC, et al. Left ventricular lead insertion using a modified transseptal catheterization technique: a totally endocardial approach for permanent biventricular pacing in end-stage heart failure. Pacing Clin Electrophysiol. 1999;22:1570–5.

Levy D, et al. Long-term trends in the incidence of and survival with heart failure. N Engl J Med. 2002;347:1397–402. [PubMed: 12409541].

Leyva F, Nisam S, Auricchio A. 20 Years of cardiac resynchronization therapy. J Am Coll Cardiol. 2014;44(5):1047–58.

Liu WH, Chen MC, Chen YL, et al. Right ventricular apical pacing acutely impairs left ventricular function and induces mechanical dyssynchrony in patients with sick sinus syndrome: a real-time three-dimensional echocardiographic study. J Am Soc Echocardiogr. 2008;21:224–9.

Loyd-Jones D, et al. Heart disease and stroke statistics—2010 update: a report from the American Heart Association. Circulation. 2010;121:e46–e215. [PubMed: 20019324].

Lustgarten DL, Calame S, Crespo EM, et al. Electrical resynchronization induced by direct His-bundle pacing. Heart Rhythm. 2010;7:15–21.

Lustgarten DL, Crespo EM, Arkhipova-Jenkins I. His-bundle pacing versus biventricular pacing in cardiac resynchronization therapy patients: a crossover design comparison. Heart Rhythm. 2015;12:1548–57.

McDonald IG. Echocardiographic demonstration of abnormal motion of the interventricular septum in left bundle branch block. Circulation. 1973;48:272–80.

McMurray JJ, Petrie MC, Murdoch DR, Davie AP. Clinical epidemiology of heart failure: public and private health burden. Eur Heart J. 1998;19(Suppl P):P9–P16. [PubMed: 9886707].

Mihalcz A, Kassai I, Geller L, et al. Alternative techniques for left ventricular pacing in cardiac resynchronization therapy. Pacing Clin Electrophysiol. 2014;37:255–61.

Moss AJ, Hall WJ, Cannom DS, et al., for the MADIT-CRT Trial Investigators. Cardiac-resynchronization therapy for the prevention of heart-failure events. N Engl J Med. 2009;361:1329–38.

Narula OS. Longitudinal dissociation in the His bundle. Bundle branch block due to asynchronous conduction within the His bundle in man. Circulation. 1977;56:996.

Oral-History: Wilson Greatbatch – engineering and technology history ... https://ethw.org/Oral-History:Wilson_Greatbatch.

Reddy VY, Knops RE, Sperzel J, et al. Permanent leadless cardiac pacing: results of the LEADLESS trial. Circulation. 2014;129:1466–71.

Reddy VY, Exner DV, Cantillon DJ, et al. LEADLESS II Study Investigators. Percutaneous implantation of an entirely intracardiac leadless pacemaker. N Engl J Med. 2015;373:1125–35.

Reddy VY, Miller MA, Neuzil P, et al. Cardiac resynchronization therapy with wireless left ventricular endocardial pacing the SELECT-LV study. JACC. 2017;69(17):2119–29.

Reynolds D, Duray GZ, Omar R, et al. Micra Transcatheter Pacing Study Group. A leadless intracardiac transcatheter pacing system. N Engl J Med. 2016;374:533–41.

Savarese G, Lund LH. Public health burden of heart failure. Card Fall Rev. 2017;3(1):7–11.

Schechter DC. Background of clinical cardiac electrostimulation. V. Direct electrostimulation of heart without thoracotomy. N Y State J Med. 1972;72:605–19.

Schneider AA, Tepper F. The lithium-iodine cell. In: Thalen HJT, Harthorne JW, editors. To pace or not to pace: controversial subjects in cardiac pacing. The Hague: M. Nijhoff; 1978. p. 116–21.

Senning Å. Cardiac pacing in retrospect. Am J Surg. 1983;145:733–9.

Spickler JW, Rasor NS, Kezdi P, et al. Totally self-contained intracardiac pacemaker. J Electrocardiol. 1970;3:325–31.

Tofield A. Earl E Bakken and Medtronic. https://academic.oup.com/eurheartj/article-pdf/39/22/2029/25015813/ehy258.pdf.

Tops LF, Schalij MJ, Bax JJ. The effects of right ventricular apical pacing on ventricular function and dyssynchrony implications for therapy. J Am Coll Cardiol. 2009;54:764–76.

Udo EO, Zuithoff NP, van Hemel NM, et al. Incidence and predictors of short and long-term complications in pacemaker therapy: the FOLLOWPACE study. Heart Rhythm. 2012;9:728–35. https://doi.org/10.1016/j.hrthm.2011.12.014.

Wieneke H, Konorza T, Erbel R, Kisker E. Leadless pacing of the heart using induction technology: a feasibility study. Pacing Clin Electrophysiol. 2009;32:177–83.

Zhang W, Huang J, Qi Y, et al. Cardiac resynchronization therapy by left bundle branch area pacing in heart failure patients with left bundle branch block. Heart Rhythm 2019;-:1–8 pii: S1547-5271(19)30827-6. https://doi.org/10.1016/j.hrthm.2019.09.006.

Zoll PM. Resuscitation of the heart in ventricular standstill by external electric stimulation. N Engl J Med. 1952;247:768–71.

When All Is Said and Done: Waiting for a Heart Transplant

Barnard CN. The operation. A human cardiac transplant: an interim report of a successful operation performed at Groote Schuur Hospital, Cape Town. S Afr Med J. 1967;41(48):1271–4.

Borel, Kis ZL, Beveridge T. The history of the discovery and development of cyclosporine. In: Merluzzi VJ, Adams J, editors. The search for anti-inflamatory drugs. Boston: Birkhauser Boston; 1995.

Carrel A, Guthrie CC. The transplantation of veins and organs. Am Med. 1905;10:1101–2.

Hunt SA, Haddad F. The changing face of heart transplantation. J Am Coll Cardiol. 2008;52(8):587–98.

Kantrowitz A, Haller JD, Joos H, Cerruti MM, Carstensen HE. Transplantation of the heart in an infant and an adult. Am J Cardiol. 1968;22(6):782–90.

Lund LH, Edwards LB, Kucheryavaya AY, et al. The registry of the International Society for Heart and Lung Transplantation: thirty-first official adult heart transplant report--2014; focus theme: retransplantation. J Heart Lung Transplant. 2014;33:996–1008.

Markus J. Wilhelm. Long-term outcome following heart transplantation: current perspective. Thorac Dis. 2015;7(3):549–51.

Najarian JS, Simmons RL. Transplantation. Philadelphia: Lea & Febiger; 1972. 797p.

Schmitto JD, Hanke JS, Rojas SV, Avsar M, Haverich A. First implantation in man of a new magnetically levitated left ventricular assist device (HeartMate III). J Heart Lung Transplant. https://doi.org/10.1016/j.healun.2015.03.001.

Stolf NAG. History of heart transplantation: a hard and glorious journey. Braz J Cardiovasc Surg. 2017;32(5):423–7.

Of Bypasses and Clot Busters

Ambrose JA, Tannenbaum MA, Alexopoulos D, Hjemdahl-Monsen CE, Leavy J, Weiss M, Borrico S, Gorlin R, Fuster V. Angiographic progression of coronary artery disease and the development of myocardial infarction. J Am Coll Cardiol. 1988;12:56–62.

Antman EM, Anbe DT, Armstrong PW, et al. ACC/AHA guidelines for the management of patients with ST-elevation myocardial infarction: executive summary: a report of the ACC/AHA Task Force on Practice Guidelines (committee to revise the 1999 guidelines on the management of patients with acute myocardial infarction). Circulation. 2004;110:588–636.

Califf RM, White HD, Van de Werf F, Sadowski Z, Armstrong PW, Vahanian A, Simoons ML, Simes RJ, Lee KL, Topol EJ. One-year results from the global utilization of streptokinase and TPA for occluded coronary arteries (GUSTO-I) trial. Circulation. 1996;94:1233–8.

Chaikhouni A. The magnificent century of cardiothoracic surgery. Heart Views. 2010;11(1):31–7.

Collen D, Lijnen HR. The tissue-type plasminogen activator story. Arterioscler Thromb Vasc Biol. 2009;29:1151–5.

Davies M, Woolf N, Robertson WB. Pathology of acute myocardial infarction with particular reference to occlusive coronary thrombi. Br Heart J. 1976;38:659–64.

DeWood MA, Spores J, Notske R, et al. Prevalence of total coronary occlusion during the early hours of transmural myocardial infarction. N Engl J Med. 1980;303:897–902.

Favaloro RG. Landmarks in the development of coronary artery bypass surgery. Circulation. 1998;98:466–78.

Fuster V, Lewis A. Conner Memorial Lecture. Mechanisms leading to myocardial infarction: insights from studies of vascular biology. Circulation. 1994;90:2126–46.

GISSI-2: a factorial randomised trial of alteplase versus streptokinase and heparin versus no heparin among 12,490 patients with acute myocardial infarction. Gruppo Italiano per lo Studio della Sopravvivenza nell'Infarto Miocardico. Lancet. 1990;336(8707):65–71.

Green G, Stertzer SH, Reppert EH. Coronary arterial bypass grafts. Ann Thorac Surg. 1968;5:443–50.

Green GE, Spencer FC, Tice DA, Stertzer SH. Arterial and venous microsurgical bypass grafts for coronary artery disease. J Thorac Cardiovasc Surg. 1970;60:491.

Hartzler GO. Electrode catheter ablation of refractory focal ventricular tachycardia. JACC. 1983;2(6):1107–13.

Hartzler GO, Rutherford BD, McConahay DR. Percutaneous transluminal coronary angioplasty: application for acute myocardial infarction. Am J Cardiol. 1984;53:117C–21C.

Hillis LD, Borer J, Braunwald E, et al. High dose intravenous streptokinase for acute myocardial infarction: preliminary results of a multicenter trial. J Am Coll Cardiol. 1985;6:957–62.

ISIS-3: a randomised comparison of streptokinase vs tissue plasminogen activator vs anistreplase and of aspirin plus heparin vs aspirin alone among 41,299 cases of suspected acute myocardial infarction. ISIS-3 (Third International Study of Infarct Survival) Collaborative Group. Lancet. 1992; 28;339(8796):753–70.

Kolesov VI. Mammary artery-coronary artery anastomosis as method of treatment for angina pectoris. J Thorac Cardiovasc Surg. 1967;45:535–44.

Lawrence S, Tillett WS. The National Academy of Sciences. Biograph Memoirs. 1993;62:383–403.

Lee TC, Laramee LA, Rutherford BD, et al. Emergency percutaneous transluminal coronary angioplasty for acute myocardial infarction in patients 70 years of age and older. Am J Cardiol. 1990;66:663–7.

Magid DJ, Calonge BN, Rumsfeld JS, et al., for the National Registry of Myocardial Infarction 2 and 3 Investigators. Relation between hospital primary angioplasty volume and mortality for patients with acute MI treated with primary angioplasty vs thrombolytic therapy. JAMA. 2000; 284:3131–8.

Ribeiro EE, Silva LA, Carneiro R, et al. Randomized trial of direct coronary angioplasty versus intravenous streptokinase in acute myo- cardial infarction. J Am Coll Cardiol. 1993;22:376–80.

Rovelli F, De Vita C, Feruglio GA, Lotto A, Selvini A, Tognoni G. GISSI trial: early results and late follow-up. Gruppo Italiano per la Sperimentazione della Streptochinasi nell'Infarto Miocardico. J Am Coll Cardiol. 1987;10(5 Suppl B):33B–9B.

Ruegsegger P, Nydick I, Hutter RC, Freiman AH, Bang NU, Cliffton EE, Ladue JS. Fibrinolytic (plasmin) therapy of experimental coronary thrombi with alteration of the evolution of myocardial infarction. Circulation. 1959;19:7–13.

Sikri N, Bardia A. A history of streptokinase use in acute myocardial infarction. Tex Heart Inst J. 2007;34(3):319–27.

Simoons ML, Serruys PW, vd Brand M, et al. Improved survival after early thrombolysis in acute myocardial infarction. A randomised trial by the Interuniversity Cardiology Institute in The Netherlands. Lancet. 1985;2:578–82.

Stefanadis C, Antoniou C-K, Tsiachris D, Pietri P. Coronary atherosclerotic vulnerable plaque: current perspectives. J Am Heart Assoc. 2017;6(3):e005543.

Streptokinase in acute myocardial infarction — European Cooperative Study Group for Streptokinase Treatment in Acute Myocardial Infarction. N Engl J Med. 1979; 301:797–802.

Vineberg AM. Development of an anastomosis between the coronary vessels and a transplanted internal mammary artery. Can Med Assoc J. 1946;55:117.

Widimsky P, Groch L, Zelízko M, et al. Multicentre randomized trial comparing transport to primary angioplasty vs immediate thrombolysis vs combined strategy for patients with acute myocardial infarction presenting to a community hospital without a catheterization laboratory: the PRAGUE study. Eur Heart J. 2000;21:823–31.

Zijlstra F, de Boer MJ, Hoorntje JC, et al. A comparison of immediate coronary angioplasty with intravenous streptokinase in acute myocardial infarction. N Engl J Med. 1993;328:680–4.

Zijlstra F, Beukema WP, van't Hof AW, et al. Randomized comparison of primary coronary angioplasty with thrombolytic therapy in low risk patients with acute myocardial infarction. J Am Coll Cardiol. 1997;29:908–12.

A Riveting New Era: The Birth of Interventional Cardiology

Anderson HV, Roubin GS, Leimgruber PP, Douglas JS, King SB, Gruentzig AR. Primary angiographic success rates of percutaneous transluminal coronary angioplasty. Am J Cardiol. 1985;56:712–7.

Aronov DM, Lupanov VP. COURAGE study results: disappointing or encouraging? Cardiovascular Therapy and Prevention. 2007;7(7):95–104.

Bredlau C, Roubin GS, Leimgruber PP, Douglas JS, King SB, Gruentzig AR. In-hospital morbidity and mortality in elective coronary angioplasty. Circulation. 1985;72:1044–52.

CABRI Trial Participants. First-year results of CABRI (Coronary Angioplasty vs Bypass Revascularisation Investigation). Lancet. 1995; 346:1179–1184.

Dangas GD, Farkouh ME, Sleeper LA, Yang M, et al., for the FREEDOM Investigators. Long-term outcome of PCI versus CABG in insulin and non–insulin-treated diabetic patients: results from the FREEDOM trial. Am Coll Cardiol. 2014;64(12):1189–97.

Douglas JS, Gruentzig AR, King SB, Hollman J, et al. Percutaneous transluminal coronary angioplasty in patients with prior coronary bypass surgery. J Am Coll Cardiol. 1983;2:745–54.

Faxon DP, Sanborn TA, Haudenschild CC. Mechanism of angioplasty and its relation to restenosis. Am J Cardiol. 1987;60(3):5B–9B.

Fischman DL, Leon MB, Baim DS. A randomized comparison of coronary-stent placement and balloon angioplasty in the treatment of coronary artery disease. N Engl J Med. 1994;331:496–501.

Fischman DL, Leon MB, Baim DS, Schatz RA, Savage MP, Penn I, Detre K, Veltri L, Ricci D, Nobuyoshi M, Cleman M, Heuser R, Almond D, Teirstein PS, Fish RD, Colombo A, Brinker J, Moses J, Shaknovich A, Hirshfeld J, Bailey S, Ellis S, Rake R, Goldberg S, for the Stent Restenosis Study Investigators. A randomized comparison of coronary-stent placement and balloon angioplasty in the treatment of coronary artery disease. N Engl J Med. 1994;331:496–501.

Goy J-J, Eeckhout E, Burnand B, Vogt P, Stauffer JC, Hurni M, Stumpe F, Ruchat P, Sadeghi H, Kappenberger L. Coronary angioplasty versus left internal mammary grafting for isolated proximal left anterior descending artery stenosis. Lancet. 1994;343:1449–53.

Gruentzig A, Turina M, Schneider J. Experimental percutaneous dilatation of coronary artery stenosis. Circulation. 1976;54:81. Abstract.

Gruentzig A, Myler R, Hanna R, Turina M. Coronary transluminal angioplasty. Circulation. 1977;56:84. Abstract.

Gruentzig A, Senning A, Siegenthaler W. Nonoperative dilatation of coronary artery stenosis: percutaneous transluminal coronary angioplasty (PTCA). N Engl J Med. 1979;301:61–8. CrossrefMedlineGoogle Scholar.

Grüntzig A. Transluminal dilatation of coronary artery stenosis. Lancet. 1978;1:263. Letters. CrossrefMedlineGoogle Scholar.

Hamid H, Coltart J. 'Miracle stents' – a future without restenosis. Mcgill J Med. 2007;10(2):105–11.

Hartzler GO, Rutherford BD, McConahay DR, McCallister SH. Simultaneous multiple lesion coronary angioplasty: a preferred therapy for patients with multiple vessel disease. Circulation. 1982;16(suppl II):II-5. Abstract.

Hollman J, Gruentzig AR, Douglas JS, King SB, Ischinger T, Meier B. Acute occlusion after percutaneous transluminal coronary angioplasty: a new approach. Circulation. 1983;68:725–35.

Hueb WA, Bellotti G, de Oliveira SA, Arie S, de Albuquerque CP, Jatene AD, Pileggi F. The Medicine, Angioplasty or Surgery Study (MASS): a prospective, randomized trial of medical therapy, balloon angioplasty or bypass surgery for single proximal left anterior descending artery stenoses. J Am Coll Cardiol. 1995;26:1600–5.

King SB 3rd. The development of interventional cardiology. J Am Coll Cardiol. 1998;31(4 Suppl B):64B–88B.

King SB III, Lembo NJ, Weintraub WS, Kosinski AS, et al, for the Emory Angioplasty versus Surgery Trial (EAST). A randomized trial comparing coronary angioplasty with coronary bypass surgery. N Engl J Med.1994; 331:1044–50.

Leimgruber PP, Roubin GS, Anderson HV, Bredlau C, Whitworth H, Douglas JS, King SB, Gruentzig AR. Influence of intimal dissection on restenosis after successful angioplasty. Circulation. 1985;72:530–5.

Leimgruber P, Roubin GS, Hollman J, Cotsonis GA, Meier B, Douglas JS, King SB, Gruentzig AR. Restenosis after successful coronary angioplasty in patients with single-vessel disease. Circulation. 1986;73:712–7.

Lev EI, Kornowski R, Vaknin-Assa H, et al. Comparison of the predictive value of four different risk scores for outcomes of patients with ST-elevation acute myocardial infarction undergoing primary percutaneous coronary intervention. Am J Cardiol. 2008;102:6–11.

Levy RI, Mock MB, William VL, Frommer PL. Percutaneous transluminal coronary angioplasty. N Engl J Med. 1979;301:101–3. Editorial.

Maron DJ, Hochman JS, Reynolds HR, Bangalore S, et al., for the ISCHEMIA Research Group. N Engl J Med. 2020;382:1395–407.

Meier B, King SB, Gruentzig AR, Douglas JS, Hollman J, Ischinger T, Galan K, Tankersley R. Repeat coronary angioplasty. J Am Coll Cardiol. 1984;4:463–6.

Meyer J, Merx W, Schmitz H, Erbel R, Kiesslich T, et al. Percutaneous transluminal coronary angioplasty immediately after intracoronary streptolysis of transmural myocardial infarction. Circulation. 1982;66:905–13.

Moses JW, Leon MB, Popma JJ, et al. Sirolimus-eluting stents versus standard stents in patients with stenosis in a native coronary artery. N Engl J Med. 2003;349:1315–23.

Proceedings of the National Heart, Lung, and Blood Institute Workshop on the Outcome of Percutaneous Transluminal Coronary Angioplasty. Am J Cardiol. 1984;53(special issue):1C–146C.

Puel J, Joffre F, Rousseau H, et al. Endo-protheses coronariennes autoexpansives dans la pre ́vention des reste ́noses apre's angioplastie transluminale. Arch Mal Coeur. 1987;8:1311–2.

Puel J, Karouny E, Marco F, Assoun B, Galinier M, Elbaz M, Alibelli MJ, Bounhoure JP. Angioplasty versus surgery in multivessel disease: immediate results and in-hospital outcome in a randomized prospective study. Circulation. 1992;86(suppl I):I-372. Abstract.

Rodriguez A, Boullon F, Perez-Balino N, Paviotti C, Liprandi MIS, Palacios I, on behalf of the ERACI Group. Argentine randomized trial of percutaneous transluminal coronary angioplasty versus coronary artery bypass surgery in multivessel disease (ERACI): in-hospital results and 1-year follow-up. J Am Coll Cardiol. 1993; 22:1060–7.

Roguin A. Stent: the man and word behind the coronary metal prosthesis. Circ Cardiovasc Interv. 2011;4:206–9.

Savage MP, Douglas JS Jr, Fischman DL, et al. Stent placement compared with balloon angioplasty for obstructed coronary bypass grafts. N Engl J Med. 1997;337:740–7.

Sedlis SP, Jurkovitz CT, Hartigan PM, Goldfarb DS, Lorin JD, Dada M, Maron DJ, Spertus JA, Mancini GBJ, Teo KK, O'Rourke RA, Boden WE, Weintraub WS, for the COURAGE Study Investigators. Optimal medical therapy with or without percutaneous coronary intervention for patients with stable coronary artery disease and chronic kidney disease. Am J Cardiol. 2009;104(12):1647–53.

Serruys PW, Rutsch W, Heyndrickx G, Danchin N, Mast G, Wijns W, Rensing BJ, for the CARPORT Study Group. Effect of long term thromboxane A2 receptor blockade on angiographic restenosis and clinical events after coronary angioplasty: the CARPORT study. J Am Coll Cardiol. 1991;17:283.

Serruys PW, de Jaegere P, Kiemeneij F, Macaya C, Rutsch W, Heyndrickx G, Emanuelsson H, Marco J, Legrand V, Materne P, Belardi J, Sigwart U, Colombo A, Goy JJ, van den Heuvel P, Delcan J, Morel M-A, for the BENESTENT Study Group. A comparison of balloon-expandable-stent implantation with balloon angioplasty in patients with coronary artery disease. N Engl J Med. 1994;331:489–95.

Serruys PW, Kutryk MJB, Ong ATL. Coronary-artery stents. N Engl J Med. 2006;354:483–95.

Sigwart U, Puel J, Mirkovitch V, Joffre F, Kappenberger L. Intravascular stents to prevent occlusion and restenosis after transluminal angioplasty. N Engl J Med. 1987;316:701–6.

Steg PG, James SK, Atar D, et al. ESC guidelines for the management of acute myocardial infarction in patients presenting with ST-segment elevation. Eur Heart J. 2012;33:2569–619.

The EPIC Investigators. Use of a monoclonal antibody directed against the platelet glycoprotein IIb/IIIa receptor in high-risk coronary angioplasty. N Engl J Med. 1994;330:956–61.

A Family Affair

Bagnall RD, et al. A prospective study of sudden cardiac death among children and young adults. N Engl J Med. 2016;374:2441–52.

Chan PS, McNally B, et al. Recent trends in survival from out-of-hospital cardiac arrest in the United States. Circulation. 2014;130:1876–82.

Cruising through Complications of a Heart Attack

Gorenek B, Lundqvist CB, Terradellas JB, et al. Cardiac arrhythmias in acute coronary syndromes: position paper from the joint EHRA, ACCA, and EAPCI task force. Europace. 2014;16:1655–73.

Heikki V, Huikuri MJ, Raatikainen P, Moerch-Joergensen R, et al. Prediction of fatal or near-fatal cardiac arrhythmia events in patients with depressed left ventricular function after an acute myocardial infarction. Eur Heart J. 2009;30(6):689–698.102.

A Missed Diagnosis: A Lifetime of Endurance

Churg J, Strauss L. Allergic granulomatosis, allergic angiitis, and periarteritis nodosa. Am J Pathol. 1951;27(2):277–301.

Ghosh S, Bhattacharya M, Dhar S. Churg–Strauss syndrome. Indian J Dermatol. 2011;56(6):718–21.

Kozak M, Gill EA, Green LS. Churg-Strauss syndrome. A case report with Angiographically documented coronary involvement and a review of the literature. Chest. 1995;107(2):578–80.

Old Age: How Long Should We Hope to Live?

Bruce Grierson. What if age is nothing but a mind-set?. https://www.nytimes.com/2014/10/26/magazine/what-if-age-is-nothing-but-a-mind-set.html.

Crimmins EM, Beltrán-Sánchez H. Mortality and morbidity trends: is there compression of morbidity. J Gerontol Soc Sci. 66B(1):75–86.

Ernest M. Gruenberg: the failures of success. The Milbank Quaterly. 2005;83(4):779–800.

Seeman TE, Merkin SS, Crimmins EM, Karlamangla AS. Disability trends among older Americans: National Health and Nutrition Examination Surveys, 1988–1994 and 1999–2004. Am J Public Health. 2010;100(1):100–7.

Some Heart Care Advice to Live By

Goldberger JJ, Basu A, Boineau R, Buxton AE, et al. Risk stratification for sudden cardiac death. A plan for the future. Circulation. 2014;129(4):516–26.

Išgum I, Rutten A, Prokop M, van Ginneken B. Detection of coronary calcifications from computed tomography scans for automated risk assessment of coronary artery disease. Med Phys. 2007;34(4):1450–61.

Linton MRF, Fazio S. A practical approach to risk assessment to prevent coronary artery disease and its complications. Am J Cardiol. 2003;92(1):19–26.

Patsouras A, Farmaki P, Garmpi A, Damaskos C, et al. Screening and risk assessment of coronary artery disease in patients with type 2 diabetes: an updated review. In Vivo. 2019;33(4):1039–49.

Pearson TA. New tools for coronary risk assessment. What are their advantages and limitations? Circulation. 2002;105(7):886–92.

Zhou P, Wang J. Genetic testing for channelopathies, more than ten years progress and remaining challenges. J Cardiovasc Dis Res. 2010;1(2):47–9.

Index